THE RISE OF VIRULENCE AND ANTIBIOTIC RESISTANCE IN *Staphylococcus aureus*

Edited by **Shymaa Enany**
and **Laura E. Crotty Alexander**

The Rise of Virulence and Antibiotic Resistance in *Staphylococcus aureus*
http://dx.doi.org/10.5772/67546
Edited by Shymaa Enany and Laura E. Crotty Alexander

Contributors

Sahra Kırmusaoğlu, Mohd Nasir Mohd Desa, Zarizal Suhaili, Abdul Rahim Abdul Rachman, Hasan Cenk Mirza, Luís Cláudio Nascimento Da Silva, Andrea De Souza Monteiro, Aleff Mendes, Bruna Pinto, Wallace Neto, Gabriella Ferreira, Ľubomír Valík, Alžbeta Medveďová, Adriana Havlíková, Dalia I. Sánchez-Machado, Ana A. Escárcega-Galaz, Fany Reffuveille, Jérome Josse, Sophie C. Gangloff, Quentin Vallé, Céline Mongaret, Juan C. Cancino-Diaz, Janet Jan-Roblero, Elizabeth García-Gómez, Sandra Rodríguez-Martínez, Mario E. Cancino-Diaz, Kazuya Morikawa, Fabio Cafini, Veronica Medrano Romero, Ricardo Mariutti, Natayme Tartaglia, Núbia Seyffert, Thiago Castro, Koji Nishifuji, Yves Le Loir, Raghuvir Arni, Vasco Azevedo, Roseane Costa Diniz, Isana Maria De Souza Feitosa Lima, Camila Itapary Dos Santos, Matheus Silva Alves, Larissa Isabela Oliveira De Souza

Published by InTech
Janeza Trdine 9, 51000 Rijeka, Croatia

Publishing Process Manager Martina Usljebrka
Technical Editor SPi Global
Cover InTech Design team

First published March, 2017
Printed in Croatia
Legal deposit, Croatia: National and University Library in Zagreb

Additional hard copies can be obtained from orders@intechopen.com

The Rise of Virulence and Antibiotic Resistance in *Staphylococcus aureus*, Edited by Shymaa Enany and Laura E. Crotty Alexander
p. cm.
Print ISBN 978-953-51-2983-7
Online ISBN 978-953-51-2984-4

For EU product safety concerns:
IN TECH d.o.o., Prolaz Marije Krucifikse Kozulić 3, 51000 Rijeka, Croatia,
info@intechopen.com or visit our website at intechopen.com.

Meet the editorss

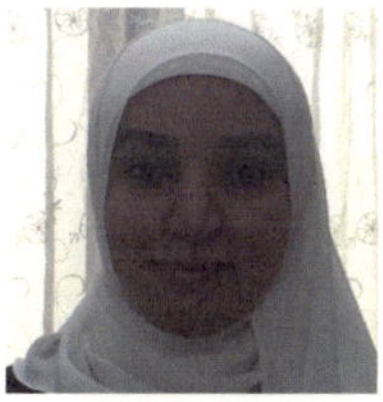

Dr. Shymaa Enany is an assistant professor of Microbiology and Immunology at the Suez Canal University, Egypt. She received her PhD degree from the School of Medical and Dental Sciences, Niigata University, Japan. Her dissertation focused on the molecular characterization of community-acquired methicillin-resistant *Staphylococcus aureus* (CA-MRSA), the leading cause of many life-threatening illnesses. For her postdoctoral work, she collaborated with many laboratories in San Diego, California, USA, and in Niigata, Japan, analyzing the proteome of *Staphylococcus aureus* and monitoring the reactions of innate immunity and airway cytokines in response to MRSA infections.

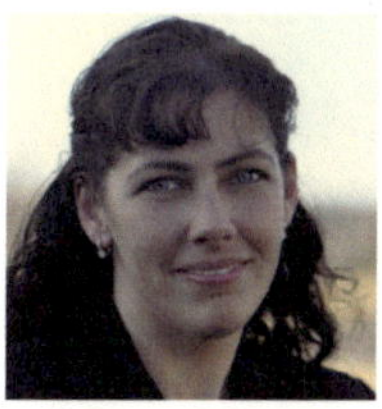

Dr. Laura E. Crotty Alexander is a Pulmonary Critical Care physician at the University of California, San Diego, and VA San Diego Healthcare System. As a biomedical basic science researcher, she studies host-pathogen interactions at molecular, cellular, organ, and organism levels and recently defined pro-virulent effects of inhalants such as cigarette smoke and e-cigarette vapor on Staphylococcal virulence. Dr. Crotty Alexander's clinical interests include bacterial pneumonia and sepsis, e-cigarette effects on innate immunity, and moderate-to-severe asthma.

Contents

Preface

Today, *Staphylococcus aureus* (*S. aureus*) is a growing issue both within hospitals and communities because of virulence determinants, including surface proteins, exotoxins, enterotoxins, and biofilm formation. Antibiotic resistance in *S. aureus*, either inherent or acquired, is considered a potential virulence factor—increasing the pathogenesis and dissemination of the bacteria. There has been rapid emergence of drug resistance in *S. aureus*, leading first to methicillin-resistant *S. aureus* (MRSA), which is causing serious public health concerns, and more recently to vancomycin-resistant *S. aureus* (VRSA), which is being reported with increasing frequency among isolates identified all over the world. The pace of antibiotic resistance development in *S. aureus*, and its extensive presence worldwide, demands that we work to obtain a comprehensive understanding of the molecular mechanisms of both *S. aureus* drug resistance and bacterial virulence.

The aim of writing "The Rise of Virulence and Antibiotic Resistance in *Staphylococcus aureus*" is to provide an unprecedented and comprehensive collection of up-to-date research about the evolution, dissemination, and mechanisms of staphylococcal antimicrobial resistance alongside bacterial virulence determinants and their impact on the medical field. This book consists of eleven review chapters, written by international leaders in their respective fields. Each chapter starts with a brief introduction, including its aim, and then goes on to provide detailed information about current research relevant to the field. Importantly, we include several review chapters to allow the readers to better understand the mechanisms of methicillin resistance, glycopeptide resistance, and horizontal gene transfer, as well as the effects of alterations in *S. aureus* membranes and cell walls on drug resistance, and induction of an SOS response by application of antibiotics. Additional chapters unveil further details of *S. aureus* pathogenicity by introducing recent research on *S. aureus* exfoliative toxins, enterotoxins, surface proteins, and biofilm.

Our timely book presents the state of the art of *S. aureus* virulence and antibiotic resistance. It is aimed at a wide range of informed readership, including clinicians, researchers, technicians, scientists, and students. We would like to thank all the authors who contributed chapters, without whose dedication, brilliant research, and keen support this book would not have been accomplished.

Dr. Shymaa Enany
Department of Microbiology and Immunology, Faculty of Pharmacy
Suez Canal University, Ismailia, Egypt

Dr. Laura E. Crotty Alexander
Department of Medicine, University of California, San Diego,
and VA San Diego Healthcare System, San Diego, CA, USA

Section 1

Resistance in *Staphylococcus aureus*

Chapter 1

The Evolution and Dissemination of Methicillin Resistance Determinant in *Staphylococcus aureus*

Abdul Rahim Abdul Rachman, Zarizal Suhaili and
Mohd Nasir Mohd Desa

Additional information is available at the end of the chapter

http://dx.doi.org/10.5772/65514

Abstract

Staphylococcus aureus is an opportunistic pathogen and is frequently associated with the antimicrobial resistance. There has been horizontal gene transfer of *Staphylococcus* chromosome cassette *mec* (SCC*mec*) among the staphylococcal species that colonize a similar colonization niche, which eventually results in emergence of new variant with enhanced survival ability in terms of antimicrobial resistance and virulence level in *S. aureus*. Evolution and dissemination of SCC*mec* structure resulted in the emergence of methicillin-resistant *S. aureus* (MRSA) clones around the world covering hospital, community, and livestock settings. MRSA also has the ability to resist different antibiotic profiles known as multidrug-resistant *S. aureus* (MDR *S. aureus*).

Keywords: *Staphylococcus aureus*, SCC*mec*, MRSA clones, multi-drug-resistant *S. aureus*

1. Introduction

Staphylococcus aureus is an opportunistic pathogen and lives as part of the animal normal flora of skin and nasopharynx. Favorably, it resides in the nasal mucosal environment posing infection threat to human as well as in domestic animals [1, 2]. In human, it is the leading agent of infection involving bloodstream, skin, and soft tissue to the lower respiratory tract [3–5]. *S. aureus* can easily colonize certain part of the body, especially the exposed area on skin due to ulcers, burns, and surgical wounds [6].

Methicillin-resistant *S. aureus* (MRSA) has been well known for being resistant to β-lactam antibiotics, which are the most common antimicrobial agents used to fight staphylococcal infection. Previous studies reported that methicillin resistance in staphylococci was carried by a specific mobile genetic element (MGE) called staphylococcal chromosome cassette *mec* (SCC*mec*), which carries with it several virulence factors as well [7]. SCC*mec* contains *mecA* gene which encodes for a low affinity penicillin-binding protein (pbp2a or pbp2′), which is currently exploited as the methicillin resistance marker in Staphylococcus species including *S. aureus* [8]. SCC*mec* contains several elements that can be categorized into several types. Genetic events such as point mutation, recombination, acquisition, and deletion, coupled with host and environmental selective pressures, make the structure evolve and disseminate in the population [9]. The emergence of certain MRSA clones, which have been disseminating worldwide since 1960, was closely related to the continuous evolution of SCC*mec* structure in *S. aureus*.

Multidrug-resistant MRSAs have also been reported that make the antibiotic regiment limited. Prevalence of MRSA is of a growing concern, particularly due to the more recent increased frequency of community-associated MRSA (CA-MRSA) and livestock-associated MRSA (LA-MRSA). Thus, this pathogen becomes a major concern in public health as well as livestock industry [10–13].

Many studies have been looking at the mechanism and dissemination pattern of MRSA and its genetic characteristics, but due to the potential, geographical, and temporal differences, a comprehensive review is needed to put the whole picture connected.

2. *Staphylococcus aureus*

S. aureus is a Gram-positive bacterium with a grape-like cluster morphology and can usually be found in skin or mucous membrane, especially in nasal of healthy person [14]. Kluytmans et al. reported that approximately 20–30% of human population carries *S. aureus* [15]. Morphologically, *S. aureus* can be observed as a 'golden' medium-size colony on solid media such as nutrient agar and can cause β-hemolysis on sheep blood agar [16].

The production of golden pigmentation of *S. aureus* colonies is closely related to the presence of carotenoids which is previously reported as virulence factor protecting *S. aureus* from the immune system [17]. Among Staphylococcus species, only *S. aureus* has the ability to ferment mannitol leading to the production of lactic acid on mannitol salt agar with yellow zones around the colonies [18]. *S. aureus* is also classified as a halophilic bacterium for being able to live in the presence of salt (sodium chloride) up to 1.7 molar. It also produces coagulase that causes blood to clot [14].

Generally, 20–30% of individuals are persistent carriers of *S. aureus* and 30% are transient or intermittent carriers [19]. *S. aureus* may live in human without any clinical symptoms, but it may infect the host when the host defense system is compromised. Individuals may acquire infection by *S. aureus* that they previously carry as commensal [15].

http://dx.doi.org/10.5772/65514

Immunocompromised patients with *S. aureus* infection may suffer several diseases such as bacteremia, ventilator-assisted pneumonia (VAP), endocarditis, and osteomyelitis, especially when the patients are frequently exposed to injections and catheter insertions [20, 21]. *S. aureus* can also cause toxin-mediated disease such as toxic shock syndrome, scalded skin syndrome, and Staphylococcal foodborne diseases (SFD) [21]. Frequently, *S. aureus* is the main cause of skin and soft tissue infection (SSTI) in human [22].

3. Methicillin-resistant *S. aureus* (MRSA)

MRSA has the ability to resist almost all available β-lactam antibiotics. Statistics showed about 40–70% of *S. aureus* nosocomial infections worldwide are caused by MRSA. MRSA was first reported in a hospital in the United Kingdom in 1961 after the introduction of methicillin to treat patient with penicillin-resistant Staphylococcus infection [23].

Generally, MRSA can be categorized into two major groups known as hospital-associated MRSA (HA-MRSA) and community-associated MRSA (CA-MRSA). Globally, the majority of MRSA infections are HA-MRSA that are acquired from healthcare facilities. Currently, MRSA isolates are subdivided into three major groups known as hospital-associated MRSA (HA-MRSA), community-associated MRSA (CA-MRSA), and livestock-associated MRSA (LA-MRSA). Previous reports revealed that both HA-MRSA and CA-MRSA isolates differ distinctly from each other, with HA-MRSA showing high antimicrobial resistance but less virulence and lack of capabilities as colonizers [23–26]. Meanwhile, CA-MRSA isolates exhibit a low antimicrobial resistance but a high virulence harboring PVL gene and numerous pathogenicity factors, as well as good colonizers [26–29].

MRSA spread in population since 1990 and become the major cause of community-associated infection [27]. The scenario worsens when multidrug MRSA emerges, in which it can resist more than two antibiotics of different classes that reduce the option for available treatment of Staphylococcal infection [30, 31].

Methicillin resistance characteristic in *S. aureus* is due to the presence of altered penicillin-binding protein (PBP2a) in the cell wall that has a reduced binding affinity to β-lactam antibiotics. PBP2a is encoded by *mecA* gene that is located in the large chromosomal cassette called staphylococcal chromosome cassette *mec* element (SCC*mec*) [32–35]. The *mecA* gene expression is controlled by *mecI-mecRI* regulatory genes encoding repressor and inducer protein, respectively [36].

4. SCC*mec* structure

Staphylococcal cassette chromosome *mec* (SCC*mec*) has a size of about 20–60 kb. The structure is unique as it carries various mobile genetic elements that are integrated in it [37]. To date, more than 80 SCC*mec* elements have been identified in several staphylococci species [38].

SCC*mec* disseminates among Staphylococcal species by horizontal gene transfer and integrates at a specific site called *att*B or ISS (integration site sequence) at the 3′ end of *orf*X gene that encodes for unknown function [39].

A single SCC*mec* carries *mec* complex and cassette chromosome recombinase (*ccr*) flanked by direct inverted repeat (DR) and inverted repeat (IR) sequences; *mec* complex consists of *mecA* gene (methicillin resistance determinant), *mecRI* (sensor inducer), and *mecI* (*mec* repressor). Both *mecRI* and *mecI* are recognized as *mec* regulator elements, while *ccr* genes encode serine recombinases (*ccr*A, *ccr*B, *ccr*C) responsible for site and orientation of specific integration and excision of SCC*mec*. In addition, SCC*mec* also harbors other elements such as insertion sequences (IS), plasmids, and transposons [24, 40, 41].

4.1. Complete SCC*mec*

To date, the International Working Group-SCC*mec* (IWG-SCC*mec*) identified eleven SCC*mec* types based on complete nucleotide sequences in Staphylococcal databases, and each SCC*mec* type is named using a roman numeral based on the unique combination of *ccr* complex and *mec* complex [40–42]. A complete SCC*mec* structure in *S. aureus* contains a *mec* complex (*mecA, mecRI* and *mecI*), a *ccr* complex (*ccrA, ccrB, ccrC*), and a J region (region other than *mec* and *ccr* complexes) [40].

Furthermore, many different SCC*mec* subtypes have also been described containing the same *ccr* and *mec* gene combination but vary in the J regions [40]. Among the eleven SCC*mec* types (I–XI) that have been reported so far, five of them (SCC*mec* I, II, III IV, and V) are globally distributed, while others only distributed in certain countries [38, 43]. Three (SCC*mec* IVa, SCC*mec* IVc, SCC*mec* V) from the 11 SCC*mec* types have been detected in MRSA isolated from animals called LA-MRSA [42]. In general, SCC*mec* type IV and V are more widely found among CA-MRSA, and the other three types (SCC*mec* I, II, III) are frequently found among HA-MRSA [44, 45, 46]. An early study by Ito et al. detected only three types of SCC*mec* structures (SCC*mec* type I, II, III) isolated from human [37], and a recent finding showed that MRSA with SCC*mec* type I, II, III is originated from animals [41].

Different types of SCC*mec* in MRSA are also observed to be geographically distributed. For example, SCC*mec* type III or IIIA was most commonly found in Asian countries, but Korea and Japan had more type II while Taiwan had more type IV [47]. SCC*mec* type IV was also commonly found in Latin and European countries [48, 49]. Similarly, in African countries, SCC*mec* type III was also predominant with SCC*mec* types II, IV, and V found in selected countries such as Egypt, Niger, Nigeria, Algeria, Tunisia, and South Africa [50].

4.2. Pseudo-SCC*mec*

Pseudo-SCC*mec* is recognized as SCC*mec* that does not carry *ccr* complexes but has *mecA* gene. Although this element is different from the complete SCC*mec* in terms of gene or operon organization, it still has some similarities in certain parts in both pseudo-SCC*mec* and complete SCC*mec* structure. Deletion is the major event as inferred by the absence of certain genes or operon in pseudo-SCC*mec* structure. For example, regions within *mec* complex and J region are absent in both pseudo-SCC*mec* II.5 and pseudo-SCC*mec*16691. It was observed that pseudo-SCC*mec*16691 lacks J1, J2 regions, and *ccr* genes, whereas missing parts were detected in pseudo-SCC*mec* II.5 and replaced by transposable elements called *Tn6012* [51, 52].

However, certain pseudo-SCC*mec* does not carry both *mec* and *ccr* complexes. An example is the arginine catabolic mobile element (ACME) for having SCC-like elements but lack in *mecA* and *ccr* genes. This could be the remnant of SCC*mec* structure that had gone through multiple mutational events. Lindqvist et al. discovered first remnant of pseudo-SCC*mec* structure in methicillin susceptible *S. aureus* (MSSA) that caused clonal outbreak in Sweden. They suggested that this pseudo-SCC*mec* structure could be derived from SCC*mec* type II [52].

ACME is found in both MRSA and MSSA, especially with sequence type ST8 (ST8), and has been disseminated in virulent *S. aureus* by horizontal gene transfer [3, 53]. Nevertheless, ACME was frequently associated with MRSA-IVa with sequence type 8 (ST8-MRSA-IVa), which was also known as CA-MRSA USA300 [3, 53]. ACME has been associated with the ability of CA-MRSA to colonize on other parts of human body such as skin and mucosal membranes rather than limited to only nostril. The acquisition of ACME may enhance the ability of CA-MRSA to survive in acidic environment of human skin by driving production of polyamine-resistant enzyme that combats excess host polyamine (toxic compound on human skin for *S. aureus*) [54].

5. Origin of SCC*mec* structure

The origin of SCC*mec* in MRSA is still in debate; *mecA* gene was believed to be originated from *Staphylococcus fleurettii* due to a high sequence similarity (>99%) with *mecA* gene of a MRSA strain N315. It was proposed that SCC*mec* is a combination of SCC elements without *mec* complex, and the *mec* gene complex was derived from *S. fleurettii* since no evidence showed that *S. fleurettii* contained SCC*mec* structure in its chromosome [55].

Several studies described coagulase-negative staphylococci (CoNS) as the primary reservoir of the SCC*mec* structure in *S. aureus*, which was considered as the recipient strain due to some reasons; a very similar SCC*mec* structure and organization was observed in both *S. aureus* and CoNS [56, 57], and the prevalence of methicillin-resistant coagulase-negative staphylococci (MRCoNS) in human is higher as compared to MRSA [35, 56–59]. Although a study discovered other non-staphylococci species called *Macrococcus* to also carry SCC*mec*-like elements, those were different with SCC*mec* in MRSA in terms of nucleotide sequences and genetic organization of the *mec* complex [55].

5.1. From coagulase-negative staphylococci species to MRSA

The existence of various forms of SCC*mec* in MRCoNS as compared to MRSA becomes the main argument why MRCoNS is suggested as the main reservoir of SCC*mec* for *S. aureus* leading to the emergence of MRSA [40, 57]. In a rapid genetic typing, polymerase chain reaction (PCR) technique is used to characterize the SCC*mec* types instead of nucleotide sequencing analysis. Consequently, SCC*mec* from MRCoNS is frequently defined as non-typeable due to a diverse combination of *ccr* and *mec* complexes that could not be assigned based on current SCC*mec* structure databases used against *S. aureus* [7]. Nevertheless, Zong et al. successfully assigned 10 SCC*mec* elements with a new combination of *ccr* and *mec* complexes in various species of MRCoNS. They assigned these untypeable SCC*mec* elements as UT1–UT10 [35]. In addition, another study also described new SCC*mec* types in *Staphylococcus hominis* and described those as NT1till NT4 [60].

Staphylococcus epidermidis, *Staphylococcus haemolyticus*, and *S. hominis* were found to carry a diverse SCC*mec* structure among CoNS. SCC*mec* type IV is the common structure found in *S. epidermidis*, while other SCC*mec* types I, II, III, V, VI and non-typeable SCC*mec* were also detected at a lower rate [61, 62]. For *S. haemolyticus*, SCC*mec* type V predominated in combination with other novel SCC*mec* types [60, 63]. In *S. hominis*, SCC*mec* types contained a combination of novel non-typeable SCC*mec*, SCC*mec* types VI, VIII, III, and other elements [35, 61].

5.2. From MSSA to MRSA

MRSA emerges when MSSA receives SCC*mec* structure elements from other MRSA or MRCoNS via horizontal gene transfer [64]. In a specific condition (high vancomycin concentration), SCC*mec* is unstable in certain MRSA that can lead to complete or partial deletion of SCC*mec* structure, which may result in the presence of certain SCC*mec* DNA fragment to remain in *S. aureus* chromosome [64–67].

Wong et al. [64] identified SCC*mec* type II with internal deletion in MSSA isolates from different geographical areas. This happened during *in vitro* exposure to vancomycin [64]. Furthermore, Vandendriessche et al. [67] described MSSA CC398 as the precursor for emergence of MRSA CC398 in livestock. They found non-SCC*mec* elements in MSSA CC398 harboring *czrC* and *tet*(K) genes generated during partial excision of SCC*mec* elements [67].

6. Clonal dissemination of MRSA

Nowadays, the dissemination of MRSA has become a major global problem that threatens human health [27]. However, only limited clones of MRSAs could be inferred to disseminate in different countries and continents through genotypic analysis using several DNA typing methods such as SCC*mec* typing, PFGE, MLST, and spa typing [27, 68, 69]. For example, more than 3000 MRSA isolates from certain continents (Europe, USA, and South America) were described to belong to only five major pandemic clones or clonal complexes (CC5, CC8, CC22, CC30, and CC45) [70]. To date, 11 clonal complexes (CC1, CC5, CC8, CC12, CC15, CC22, CC25, CC30, CC45, CC51, and CC121) have been detected in which 5 of them (CC8, CC15, CC22, CC30, and CC45) were isolated from human [71, 72]. These successful clones may transmit their genetic elements into other *S. aureus*, which are well adapted to hospital environment [73].

MRSA strain COL was the first MRSA clone detected carrying SCC*mec* type I with sequence type 250 (ST 250) and belonged to clonal complex 8 (CC8). Then, other MRSA clones with SCC*mec* type II and III were reported and recognized as EMRSA-1 (ST239), EMRSA-5 (ST247), and New York/Japan clone (ST5, USA100) [74]. Certain MRSA clones were originated from community setting. For example, Wang and co-workers (2007) detected the spread of community-associated SCC*mec* type IV and V MRSA in hospital setting in Taiwan between 1999 and 2005. They concluded that SCC*mec* types IV and V are carried by both CA-MRSA and HA-MRSA [75–77].

The popular human MRSA pandemic clones, the EMRSA-15 and EMRSA-16, were identified in the United Kingdom (UK) around early 1990s. Since then, the clones become predominant healthcare-associated MRSA in UK [78, 79] and several European countries such as Denmark [80], Sweden [81], Belgium [79], and Spain [82]. Studies in Kuwait [83] and USA [84] also reported the spread of EMRSA-15 and 16 clones in hospital setting in the countries. To date, these clones have already been widespread in 15 countries around the world [85]. Both MRSAs belong to SCC*mec* type IV with sequence type 22 (ST 22) for EMRSA-15 and sequence type 30 (ST 30) for EMRSA-16 and originated from hospital setting. EMRSA-15 and 16 have high surviving and spreading rate in hospital compared to other EMRSA in UK [78]. In 2013, MRSA clone with a rare sequence type, ST 779, was identified in eleven Irish hospitals from 2006 until 2011 harboring a novel pseudo (SCC*mec*)-SCC-SCC_{CRISPR} composite element. This clone contained novel *mec* class region, a fusidic acid resistance gene (*fusC*), and two copper resistance genes (*copB* and *copC*) but lacking *ccr* genes [86].

CA-MRSA clones have also been observed to disseminate worldwide particularly with sequence types ST80 and ST30. MRSA clone with ST80 is the most common CA-MRSA clone in European countries and usually carries PVL genes. Moreover, ST80 clone also showed resistance toward fluoroquinolones, tetracyclines, and fusidic acid [87]. CA-MRSA clone with sequence type ST30 was observed to disseminate in Asian and Oceanic countries. An example is the multidrug USA300 clone, known as West Pacific clone. It was first identified in the USA and carried plasmid that encodes several antibiotic resistance genes [88]. Enany et al. identified novel clones with sequence types ST1010 (121)c and ST1009 (1153)c isolated from Egypt after they analyzed different genetic patterns of PVL+CA-MRSA isolates from different countries [89].

In certain countries, it was found that MRSA can also spread among livestock, known as LA-MRSA. LA-MRSA CC398 is the popular clonal complex among livestock and has already been reported to spread in several European farms in Netherland, Denmark, Germany, France, and Italy [90]. MRSA CC398 was originated from pigs and spread among dairy cattle and turkey [91, 92]. In Netherlands, MRSA contamination on meat was reported after 2217 meat samples were analyzed covering 35.3% turkey, 15.2% beef, 15.2% veal, 10.7% pork, and 6.2% lamb meat [93]. LA-MRSA can be transmitted to human by physical contact with livestock contaminated with MRSA [94]. LA-MRSA may have equal virulence ability as compared to CA-MRSA and HA-MRSA toward human. Therefore, persons with continuous exposure to livestock carrying LA-MRSA are at high risk [95]. Other than meat, LA-MRSA can also be found in dairy milk. Recently, 11 sequence types were detected from LA-MRSA isolated from 15 Brazilian dairy farms (n = 552) with four of them contain novel sequence types (ST1622, ST1623, ST1624, and ST1625) [96].

7. Multidrug-resistant (MDR) MRSA

Antibiotic or antimicrobial drugs are the most effective therapeutic agents used in treating microbial infections through either one or both bactericidal and bacteriostatic effects. Nevertheless, antibiotic or antimicrobial drug resistance has been a major problem worldwide, with incidence of MRSA reported in healthcare facilities in Asia to reach its peak in late 1990s, and stayed at plateau level during 2000s [97]. The heavy usage of drugs in treatment hastens the selection of bacteria that harbor multidrug resistance genes particularly *S. aureus* to proliferate and dominate [98, 99]. Moreover, over-crowded community creates environment that is suitable for the rapid spread of numerous multidrug-resistant pathogens, particularly the airborne organisms such as *S. aureus*.

The emergence of multidrug-resistant *S. aureus* in both hospitals and community invokes a tremendous financial burden due to the persistence of hard-to-treat infections [97, 100–102]. Until present, it was reported that <90% of *S. aureus* strains are resistant to penicillin as well as ordinary antimicrobial agents such as drug from categories of aminoglycosides, ansamycins, anti-staphylococcal β-lactams (or cephamycins), chloramphenicols, fusidanases, fluoroquinolones, glycopeptides, lincosamides, macrolides, phenicols, and tetracyclines [103–105]. We are now observing the emergence of multidrug-resistant *S. aureus* and MDR-MRSA with broad spectrum of resistance with a distinct ability to survive and spread in the hospital environment, community setting, as well as livestock sectors.

There has been a dramatic increase in the incidence of nosocomial infections as well as community-associated MRSA and livestock-associated MRSA caused by strains of *S. aureus* that are resistant to multiple antibiotics [106]. At present, there have been reports that some strains demonstrate resistance to as many as 20 antimicrobial compound types, including antiseptics and disinfectants [107, 108]. Central Asian surveillance studies found that the prevalence of MRSA infection in tertiary hospital was reported in 10 among 1000 hospital admissions [109] and incidence reported previously in Japan was between 0.7 and 0.8 per 100 admission from 1999 to 2003 with a total rate among hospitalized patients in the Asia-Pacific region at 45.9% [110, 111]. Previous surveillance also reported that Asia is among the highest for the incidence of MRSA in the world, and interestingly a novel MRSA strain with glycopeptides resistance had spread in livestock animals making it as a potential human pathogen in this region [112].

Several studies attempted to profile all possible multidrug-resistant MRSA since 1987, encompassing samples from hospitals, community, as well as veterinary settings [113, 114]. Lim et al. (2013) carried out temporal comparative surveillance of antibiograms from clinical samples in 2003–2008 and showed a significant increase in resistance rates (from 1 to 96%), as well as multidrug-resistant phenotypes (96%). This study also indicated the prevalence of multidrug-resistant MRSA with SCC*mec* type III and ST239 [99]. Another study also reported the prevalence of resistance against other important antibiotics such as mupirocin, whose resistance rate in Malaysia is still low, but still higher than previous reports in Malaysia [107]. Another cross-sectional studies at a few major medical centers in Malaysia found that the occurrence of MRSA infection increased gradually with years, from 25.7 to 28.7% in 1996, 27.9% in 1998, and 33% in 2000 [115, 117, 118]. Meanwhile, a study done at a single Malaysian hospital found a gradual reduction in MRSA prevalence from 2002 to 2006, most likely due to the improvement in the quality of healthcare systems [103, 109, 116 118].

The first international surveillance study on epidemiology of CA-MRSA in Asian countries revealed important findings with regard to the current epidemiology of MRSA infections in the community and hospitals within Asia with multidrug-resistance rates at 73.1 and 83.7% for CA-MRSA and HA-MRSA, respectively [119]. At least, 357 isolates of CA-MRSA were analyzed with resistance rates of gentamicin, ciprofloxacin, and trimethoprim/sulfamethoxazole being significantly lower than those of HA-MRSA isolates, whereas resistance rates of clindamycin, erythromycin, and tetracycline were similarly high in both CA-MRSA and HA-MRSA [119, 120].

8. Conclusion

S. aureus and MRSA evolve and adapt the changing environment. Therefore, dissemination of MRSA should be continuously monitored for the antibiotic susceptibility pattern and molecular epidemiology comprising hospital, community, and livestock settings. The origin and dissemination of SCC*mec* are also important to be tracked in the diverse staphylococcal population. With the advancement in molecular methods such as next-generation sequencing, the pattern of the genetic evolution, spread of the bacteria, and the resistance determinants can be further explored and understood.

Author details

Abdul Rahim Abdul Rachman[1], Zarizal Suhaili[1,2] and Mohd Nasir Mohd Desa[1,3*]

*Address all correspondence to: mnasir@upm.edu.my

1 Department of Biomedical Science, Faculty of Medicine and Health Sciences, Universiti Putra Malaysia, Serdang, Selangor, Malaysia

2 School of Animal Sciences, Faculty of Bioresources and Food Industry, Universiti Sultan Zainal Abidin, Besut, Terengganu, Malaysia

3 Halal Products Research Institute, Universiti Putra Malaysia, Serdang, Selangor, Malaysia

References

[1] Azis MA, AB Hamid A, Pung H., Abdul PA, Suhaili Z, Mohd Nasir MD: *Staphylococcus aureus* infection risk in a population of health sciences students at a public university. Iranian Journal of Public Health, 2014; 43(3): 112–116.

[2] ChengAG, Kim HK, Burts ML, Krausz T, Schneewind O, Missiakas DM: Genetic requirements for *Staphylococcus aureus* abscess formation and persistence in host tissues. FASEB Journal: Official Publication of the Federation of American Societies for Experimental Biology, 2009; *23*(10): 3393–3404. doi:10.1096/fj.09-135467

[3] Diep BA, Sensabaugh GF, Somboonna N, Somboona NS, Carleton HA, Perdreau-Remington F: Widespread skin and soft-tissue infections due to two methicillin-resistant *Staphylococcus aureus* strains harboring the genes for Panton-Valentine leucocidin. Journal of Clinical Microbiology, 2004; 42(5): 2080–2084. doi:10.1128/JCM. 42.5

[4] Forbes, Forbes GB: Infection with penicillin-resistant staphylococci in hospital and general practice. British Medical Journal, 1949; 2(4627): 569–571. doi:10;2(4627)

[5] Gehanno JF, Louvel A, Nouvellon M, Caillard JF,Pestel-Caron M: Aerial dispersal of methicillin-resistant *Staphylococcus aureus* in hospital rooms by infected or colonised patients. The Journal of Hospital Infection, 2009; 71(3): 256–262. doi:10.1016/j.jhin. 2008.11.015

[6] Dryden MS: Skin and soft tissue infection: microbiology and epidemiology. International Journal of Antimicrobial Agents, 2009; 34 Suppl 1(1872–7913 (Electronic): S2–S7. doi:10.1016/S0924-8579(09)70541-2

[7] Shore AC, Coleman DC: Staphylococcal cassette chromosome *mec*: Recent advances and new insights. International Journal of Medical Microbiology, 2003; 303(6–7): 350–359. doi:10.1016/j.ijmm.2013.02.002

[8] Al-Abbas MA: Antimicrobial susceptibility of *Enterococcus faecalis* and a novel Planomicrobium isolate of bacteraemia. International Journal of Medicine and Medical Sciences, 2012; 4: 19–27. doi:10.5897/IJMMS11.130

[9] Deurenberg RH, Vink C, Kalenic S, Friedrich AW, Bruggeman CA, Stobberingh EE: The molecular evolution of methicillin-resistant *Staphylococcus aureus*. Clinical Microbiology and Infection: The Official Publication of the European Society of Clinical Microbiology and Infectious Diseases, 2007; 13(3): 222–235. doi: 10.1111/j.1469-0691.200 6.01573.x

[10] Graveland H, Duim B, van Duijkeren E, Dick Heederik JAW: Livestock-associated methicillin-resistant in animals and humans. International Journal of Medical Microbiology, 2011; 301(8): 630–634. doi:10.1016/j.ijmm.2011.09.004

[11] Michalopoulos AS, Livaditis IG, Gougoutas V: The revival of fosfomycin. International Journal of Infectious Diseases: IJID: Official Publication of the International Society for Infectious Diseases, 2011; 15(11): e732–739. doi:10.1016/j.ijid.2011.07.007

[12] Roberts MC, Soge OO, No D. Comparison of multi-drug resistant environmental methicillin-resistant *Staphylococcus aureus* isolated from recreational beaches and high touch surfaces in built environments. Frontiers in Microbiology, 2013; 4: 74. doi:10.3389/fmicb.2013.00074.

[13] Uzunovi S, Ibrahimagi A, Kamberovi F, Rijnders MIA, Stobberingh EE: Molecular characterization of methicillin-susceptible and methicillin-resistant *Staphylococcus aureus* in food handlers in Bosnia and Herzegovina. The Open Infectious Diseases Journal, 2013; 7: 15–20. doi:10.1007/s10354-012-0142-8

[14] Crossley KB, Archer GL. Jefferson KK: Staphylococci in Human Disease, Hoboken, NJ: John Wiley & Sons, Inc., 2009; doi:10.1002/9781444308464

[15] Kluytmans J, van Belkum A, Verbrugh H: Nasal carriage of *Staphylococcus aureus*: epidemiology, underlying *mec*hanisms, and associated risks. Clinical Microbiology Reviews, 1997; 10(3): 505–520.

[16] Sasaki T, Kikuchi K, Tanaka Y, Takahashi N, Kamata S. Hiramatsu K: reclassification of phenotypically identified *Staphylococcus intermedius* strains. Journal of Clinical Microbiology, 2007; 45: 2770–2778. doi:10.1128/JCM.00360-07

[17] Liu D, Chai T, Xia X, Gao Y, Cai Y, Li X., Miao Z, Hao H, Roesler U, Wang, J: Formation and transmission of *Staphylococcus aureus* (including MRSA) aerosols carrying antibiotic-resistant genes in a poultry farming environment. Science of the Total Environment, 2012; 426: 139–145. doi:10.1016/j.scitotenv.2012.03.060

[18] Pai V, Rao VI, Rao SP: Prevalence and antimicrobial susceptibility pattern of methicillin-resistant *Staphylococcus aureus* (MRSA) isolates at a tertiary care hospital in Mangalore, South India. Journal of Laboratory Physicians, 2010; 2(2): 82–84. doi:10.4103/0 974-27 27.72155

[19] Wertheim HFL, Melles DC, Vos MC, van Leeuwen W, van Belkum A, Verbrugh HA, Nouwen JL: The role of nasal carriage in *Staphylococcus aureus* infections. The Lancet. Infectious Diseases, 2005; 5(12): 751–762. doi:10.1016/S1473-3099(05)70295-4

[20] Schito GC. The importance of the development of antibiotic resistance in *Staphylococcus aureus*. Clinical Microbiology and Infection: The Official Publication of the European Society of Clinical Microbiology and Infectious Diseases, 2006; 12 Suppl 1: 3–8. doi:10.1111/j.1469-0691.2006.01343.x

[21] Lindsay JA, Holden MTG: Understanding the rise of the superbug: Investigation of the evolution and genomic variation of *Staphylococcus aureus*. Functional and Integrative Genomics, 2006; 6: 186–201. doi:10.1007/s10142-005-0019-7

[22] Diekema DJ, Pfaller MA, Schmitz FJ, Smayevsky J, Bell J, Jones RN, Beach M: Survey of infections due to staphylococcus species: frequency of occurrence and antimicrobial susceptibility of isolates collected in the United States, Canada, Latin America, Europe, and the Western Pacific Region for the SENTRY Antimicrobial Surveillance. Clinical Infectious Diseases, 2001; 32(s2): S114–S132. doi:10.1086/320184

[23] Chambers HF. DeLeo FR: Waves of resistance: *Staphylococcus aureus* in the antibiotic era. Nature Revision Microbiology. 2009; 7: 629–641. doi:10.1038/nrmicro2200

[24] Chongtrakool P, Ito T, Ma XX, Kondo Y, Trakulsomboon S, Tiensasitorn C, Jamklang M, Chavalit T, Song JH, Hiramatsu K: Staphylococcal cassette chromosome *mec* (SCC*mec*) typing of methicillin-resistant *Staphylococcus aureus* strains isolated in 11 Asian countries: a proposal for a new nomenclature for SCC*mec* elements. Antimicrobial Agents and Chemotherapy, 2006; 50(3): 1001–1012. doi:10.1128/AAC.50.3.1001-1012.2006

[25] Afroz S, Kobayashi N, Nagashima S, Alam MM, Hossain AB, Rahman MA, Islam MR, Lutfor AB, Muazzam N, Khan MA, Paul SK, AK, Mahmud MC, Musa AK, Hossain, MA: Genetic characterization of *Staphylococcus aureus* isolates carrying Panton-Valentine leukocidin genes in Bangladesh. Japanese Journal of Infectious Diseases, 2008; 61(5): 393–396.

[26] Berglund C, Prévost G, Laventie BJ, Keller D, Söderquist B: The genes for Panton Valentine leukocidin (PVL) are conserved in diverse lines of methicillin-resistant and methicillin-susceptible *Staphylococcus aureus*. Microbes and Infection, 2008; 10(8): 878–884. doi:10.1016/j.micinf.2008.04.018

[27] Deleo FR, Chambers HF: Review series re-emergence of antibiotic-resistant *Staphylococcus aureus* in the genomics era. Journal of Clinical Investigation, 2009; 119(9): 2464–2474. doi:10.1172/JCI38226

[28] Gonzalez BE, Rueda AM, Shelburne SA, Musher DM, Hamill RJ, Hulten KG: Community-associated strains of methicillin-resistant *Staphylococcus aureus* as the cause of healthcare-associated infection. Infection Control and Hospital Epidemiology: The Official Journal of the Society of Hospital Epidemiologists of America, 2006; 27(10): 1051–1056. doi:10.1086/507923

[29] Suhaili Z, Lean SS, Yahya A, Mohd Desa MN, AliAM, Yeo CC: Draft genome sequence of methicillin-resistant *Staphylococcus aureus* KT/Y21, a sequence type 772 (ST772) strain isolated from a pediatric blood sample in Terengganu, Malaysia. Genome Announcements, 2014; 2(2): 2–3. doi:10.1128/genomeA.00271-14

[30] Oliveira DC, de Lencastre H: Methicillin-resistance in *Staphylococcus aureus* is not affected by the overexpression in trans of the *mecA* gene repressor: a surprising observation. PLoS One, 2011; 6(8): e23287. doi:10.1371/journal.pone.0023287

[31] Tong SYC, Steer AC, Jenney AW, Carapetis JR: Community-associated methicillin-resistant *Staphylococcus aureus* skin infections in the tropics. Dermatologic Clinics, 2011; 29(1): 21–32. doi:10.1016/j.det.2010.09.005

[32] Song MD, Wachi M, Doi M, Ishino F, Matsuhashi M: Evolution of an inducible penicillin target protein in MRSA by gene fusion. FEBS Letters, 1987; 221(I): 167. doi: 10.1016/0014-5793(87)80373-3

[33] Hartmann FA, Trostle SS, Klohnen AAO: Isolation of methicillin-resistant *Staphylococcus aureus* from a postoperative wound infection in a horse. Journal of the American Veterinary Medical Association, 1997; 211(5): 590–592.

[34] Ito T, Katayama Y, Hiramatsu K: Cloning and nucleotide sequence determination of the entire *mec* DNA of pre-methicillin-resistant *Staphylococcus aureus* N315. Antimicrobial Agents and Chemotherapy, 1999; 43(6): 1449–1458.

[35] Zong Z, Peng C, Lü X: Diversity of SCC*mec* elements in methicillin-resistant coagulase-negative staphylococci clinical isolates. PLoS One, 2011; 6(5): 1–6. doi:10.1371/journal.pone.0020191

[36] Hiramatsu K, Asada K, Suzuki E, Okonogi K, Yokota T: Molecular cloning and nucleotide sequence determination of the regulator region of *mecA* gene in methicillin-resistant *Staphylococcus aureus* (MRSA). FEBS Letters. 1992; 298: 133–136. doi: 10.1016/0014-5793(92)80039-J

[37] Ito T, Katayama Y, Asada K, Mori N, Tsutsumimoto K, Tiensasitorn C, Hiramatsu K: Structural comparison of three types of staphylococcal cassette chromosome *mec* integrated in the chromosome in methicillin-resistant *Staphylococcus aureus*. Antimicrobial Agents and Chemotherapy, 2001; 45(5): 1323–1336. doi:10.1128/AAC.45.5.1323-1336.2001

[38] Ito T, Kuwahara-Arai K, Katayama Y, Uehara Y, Han X, Yoko Kondo KH: Staphylococcal cassette chromosome *mec* (SCC*mec*) analysis of MRSA. Methods in Molecular Biology, 2014; 1085: 131–148. doi:10.1007/978-1-62703-664-1_8

[39] Boundy S, Safo MK, Wang L, Musayev FN, O'Farrell HC, Rife JP, Archer GL: Characterization of the *Staphylococcus aureus* rRNA methyltransferase encoded by orfX, the gene containing the staphylococcal chromosome Cassette *mec* (SCC*mec*) insertion site. The Journal of Biological Chemistry, 2013; 288: 132–140. doi:10.1074/jbc.M112.385138

[40] International Working Group on the Classification of Staphylococcal Cassette Chromosome Elements (IWG-SCC), & IWG: CLASSIFICATION of Staphylococcal Cassette Chromosome *mec* (SCC*mec*): Guidelines for reporting novel SCC*mec* Elements. Antimicrobial Agents and Chemotherapy, 2009; 53(12): 4961–4967. doi:10.1128/AAC.00579-09

[41] Shore AC, Deasy EC, Slickers P, Brennan G, O'Connell B, Monecke S, Ehricht R, Coleman DC: Detection of staphylococcal cassette chromosome *mec* type XI carrying highly divergent *mecA, mecI, mecR1, blaZ,* and *ccr* genes in human clinical isolates of

clonal complex 130 methicillin-resistant *Staphylococcus aureus*. Antimicrobial Agents and Chemotherapy, 2011; 55(8): 3765–3773. doi:10.1128/AAC.00187-11

[42] García-Álvarez L, Holden MTG, Lindsay H, Webb CR, Brown DFJ, Curran MD, Walpole E, Brooks K, Pickard DJ, Teale C, Parkhill J, Bentley SD, Edwards GF, Girvan EK, Kearns AM, Pichon B, Hill RL, Larsen AR, Skov RL, Peacock SJ, Maskell DJ, Holmes MA: Methicillin-resistant *Staphylococcus aureus* with a novel *mecA* homologue in human and bovine populations in the UK and Denmark: a descriptive study. The Lancet Infectious Diseases, 2011; 11(8): 595–603. doi:10.1016/S1473-3099(11)70126-8

[43] Ghaznavi-Rad E, Nor Shamsudin M, Sekawi Z, Khoon LY, Aziz MN, Hamat RA, Othman N, Chong PP, van Belkum A, Ghasemzadeh-Moghaddam H, Neela V: Predominance and emergence of clones of hospital-acquired methicillin-resistant *Staphylococcus aureus* in Malaysia. Journal of Clinical Microbiology, 2010; 48(3): 867–872. doi: 10.1128/JCM.01112-09

[44] Oliveira DC, Milheiriço C, de Lencastre H: Redefining a structural variant of staphylococcal cassette chromosome *mec*, SCC*mec* type VI. Antimicrobial Agents and Chemotherapy, 2006; 50(10): 3457–3459. doi:10.1128/AAC.00629-06

[45] Hiramatsu K, Okuma K, Ma XX, Yamamoto M, Hori S, Kapi M: New trends in *Staphylococcus aureus* infections: glycopeptide resistance in hospital and methicillin resistance in the community. Current Opinion in Infectious Diseases, 2002; 15(4): 407–413.

[46] Ma XX, Ito T, Tiensasitorn C, Jamklang M, Chongtrakool P, Boyle-Vavra S, Daum RS, Hiramatsu K: Novel type of staphylococcal cassette chromosome *mec* identified in community-acquired methicillin-resistant *Staphylococcus aureus* strains. Antimicrobial Agents and Chemotherapy, 2002; 46(4): 1147–1152. doi:10.1128/AAC.46.4.1147-1152. 2002

[47] Ko KS, Lee Ji-Y, Suh JY, Oh WS, Peck KR, Lee NY, Song Jae-H: Distribution of major genotypes among methicillin-resistant *Staphylococcus aureus* clones in Asian countries. Journal of Clinical Microbiology, 2005; 43(1), 421–426. doi:10.1128/JCM.43.1.42 1-426. 2005

[48] Jiménez JN, Ocampo AM, Vanegas JM, Rodriguez EA, Mediavilla JR, Chen L, Muskus CE, Vélez LA, Rojas C, Restrepo AV, Ospina S, Garcés C, Franco L, Bifani P, Kreiswirth BN, Correa MM: CC8 MRSA strains harboring SCCmec type ivc are predominant in Colombian hospitals. 2012; 7(6), e38576. doi: 10.1371/journal.pone.003857631

[49] Berglund, C. Mölling, P. Sjöberg, L. Söderquist, Bo: Predominance of staphylococcal cassette chromosome mec (SCCmec) type IV among methicillin-resistant *Staphylococcus aureus* (MRSA) in a Swedish county and presence of unknown SCCmec types with Panton-Valentine leukocidin genes. Clinical Microbiology and Infection, 2005; 11(6), 447–456. doi:10.1111/j.1469-0691.2005.01150.x

[50] Abdulgader SM, Shittu AO, Nicol MP, Kaba M: Molecular epidemiology of methicillin-resistant *Staphylococcus aureus* in Africa: a systematic review. Frontier Microbiology, 2015; 6, 348. doi:10.3389/fmicb.2015.00348

[51] Shore AC, Rossney AS, O'Connell B, Herra CM, Sullivan DJ, Humphreys H, Coleman DC: Detection of staphylococcal cassette chromosome *mec*-associated DNA segments in multiresistant methicillin-susceptible *Staphylococcus aureus* (MSSA) and identification of *Staphylococcus epidermidisccrAB4* in both methicillin- resistant *S. aureus* and MSSA. Antimicrobial Agents and Chemotherapy, 2008; 52: 4407–4419. doi:10.1128/AAC.00447-08

[52] Lindqvist M, Isaksson B, Grub C, Jonassen TO, Hällgren A: Detection and characterisation of SCC*mec* remnants in multiresistant methicillin-susceptible *Staphylococcus aureus* causing a clonal outbreak in a Swedish county. European Journal of Clinical Microbiology and Infectious Diseases, 2012; 31: 141–147. doi:10.1007/s10096-011-12 86-y

[53] Ghasemzadeh-Moghaddam H, Neela V, Goering R, Mariana NS: Methicillin sensitive *Staphylococcus aureus* (MSSA) isolates as a potential source for the emergence of USA 300 methicillin resistant *Staphylococcus aureus* (MRSA) in Malaysia. Tropical Biomedicine, 2012; 29(3): 429–433.

[54] Thurlow LR, Joshi GS., Clark JR., Spontak JS., Neely CJ, Maile R., Richardson AR.: Functional modularity of the arginine catabolic mobile element contributes to the success of USA300 methicillin-resistant *Staphylococcus aureus*. Cell Host and Microbe, 2013; 13(1): 100-107. doi:10.1016/j.chom.2012.11.012

[55] Tsubakishita S, Kuwahara-Arai K, Sasaki T, Hiramatsu K: Origin and molecular evolution of the determinant of methicillin resistance in staphylococci. Antimicrobial Agents and Chemotherapy, 2010; 54(10): 4352–4359. doi:10.1128/AAC.00356-10

[56] Hanssen AM, Ericson Sollid JU: SCC*mec* in staphylococci: Genes on the move. FEMS Immunology and Medical Microbiology, 2006; 46(1): 8–20. doi:10.1111/j.1574-695X.2005.00009.x.

[57] Tulinski P, Fluit AC, Wagenaar JA, Mevius D, van de Vijver L, Duim B: Methicillin-resistant coagulase-negative staphylococci on pig farms as a reservoir of heterogeneous staphylococcal cassette chromosome *mec* elements. Applied and Environmental Microbiology, 2012; 78(2):, 299–304. doi:10.1128/AEM.05594-11

[58] McGavin MJ: Genome comparisons of diverse *Staphylococcus aureus* strains. Bacterial Genomes and Infectious Diseases, 2006; 5: 191–212. doi:10.1007/978-1-59745-152-9_11

[59] Wielders CL, Vriens MR, Brisse S, Al, E: In-vivo transfer of *mec*A DNA to *Staphylococcus aureus*. Lancet, 2001; 357: 1674–1675. doi: 10.1016/S0140-6736(00)04832-7

[60] Bouchami O, Ben Hassen A, de Lencastre H, Miragaia M: Molecular epidemiology of methicillin-resistant *Staphylococcus hominis* (MRSHo): low clonality and reservoirs of

SCC*mec* structural elements. PLoS One, 2011; 6(7): e21940. doi:10.1371/journal.pone.0021940

[61] Lebeaux D, Barbier F, Angebault C, Benmahdi L, Ruppé E, Felix B, Gaillard K, Djossou F, Epelboin L, Dupont C, Renard M, Peroz G, Vandenesch F, Wolff M, Andremont A, Ruimy R: Evolution of nasal carriage of methicillin-resistant coagulase-negative staphylococci in a remote population. Antimicrobial Agents and Chemotherapy, 2012; 56(1): 315–323. doi:10.1128/AAC.00547-11

[62] Rolo J, de Lencastre H, Miragaia M: Strategies of adaptation of *Staphylococcus epidermidis* to hospital and community: amplification and diversification of SCC*mec*. The Journal of Antimicrobial Chemotherapy, 2012; 67(6): 1333–1341. doi:10.1093/jac/dks068

[63] Ruppé E, Barbier F, Mesli Y, Maiga A, Cojocaru R, Benkhalfat M, Benchouk S, Hassaine H, Maiga I, Diallo A, Koumaré AK, Ouattara K, Soumaré S, Dufourcq JB, Nareth C, Sarthou JL, Andremont A, Ruimy R: Diversity of staphylococcal cassette chromosome *mec* structures in methicillin-resistant *Staphylococcus epidermidis* and *Staphylococcus haemolyticus* strains among outpatients from four countries. Antimicrobial Agents and Chemotherapy, 2009; 53(2): 442–449. doi:10.1128/AAC.00724-08

[64] Wong H, Louie L, Lo RYC, Simor AE: Characterization of *Staphylococcus aureus* isolates with a partial or complete absence of staphylococcal cassette chromosome elements. Journal of Clinical Microbiology, 2010; 48(10): 3525–3531. doi:10.1128/JCM.00775-10

[65] Donnio PY, Février F, Bifani P, Dehem M, Kervégant C, Wilhelm N, Gautier-Lerestif AL, Lafforgue N, Cormier M; MR-MSSA study group of the Collège de Bactériologie-Virologie-Hygiène des Hôpitaux de France, Le Coustumier A. Molecular and epidemiological evidence for spread of multiresistant methicillin-susceptible *Staphylococcus aureus* strains in hospitals. Antimicrobial Agents and Chemotherapy, 2007; 51(12): 4342–4350. doi:10.1128/AAC.01414-06

[66] Chlebowicz MA, Nganou K, Kozytska S, Arends JP, Engelmann S, Grundmann H, Ohlsen K, van Dijl JM, Buist G: Recombination between *ccr*C genes in a type V (5C2&5) staphylococcal cassette chromosome *mec* (SCC*mec*) of *Staphylococcus aureus* ST398 leads to conversion from methicillin resistance to methicillin susceptibility in vivo. Antimicrobial Agents and Chemotherapy, 2010; 54(2): 783–791. doi:10.1128/AAC.00696-09

[67] Vandendriessche S, Vanderhaeghen W, Larsen J, de Mendonça R, Hallin M, Butaye P, Hermans K, Haesebrouck F, Denis O: High genetic diversity of methicillin-susceptible *Staphylococcus aureus* (MSSA) from humans and animals on livestock farms and presence of SCC*mec* remnant DNA in MSSA CC398. The Journal of Antimicrobial Chemotherapy, 2014; 69(2): 355–362. doi:10.1093/jac/dkt366

[68] Aires de Sousa M, de Lencastre H: Bridges from hospitals to the laboratory: genetic portraits of methicillin-resistant *Staphylococcus aureus* clones. FEMS Immunology and Medical Microbiology, 2004; 40(2): 101–111. doi:10.1016/S0928-8244(03)00370-5

[69] Crisóstomo MI, Westh H, Tomasz A, Chung M, Oliveira DC, de Lencastre H: The evolution of methicillin resistance in *Staphylococcus aureus*: similarity of genetic

backgrounds in historically early methicillin-susceptible and resistant isolates and contemporary epidemic clones. Proceedings of the National Academy of Sciences of the United States of America, 2001; 98(17): 9865–9870. doi:10.1073/pnas.161272898

[70] Oliveira DC, de Lencastre H: Multiplex PCR strategy for rapid identification of structural types and variants of the *mec* element in methicillin-resistant *Staphylococcus aureus*. Antimicrobial Agents and Chemotherapy, 2002; 46(7): 2155–2161. doi:10.1128/AAC.46.7.2155-2161

[71] Witte W, Strommenger B, Stanek C, Cuny C: Methicillin-resistant *Staphylococcus aureus* ST398 in Humans and Animals, Central Europe. Emerging Infectious Diseases, 2007; 13(2): 255–258. doi:10.3201/eid1302.060924

[72] Cuny C, Wieler L, Witte W: Livestock-associated MRSA: the impact on humans. Antibiotics, 2015; 4(4): 521–543. doi:10.3390/antibiotics4040521

[73] Blanc DS, Petignat C, Moreillon P, Entenza JM, Eisenring M, Kleiber H, Wenger A, Troillet N, Blanc C, Francioli P: Unusual spread of a penicillin-susceptible methicillin-resistant *Staphylococcus aureus* clone in a geographic area of low incidence. Clinical Infectious Diseases: An Official Publication of the Infectious Diseases Society of America, 1999; 29(6): 1512–1518. doi:10.1086/313522

[74] Otto M: MRSA virulence and spread. Cellular Microbiology, 2012; 14(10): 1513–1521. doi:10.1111/j.1462-5822.2012.01832.x

[75] Wang JT, Fang CT, Chen YC, Wu CL, Chen ML, Chang SC: Staphylococcal cassette chromosome *mec* in MRSA, Taiwan. Emerging Infectious Diseases, 2007; 13(3): 494–497.

[76] Ahmad N, Ruzan IN, Abd Ghani MK, Hussin A, Nawi S, Aziz MN, Maning N, Eow VL: Characteristics of community and hospital-acquired methicillin-resistant *Staphylococcus aureus* strains carrying SCC*mec* type IV isolated in Malaysia. Journal of Medical Microbiology, 2009; 58(9): 1213–1218. doi:10.1099/jmm.0.011353-0

[77] Brennan GI, Shore A C, Corcoran S, Tecklenborg S, Coleman DC, O'Connell B: Emergence of hospital and community-associated Panton-valentine leukocidin-positive methicillin-resistant *Staphylococcus aureus* genotype ST772-MRSA-V in Ireland and detailed investigation of an ST772-MRSA-V cluster in a neonatal intensive care unit. Journal of Clinical Microbiology, 2012; 50(3): 841–847. doi:10.1128/JCM.06354-11

[78] Moore PCL, Lindsay JA: Molecular characterisation of the dominant UK methicillin-resistant *Staphylococcus aureus* strains, EMRSA-15 and EMRSA-16. Journal of Medical Microbiology, 2002; 51(6): 516–521. doi:10.1099/0022-1317-51-6-516

[79] Murchan S, Kaufmann ME, Deplano A, de Ryck R, Struelens M, Zinn CE, Fussing V, Salmenlinna S, Vuopio-Varkila J, El Solh N, Cuny C, Witte W, Tassios PT, Legakis N, van Leeuwen W, van Belkum A, Vindel A, Laconcha I, Garaizar J, Haeggman S, Olsson-Liljequist B, Ransjo U, Coombes G, Cookson B: Harmonization of pulsed-field gel electrophoresis protocols for epidemiological typing of strains of methicillin-resistant

Staphylococcus aureus: a single approach developed by consensus in 10 European laboratories and its application for tracing the spread of related strains. Journal of Clinical Microbiology, 2009; 41(4): 1574–1585. doi:10.1128/JCM.41.4.1574-1585.2003

[80] Faria NA, Oliveira DC, Westh H, Monnet DL, Larsen AR, Skov R, de Lencastre H: Epidemiology of emerging methicillin-resistant *Staphylococcus aureus* (MRSA) in Denmark: a nationwide study in a country with low prevalence of MRSA infection. Journal of Clinical Microbiology, 2005; 43(4): 1836–1842. doi:10.1128/JCM.43.4.1836-18 42.2005

[81] Seeberg S, Larsson L, Welinder-Olsson C, Sandberg T, Skyman E, Bresky B, Lindqvist A, van Raalte M: How an outbreak of MRSA in gothenburg was eliminated: by strict hygienic routines and massive control-culture program. Läkartidningen, 2002; 99(32–33): 3198–3204.

[82] Montesinos I, Delgado T, Riverol D, Salido E, Miguel MA, Jimenez A, Sierra A: Changes in the epidemiology of methicillin-resistant *Staphylococcus aureus* associated with the emergence of EMRSA-16 at a university hospital. Journal of Hospital Infection, 2006; 64(3): 257–263. doi:10.1016/j.jhin.2006.07.004

[83] Udo EE, Al-Sweih N, Noronha B: Characterisation of non-multiresistant methicillin-resistant *Staphylococcus aureus* (including EMRSA-15) in Kuwait hospitals. Clinical Microbiology and Infection, 2006; 12(3): 262–269. doi:10.1111/j.1469-0691.2005.01350.x

[84] McDougal LK, Steward CD, Killgore GE, Chaitram JM, McAllister SK, Tenover FC: Pulsed-field gel electrophoresis typing of oxacillin-resistant *Staphylococcus aureus* isolates from the United States: establishing a national database. Journal of Clinical Microbiology, 2003; 41(11): 5113–5120. doi:10.1128/JCM.41.11.5113-5120.2003

[85] Grundmann H, Aanensen DM, van den Wijngaard CC, Spratt BG, Harmsen D, Friedrich AW: Group the European staphylococcal reference laboratory working group. geographic distribution of *Staphylococcus aureus* causing invasive infections in Europe: A molecular-epidemiological analysis. PLoS Medicine, 2010;7(1): e1000215. doi:10.1371/journal.pmed.1000215

[86] Kinneveya PM., Shore AC., Brennan GI, Sullivana DJ, Ehrichtd R, Monecke S, Slickers P., Coleman DC: Emergence of sequence type 779 methicillin-resistant *Staphylococcus aureus* harboring a novel pseudo staphylococcal cassette chromosome mec (SCCmec)-SCC-SCC_{CRISPR} composite element in irish hospitals. Antimicrobial Agents and Chemotherapy, 2013;57(1), 524–531. doi:10.1128/AAC.01689-12

[87] Vandenesch F, Naimi T, Enright MC, et al: Community-acquired methicillin-resistant *Staphylococcus aureus* carrying Panton-Valentine leukocidin genes: worldwide emergence. Emerging Infectious Diseases, 2003;9:978–984. doi:10.3201/eid0908.030089

[88] Y. Takizawa, I. Taneike, S. Nakagawa, T. Oishi, Y. Nitahara, N. Iwakura: A Panton-Valentine leucocidin (PVL)-positive community-acquired methicillin-resistant *Staphylococcus aureus* (MRSA) strain, another such strain carrying a multiple-drug resistance

plasmid, and other more-typical PVL-negative MRSA strains found in Japan. Journal of Clinical Microbiology, 2005; 43, 3356–3363. doi:10.1128/JCM.43.7.3356-33 63.2005

[89] Enany S., Yaoita E., Yoshida Y., Enany M., Yamamoto T: Molecular characterization of Panton-Valentine leukocidin-positive community-acquired methicillin-resistant *Staphylococcus aureus* isolates in Egypt. Microbiological Research. 2010; 165(2); 152–162. doi:10.1016/j.micres.2009.03.005

[90] Olivier Andreoletti, Herbert Budka, Sava Buncic, Pierre Colin, John D Collins, Aline De Koeijer, John Griffin, Arie Havelaar, James Hope, Günter Klein, Hilde Kruse, Simone Magnino, Antonio, Martínez López, James McLauchlin, Christophe Nguyen-The, Karsten Noeckler, Birgit Noerrung, Miguel Prieto Maradona, Terence Roberts, Ivar Vågsholm, Emmanuel Vanopdenbosch: Assessment of the public health significance of methicillin resistant *Staphylococcus aureus* (MRSA) in animals and foods. scientific opinion of the panel on biological hazards adopted on 5 March 2009. The EFSA Journal, 2009; 993: 1–73. doi:10.2903/j.efsa.2009.993

[91] Vanderhaeghen W, Cerpentier T, Adriaensen C, Vicca J, Hermans K, Butaye P: Methicillin-resistant *Staphylococcus aureus* (MRSA) ST398 associated with clinical and subclinical mastitis in Belgian cows. Veterinary Microbiology, 2010; 144(1–2): 166–171. doi:10.1016/j.vetmic.2009.12.044

[92] Richter A, Sting R, Popp C, Rau J, Tenhagen BA, Guerra B, Hafez HM, Fetsch A: Prevalence of types of methicillin-resistant *Staphylococcus aureus* in turkey flocks and personnel attending the animals. Epidemiology and Infection, 2012; 140(12): 2223–2232. doi:10.1017/S095026881200009X

[93] de Boer E, Zwartkruis-Nahuis JT, Wit B, Huijsdens XW, de Neeling AJ, Bosch T, van Oosterom RA, Vila A, Heuvelink AE: Prevalence of methicillin-resistant *Staphylococcus aureus* in meat. International Journal of Food Microbiology, 2009; 134(1–2): 52–56. doi: 10.1016/j.ijfoodmicro.2008.12.007

[94] Schulz J, Friese A, Klees S, Tenhagen BA, Fetsch A, Rösler U, Hartung J: Longitudinal study of the contamination of air and of soil surfaces in the vicinity of pig barns by livestock-associated methicillin-resistant *Staphylococcus aureus*. Applied and Environmental Microbiology, 2012; 78(16): 5666–5671. doi:10.1128/AEM.00550-12

[95] Layer F, Cuny C, Strommenger B, Werner G, Witte W: Current data and trends on methicillin-resistant *Staphylococcus aureus* (MRSA). Bundesgesundheitsblatt, Gesundheitsforschung, Gesundheitsschutz, 2012; 55(11–12):1377–1386. doi:10.1007/s00103-0 12-1560-x

[96] Oliveira CJ. Tiao N, de Sousa F.G, de Moura J.F, Santos Filho L, Gebreyes WA: Methicillin-resistant *Staphylococcus aureus* from Brazilian dairy farms and identification of novel sequence types. Zoonoses Public Health. 2016;63(2):97–105. doi:10.1111/zph.12209

[97] Chen CJ, Huang YC: New epidemiology of *Staphylococcus aureus* infection in Asia. Clinical Microbiology and Infection., 2014; 20(7): 605–623. doi:10.1111/1469-0691.12705

[98] Levy SB, Marshall B: Antibacterial resistance worldwide: causes, challenges and responses. Nature Medicine, 2004; 10(1078–8956 (Print): S122–S129. doi:10.1038/nm1145

[99] Lim KT, Hanifah YA, Mohd Yusof MY, Ito T, Thong KL: Comparison of methicillin-resistant *Staphylococcus aureus* strains isolated in 2003 and 2008 with an emergence of multidrug resistant ST22: SCC*mec* IV clone in a tertiary hospital, Malaysia. Journal of Microbiology, Immunology and Infection, 2013; 46(3): 224–33. doi:10.1016/j.jmii. 2013.02.001.

[100] Cosgrove SE, Sakoulas G, Perencevich EN, Schwaber MJ, Karchmer AW, Carmeli Y: Comparison of mortality associated with methicillin-resistant and methicillin-susceptible *Staphylococcus aureus* bacteremia: a meta-analysis. Clinical Infectious Diseases®: An Official Publication of the Infectious Diseases Society of America, 2003; 36(1): 53–59. doi:10.1086/345476

[101] Suhaili Z, Johari SA, Mohtar M, Abdullah ART, Ahmad A, Ali AM: Detection of Malaysian methicillin-resistant *Staphylococcus aureus* (MRSA) clinical isolates using simplex and duplex real-time PCR. World Journal of Microbiology and Biotechnology, 2009; 25(2): 253–258. doi:10.1007/s11274-008-9887-z

[102] Lyon BR, Skurray R: Antimicrobial resistance of *Staphylococcus aureus*: genetic basis. Microbiological Reviews, 1987; 51(1): 88–134.

[103] Al-Talib H, Alyaa Al-Khateeb HH: Antimicrobial resistance of *Staphylococcus aureus* isolates in Malaysian tertiary hospital. International Medical Journal, 2015; 22(1): 1–3.

[104] Magiorakos AP, Srinivasan A, Carey RB, Carmeli Y, Falagas ME, Giske CG, Harbarth S, Hindler JF, Kahlmeter G, Olsson-Liljequist B, Paterson DL, Rice LB, Stelling J, Struelens MJ, Vatopoulos A, Weber JT, Monnet DL: Multidrug-resistant, extensively drug-resistant and pan-drug-resistant bacteria: an international expert proposal for interim standard definitions for acquired resistance. Clinical Microbiology and Infection, 2012; 18(3): 268–281. doi:10.1111/j.1469-0691.2011.03570.x

[105] Ullah A, Qasim M, Rahman H, Khan J, Haroon M, Muhammad N, Khan A, Muhammad N: High frequency of methicillin-resistant *Staphylococcus aureus* in Peshawar Region of Pakistan. Springerplus, 2016; 5(1): 600. doi:10.1186/s40064-016-2277-3

[106] Nickerson EK, Wuthiekanun V, Kumar V, Amornchai P, Wongdeethai N, Chheng K, Chantratita N, Putchhat H, Thaipadungpanit J, Day NP, Peacock SJ: Emergence of community-associated methicillin-resistant *Staphylococcus aureus* carriage in children in Cambodia. American Journal of Tropical Medicine and Hygiene, 2011; 84(2): 313–317. doi:10.4269/ajtmh.2011.10-0300

[107] Lim SK, Nam HM, Park HJ, Lee HS, Choi MJ, Jung SC, Lee JY., Kim YC, Song SW, Wee SH: Prevalence and characterization of methicillin-resistant *Staphylococcus aureus* in raw meat in Korea. Journal of Microbiology and Biotechnology, 2010; 20(4): 775–778.

[108] Lim KT, Hanifah YA, Yusof M, Thong KL: *erm*A, *erm*C, *tet*M and *tet*K are essential for erythromycin and tetracycline resistance among methicillin-resistant *Staphylococcus aureus* strains isolated from a tertiary hospital in Malaysia. Indian Journal of Medical Microbiology, 2012; 30(2): 203–207. doi:10.4103/0255-0857.96693

[109] Al-Talib HI, Yean CY, Al-Jashamy K, Hasan H: Methicillin-resistant *Staphylococcus aureus* nosocomial infection trends in hospital Universiti Sains Malaysia during 2002–2007. Annals of Saudi Medicine, 2010; 30(5): 358–363. doi:10.4103/0256-4947.67077

[110] Bell JM, Turnidge JD: SENTRY APAC. High prevalence of oxacillin-resistant *Staphylococcus aureus* isolates from hospitalized patients in Asia-Pacific and South Africa: results from SENTRY antimicrobial surveillance program, 1998–1999. Antimicrobial Agents and Chemotherapy. 2002; 46(3): 879–881. doi:10.1128/AAC.46.3.880-882.2002

[111] Kobayashi H: National hospital infection surveillance on methicillin-resistant *Staphylococcus aureus*. The Journal of Hospital Infection, 2005; 60(2): 172–175.

[112] Kang Cheol-I, Song Jae-H: Antimicrobial resistance in Asia: Current epidemiology and clinical implications. Infection and Chemotherapy, 2013; 45(1): 22–31. doi:10.3947/ic.2013.45.1.22

[113] Saleha AA, Zunita Z: Methicillin resistant *Staphylococcus aureus* (MRSA): An emerging veterinary and zoonotic pathogen of public health concern and some studies in Malaysia. Journal of Animal and Veterinary Advances, 2010; 9(7): 1094–1098. doi:10.3923/javaa.2010.1094.1098

[114] Choi CS, Yin CS, Bakar AA, Sakewi Z, Naing NN, Jamal F, Othman N: Nasal carriage of *Staphylococcus aureus* among healthy adults. Journal of Microbiology, Immunology and Infection, 2006; 39(6): 458–464.

[115] Lim VK, Zulkifli HI: Methicillin resistant *Staphylococcus aureus* in a Malaysian neonatal unit. Singapore Medical Journal, 1987; 28(2): 176–179.

[116] Norazah A, Lim VK, Koh YT, Rohani MY, Zuridah H, Spencer K, Ng PP, Kamel AG: Molecular fingerprinting of fusidic acid- and rifampicin-resistant strains of methicillin-resistant *Staphylococcus aureus* (MRSA) from Malaysian hospitals. Journal of Medical Microbiology, 2002; 51(12): 1113–1116. doi:10.1099/0022-1317-51-12-1113

[117] Ong WHS, Lai QX, Azhan F, Sapiee NA, Mohd Zaidi SH, Zahir ME, Harun SN: Choices of antibiotics for MRSA infection in choices of antibiotics for MRSA infection in Malaysia. Web Medical Central, 2011; 2(12): 1–12. doi:10.9754/journal.wmc.2011.002675

[118] Asmat A, Zulkifli A, Usup G: Detection of methicillin resistant *Staphylococcus aureus* (MRSA) isolated from Bagan Lalang recreational beach, Malaysia. Malaysian Journal of Microbiology, 2013; 9(2): 166–175.

[119] Song JH, Hsueh PR, Chung DR, Ko KS, Kang CI, Peck KR, Yeom JS, Kim SW, Chang HH, Kim YS, Jung SI, Son JS, So TM, Lalitha MK, Yang Y, Huang SG, Wang H, Lu Q,

Carlos CC, Perera JA, Chiu CH, Liu JW, Chongthaleong A, Thamlikitkul V, Van PH; ansorp study group. Spread of methicillin-resistant *Staphylococcus aureus* between the community and the hospitals in Asian countries: An ANSORP study. Journal of Antimicrobial Chemotherapy, 2011; 66(5), 1061–1069. doi:10.1093/jac/dkr024

[120] Song JH, Hiramatsu K, Suh JY, Ko KS, Ito T, Kapi M, Kiem S, Kim YS, Oh WS, Peck KR, Lee NY: Asian network for surveillance of resistant pathogens study group. Emergence in Asian countries of *Staphylococcus aureus* with reduced susceptibility to vancomycin. Antimicrobial Agents and Chemotherapy, 2004; 48(12): 4926–4928. doi:10.1128/AAC.48.12.4926-4928.2004

Chapter 2

MRSA and MSSA: The Mechanism of Methicillin Resistance and the Influence of Methicillin Resistance on Biofilm Phenotype of *Staphylococcus aureus*

Sahra Kırmusaoğlu

Additional information is available at the end of the chapter

http://dx.doi.org/10.5772/65452

Abstract

Staphylococcus aureus (*S. aureus*), which is one of the most common causes of indwelling device–associated, nosocomial, and community-acquired infections, can produce biofilm as a virulence factor. Methicillin-resistant *S. aureus* (MRSA) that is resistant to β-lactam antibiotics causes life-threatening infections. Biofilm producer strains of *S. aureus* that causes indwelling device–associated infections resist to antimicrobials and immune system. The combination of methicillin resistance and the ability of biofilm formation of *S. aureus* makes treatment difficult. Methicillin resistance of *S. aureus* can affect biofilm phenotype of *S. aureus*; the *mec*A gene of MRSA increases biofilm production by inactivating accessory gene regulator (agr) quorum sensing regulator system, which is a two-component regulator system of virulence factor production. The aim of this review is to determine virulence factors of *S. aureus*, resistance mechanisms of methicillin, and the influence of methicillin resistance on biofilm phenotype of *S. aureus*.

Keywords: *Staphylococcus aureus*, MRSA, MSSA, biofilm, methicillin resistance, virulence, influence of methicillin resistance on biofilm

1. Introduction

The biofilm has an important role in the pathogenesis of certain bacterial infections such as staphylococcal indwelling device–associated infections, wound infections, chronic urinary tract infections (UTI), cystic fibrosis pneumonia, chronic otitis media (OM), chronic rhinosinusitis, periodontitis, and recurrent tonsillitis [1].

The biofilm infections such as *Staphylococcus aureus* (*S. aureus*) infections are the important problems in hospitalized and immunosuppressed patients worldwide due to their tough and nonresponsive treatment by antibiotics. Biofilm-producing bacteria are resistant to immune defense, antibiotics, and many antimicrobial agents [2, 3].

The *mecA* gene, which is located in the staphylococcal chromosomes, enhances virulence of *Staphylococcus* by causing resistant to methicillin antibiotics. Methicillin-resistant *S. aureus* (MRSA) causes hospital-associated (HA-MRSA) and community-associated (CA-MRSA) infections. Methicillin resistance of *S. aureus* causes treatment of *S. aureus* tough by antibiotics due to its resistance to all β-lactam antibiotics. Mechanisms of resistance to β-lactam antibiotics such as methicillin are regulated by regulatory genes in the presence of such antibiotics. *S. aureus* biofilm formation is regulated globally by the accessory gene regulator (agr) quorum sensing system that is also inactivated by the *mec*A gene of MRSA [2–4]. The virulence of *S. aureus*, mechanisms of methicillin resistance, role of methicillin resistance on biofilm, and alteration of biofilm formation of *S. aureus* in methicillin resistance are discussed in this review.

2. *Staphylococcus aureus* and virulence

2.1. Staphylococcus aureus

S. aureus, a Gram-positive coccus, produces catalase enzyme and coagulase enzyme, which coagulates blood by reacting with prothrombin, which converts fibrinogen to fibrin [5]. While *S. aureus* is a commensal bacterium and colonizes primary anterior nares of healthy staphylococcal nasal carrier individuals, *S. aureus* causes a wide range of infections such as skin infections, including abscesses, impetigo, and necrotizing fasciitis; tissue infections, including osteomyelitis and endocarditis; and toxinoses, including toxic shock syndrome, when immunity of the staphylococcal nasal carrier is suppressed [6, 7]. If MRSA is colonized in nares of healthy person, 29% potential risk appears for MRSA infections [8].

While antibiotics such as methicillin are used frequently in patients, antibiotic-resistant strains may develop. After penicillin usage had become widespread to treat infections, penicillin-resistant *S. aureus* strains arose. Only a few years after following the usage of penicillin, penicillin-resistant *S. aureus* strains had arisen, and penicillinase-resistant methicillin usage had introduced for the treatment of penicillin-resistant *S. aureus* strains. After methicillin usage was introduced in 1961, MRSA strains that were also multidrug-resistant arose within a year. Methicillin that has been providing widespread of MRSA and becomes useless drug has not being used in recent years [7].

MRSA has become epidemic not only in nosocomial infections but also in community-associated infections [9]. MRSA that has been a common cause of nosocomial infections worldwide also has been arising in the community in recent years [10]. Invasive infections of MRSA have high morbidity and mortality rates [11]. Most of invasive staphylococcal and community-acquired MRSA (CA-MRSA) infections are related to the nasal carriage of *Staphylococcus* [6].

http://dx.doi.org/10.5772/65452

2.2. Biofilm and pathogenesis

Biofilm plays a role in the pathogenesis of staphylococcal infections. When microorganisms exposed to stress conditions, gene expression of biofilm is induced as a stress response. The biofilm that is a slime-like glycocalyx causes bacteria to survive in the stress conditions, causes bacterial attachment and colonization on biotic or abiotic surfaces such as prosthetic surfaces that may act as a substrate for microbial adhesion, and causes bacterial spread to whole body [12–14]. The biofilm producer *S. aureus* causes chronic infections such as indwelling device-related infections and chronic wound infections. Indwelling device-associated infections are mainly caused by biofilm producer *Staphylococci* including *S. aureus* and *Staphylococcus epidermidis*. The treatment of biofilm-embedded bacteria that are not eliminated completely by antimicrobials even at the high doses is tough and irresponsive. The patients whose indwelling device is infected by biofilm producers have higher risk of mortality. Infected implants that cannot be treated by antibiotics are removed out of the body to prevent biofilm-related infections [14].

2.3. Virulence of *S. aureus* Biofilm

Biofilm that is a slime-like glycocalyx embedded sessile community of microorganism inside. Polysaccharide matrix, staphylococcal surface proteins, extracellular DNA (eDNA), and teichoic acids construct biofilm of *S. aureus* that is an extracellular polymeric substance. Surface proteins of *S. aureus* also contribute biofilm formation, whereas polysaccharide intracellular adhesin (PIA) is the main component of biofilm formation in *S. aureus*. Extracellular DNA (eDNA) that plays a role in resistance and channels that store antibiotic-degrading enzymes such as β-lactamases construct extracellular polysaccharide matrix [14].

3. Mechanisms of biofilm formation and regulation by MRSA and MSSA

Biofilm is produced by distinct mechanisms in MRSA and Methicillin-sensitive Staphylococcus aureus (MSSA). Fitzpatrick et al. revealed that biofilm formation of the *icaADBC* operon deleted MRSA mutants was not affected, whereas biofilm formation of the *icaADBC* operon deleted MSSA mutants was impaired. This study showed that *ica*-independent biofilm formation is strain specific [15].

Biofilm is constructed not only by polysaccharide intracellular adhesin (PIA) but also by surface proteins. In the catheter infection, biofilm formation of clinical isolates of *S. aureus* of which *ica* operon is mutated is not reduced [13]. Biofilm of MSSA is formed in *ica*-dependent manner (PIA-dependent) by PIA that is encoded by *icaADBC* gene, whereas biofilm of MRSA is formed in *ica*-independent manner (PIA-independent) by surface proteins containing LPXTG anchoring domain that are anchored to peptidoglycan by sortase as a transpeptidase coded by *srtA* gene. Adherence to surfaces and intercellular aggregations of MSSA and MRSA cells are contributed by PIA in *ica*-dependent manner and surface proteins in *ica*-independent manner, respectively [4, 14]. Initial adherence of *S. aureus* to surfaces is contributed by Autolysin Atl that lyses cell causes release of eDNA and accumulation of cells in *ica*-independent manner [14, 16]. Especially, clinical MRSA adheres to polystyrene abiotic surfaces with Atl [16]. Intercellular accumulation of HA-MRSA and CA-MRSA is formed by FnBPA, FnBPB, Bap proteins, SasG, and protein A [4, 17, 18].

Three stages of *ica*-dependent and *ica*-independent biofilm formation that are adherence (adhesion, attachment), aggregation (maturation, accumulation), and detachment (dispersal) are regulated by *ica* operon and accessory gene regulator (agr) quorum sensing two-component signal transduction system, respectively [14].

Not only biofilm formation but also virulence factors such as phenol-soluble modulins (PSMs), toxins, and degradation enzymes production are regulated by agr quorum sensing two-component regulatory system [14, 19, 20]. Activation of *agr* system causes reduction in biofilm production due to the production of phenol-soluble modulins (PSMs) as surfactants, proteases, and nucleases that disperse microorganisms embedded in biofilm by enzymatic degradation of the biofilm matrix [14, 21, 22].

Accessory gene regulator (*agr*) system, which includes *agr* locus, regulates cell density, virulence, and biofilm formation of bacteria. RNAII and RNAIII are transcribed by binding of activated AgrA to P2 and P3 promoters in *agr* operon (*agr*BDCA), respectively. RNAII transcript that contains *agrB, D,* C, *A* genes encodes AgrB, D, C, A as a component of agr system, whereas RNAIII transcript that contains the *hld* gene encodes the δ-PSM (δ-phenol-soluble modulins or termed δ-hemolysin). RNAIII regulates virulence factors such as surface proteins that cause biofilm formation and exotoxins (RNAIII dependent control). In RNAIII independent control of *S. aureus*, synthesis of α-PSMs and β-PSMs is regulated by binding of AgrA to promoters of α-PSMs and β-PSMs in *psm* operon [14].

Supplementations of certain chemicals to growth media affect biofilm formation of *S. aureus* strains by regulating of gene expressions or breaking bonds that construct biofilm. Sodium chloride (NaCI) that induces expression of *ica* operon increases biofilm formation of MSSA [4, 23, 24]. Sodium metaperiodate that degrades polysaccharide bonds decreases biofilm formation of MSSA, whereas biofilms of MRSA are not affected. Proteinase A does not affect biofilm formation of MSSA [24, 4], whereas biofilm formation of MRSA is affected. pH of growth media that is decreased by glucose degradation represses agr regulator system. So, glucose supplementation of growth media that represses agr regulator system increases biofilm formation [4, 25]. Phenyl-methylsulfonyl fluoride (PMSF) that is a serine protease inhibitor increases biofilm formation by preventing *agr*-related biofilm detachment [21] and enhancing secretion of autolytic enzymes [26]. In early biofilm formation of HA-MRSA, biofilm formation is inhibited by polyanethole sodium sulfanate of which effect is not only preventing autolytic activity but also maintaining growth [16].

4. *Staphylococcus aureus* genome

Staphylococcus aureus genome contains core genome, accessory component, and foreign genes. Core genome that constructs backbone of genome has main metabolic function. Core genome

http://dx.doi.org/10.5772/65452

is highly conserved, and similarity of genes among isolates is ~98–100%. Accessory component that constructs 25% of *S. aureus* genome contains mobile genetic elements (MGEs) such as transposons (Tn), chromosomal cassettes, pathogenicity islands (PIs), genomic islands, and prophages acquired horizontally between strains [5] (**Figure 1**). MGEs carry virulence genes that are acquired horizontally by other strains (bacterial horizontal gene transfer (HGT)) [7, 27].

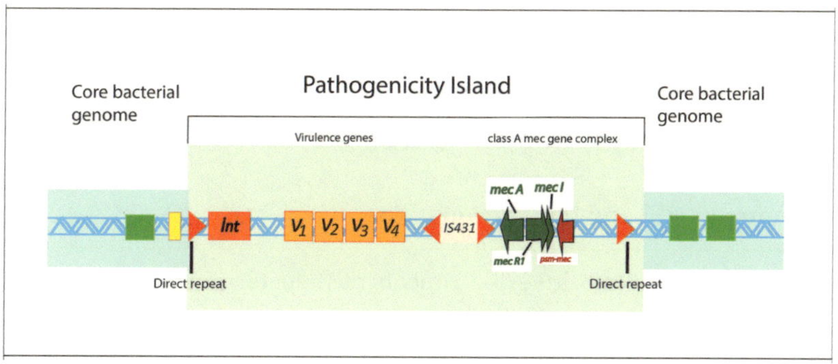

Figure 1. Staphylococcal genome.

Each strain of *S. aureus* has virulence varied according to having mobile genetic elements (MGEs) of which genes encode for varied virulence factors and toxins [9]. Genes of many secreted virulence factors such as exfoliative toxin A and B, superantigen toxins (SaPIs), toxic shock syndrome toxin (TSST), and enterotoxins are located in accessory genetic elements such as transposons, plasmids, prophages, and pathogenicity islands (PIs) that are also referred as MGEs, whereas genes that encode toxins such as α-toxins present in whole *S. aureus* strains and are located in core genome [7, 9]. Phenol-soluble modulins (PSMs) that are surfactant and encoded in core genome lyse immune cells such as neutrophils in inflammation and disperse biofilm [9, 14]. Cytolytic activity is present in shorter PSM-α type, while longer PSM-β type does not have cytolytic activity. It is seen that virulence of *S. aureus* is reduced by removing *psm-α* operon [7].

4.1. Prophages

Prophages have an effective role in pathogenicity of *S. aureus* due to causing horizontal gene transfer (HGT) by transferring virulence genes of which products are staphylokinase, enterotoxin A, G, K, Panton-Valentine leukocidin (PVL), and exfoliative toxin [5].

4.2. Pathogenicity islands (PIs)

The gene of superantigen toxins (SaPIs), which is one of the secreted virulence factors of *S. aureus*, is located in pathogenicity islands (PIs) that is also located in chromosome. SaPIs contain bacteriophage-associated genes that encode helicases and terminases involved in replication, integrases involved in integration, recombination and excition of MGE, and certain direct repeats [5, 28, 29].

The most known PI of *S. aureus* is SaPI1 that contains the *tst* gene encoding for TSST [7]. High-frequency transduction of SaPI1 is mediated by encapsulating SaPI1 by staphylococcal phage 80α that is own phage of *S. aureus* to transfer its genes in transduction process. Enterotoxin B is encoded by SaPI3 that is one of the SaPIs and encapsulated by phage 29 that is phage of *S. aureus* to transfer its genes in transduction process [5, 28].

S. aureus not only carry SaPIs but also carry vSa family genomic islands that encode ~50% of toxin and virulence factors of *S. aureus*. Conserved genes are present in this family. Among this family, vSa1 contains genes encoding for enterotoxin such as *seb, tsst,* and *ear,* whereas vSa2 contains genes encoding for enterotoxin such as *sec* and TSST (*tsst*). vSaα and vSaβ that are also present among vSa family genomic islands contain leukocidin genes [5].

4.3. Insertion sequence (IS) and transposons (Tn)

Insertion sequences (ISs) contain inverted repeats at their terminals and the integrases gene that causes transposition. Transposons (Tn) not only contain the transposase gene but also may contain ISs that induce movement of Tn and certain genes such as antibiotic resistance genes [5]. These elements provide a mechanism to transfer of virulence and resistance genes such as antibiotic resistance genes from place to place within the same cell or to other cell. These movable elements are excised from paired inverted repeats by transposase enzyme. While these elements are excised and inserted to new location such as within a gene that may be located within the same cell or other cell, the gene is disrupted [30].

4.4. Plasmids

Plasmids that are extrachromosomal genetic elements carry resistance genes causing antibiotic or heavy metal resistance, and virulence genes encoding for virulence factors, rather than genes involved in metabolic processes having vital functions [5]. There are three types of plasmids of *S. aureus* according to their size. Type I plasmids that are the smallest plasmids contain just one antibiotic-resistant determinant. Type II plasmids of which sizes are intermediate contain β-lactamase gene. The largest one is type III plasmids containing multiple resistant determinants such as gentamycin, trimethoprim, and ethidium bromide resistance [31]. Conjugative plasmids that are also type III plasmids are transferred horizontally to other cell by their own *tra* genes [5].

4.5. SCCmec

MGEs contain the *mecA* gene causing methicillin and other β-lactam resistance and occur in chromosome of methicillin-resistant *Staphylococcus* such as MRSA, and methicillin-resistant *S. epidermidis* MRSE is called staphylococcal cassette chromosome *mec* (*SCCmec*) [7, 9]. Inverted repeats that are localized at both terminals of *SCCmec* are the recognizing sequences for *SCCmec*-specific recombinase in the processes of excision of *SCCmec* from chromosome and integration of *SCCmec* to either other parts of chromosome or chromosome of other strain (**Figure 1**) [32].

SCCmec is composed of variable and conserved genetic elements. *SCCmec* carries *mec* operon that contains *mecA*, and regulatory genes such as *mecI* and *mecRI*, and cassette chromosome recombinase genes *ccrA*, *ccrB*, and *ccrC* that are localized in *ccr* locus and contribute excision from *SCCmec* and integration to chromosome. All these elements are highly conserved among *Staphylococcus*. J-region that is a variable region of *SCCmec* composed of genetic elements integrated such as ISs, Tns, and plasmids. In addition to methicillin resistance that is caused by *mecA* in a strain, if these integrated elements include additional genes encoding for antibiotic resistance, rather than methicillin, multiple resistance arises in this strain [5]. Just a year later on the first usage of methicillin for treatment of MRSA, clinical MRSA isolates that have multiple resistant to antibiotics were reported [33].

Variants of *mec* operon that are located in *SCCmec* are present according to whether *mecI* and *mecRI* genes are intact or having deletions. The variants of *mec* complex are class A, B, C, D, and E *mec*. IS431 that is related to the *mecA* gene are present in all *mec* operon classes. All classes except A consist of deleted portions that are happened in *mecI* and may run through to a portion of *mecRI* gene. Eight types of *SCCmec* were found according to having combinations of distinct variants of *mec* and *ccr* [5]. Multidrug-resistant strains have *SCCmec* type II and III that contain additional resistance genes. While MRSA is characterized by containing *SCCmec* type I or III and II in recent years, CA-MRSA strains are characterized by containing *SCCmec* type IV. Other *SCCmec* types are seen in strains very rare [7].

Methicillin-resistant strains of *Staphylococcus* have *mec* operon, whereas methicillin-sensitive strains of *Staphylococcus* do not have *mec* operon [34]. HGT of *mecA* from one to another strain is proved by researchers; the *mecA* gene of MRSA and *mecA* homolog of *Staphylococcus sciuri* revealed 88% identity. But *S. sciuri* containing *mecA* homolog is susceptible to methicillin. This supported that MRSA strains are descendents of ancestral strains in evolutionary process [35, 36]. *Staphylococcus haemolyticus* (*S. haemolyticus*) genome carries intact IS*1272* element, whereas the gene of *S. aureus* and *S. epidermidis* carries IS*1272* element deleted [37]. This revealed that horizontal gene transfer (HGT) is happened by acquisition of IS1272 from *S. haemolyticus* to *S. aureus* and *S. epidermidis*. HGT of *mecA* that is happened from *S. epidermidis* to *S. aureus* causes arising of MRSA during treatment with antibiotic [38]; *mecA* is transferred to methicillin-resistant *Staphylococcus* by the way that having inverted repeats at terminals of the *mec* gene complex and IS*431* of which location is especially within gene complexes encoding various resistance factors such as the *mec* gene complex.

Methicillin resistance is not only seen in isolates of *S. aureus* but also seen more common in isolates of *S. epidermidis*. Approximately, 70% of whole hospital-acquired methicillin-resistant *Staphylococcus* isolates is S. *epidermidis* [5].

5. The relationship between methicillin resistance and biofilm formation

The association between methicillin resistance and biofilm phenotype is taken attention according to studies executed [39–41]. Researchers determined that biofilm formation of HA-

MRSA BH1CC strain is decreased by removing *SCCmec* that results up-regulation of protease activity [4, 42, 43].

Biofilm formation of MRSA is enhanced by both phenol-soluble modulin mec (PSMmec) encoded by *psm-mec* and penicillin-binding protein 2a (PBP2a) encoded by *mecA* that also repress virulence of MRSA [42].

5.1. psm-mec

SCCmec not only contains genes encoding methicillin resistance and recombination but also contains genes encoding other antibiotics and heavy metal resistance; the *psm-mec* gene that is located near *mecA* in *SCCmec* especially type II, III, and VIII encodes PSMmec peptide. The PSMmec that is a cytolysin is the only staphylococcal toxin of which the gene is colocated with antibiotic-resistant determinant in MGEs of *S. aureus* rather than core genome; the *psm-mec* gene is conserved region of class A *mec* gene complex (**Figure 1**) [9].

Like many virulence toxins of *S. aureus* such as α-toxin and other PSMs, expression of PSMmec is also regulated by Agr two-component signal transport system [14, 44]. Many virulence toxins are regulated by RNAIII-dependent manner, whereas other PSMs and *psm-mec* are regulated by RNAIII independent manner (**Figure 2**) [14].

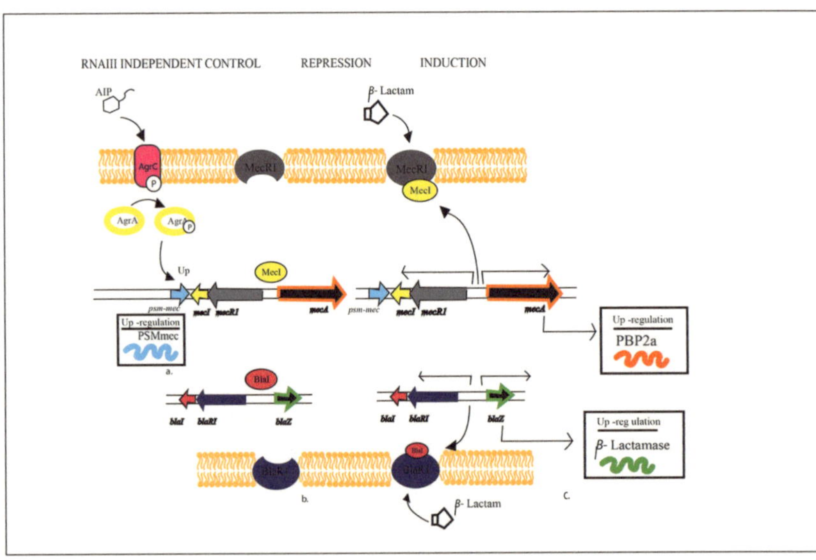

Figure 2. Mechanisms of *PSMmec*, PBP2a, and β-lactamase regulations. (a) Up-regulation of *psm-mec* by RNAIII independent Agr regulator system. (b) Repression of *mecA* and *blaZ* genes: In lack of β-lactams no transcription occurs. (c) Induction of genes: PBP2a and β-lactamase are transcribed by expression of *mecA* and *blaZ* in the presence of β-lactams, respectively.

Biofilm formation is increased by the repression of Agr system that downregulates *psm-mec* in MRSA [4] and PSMs [14]; the *psm-mec* gene of MRSA also has pleiotropic effect by changing biofilm phenotype and regulation of *psm* gene, decreasing toxin production, and the way

http://dx.doi.org/10.5772/65452

decreasing virulence, and the *psm-mec* gene that is up-regulated by Agr regulator system promotes biofilm formation of MRSA by reducing expression of PSMα toxin that is encoded in chromosome. As a result of reduced expression of PSMα toxin, virulence of *S. aureus* is reduced by PSMmec (**Figure 3**) [45, 46].

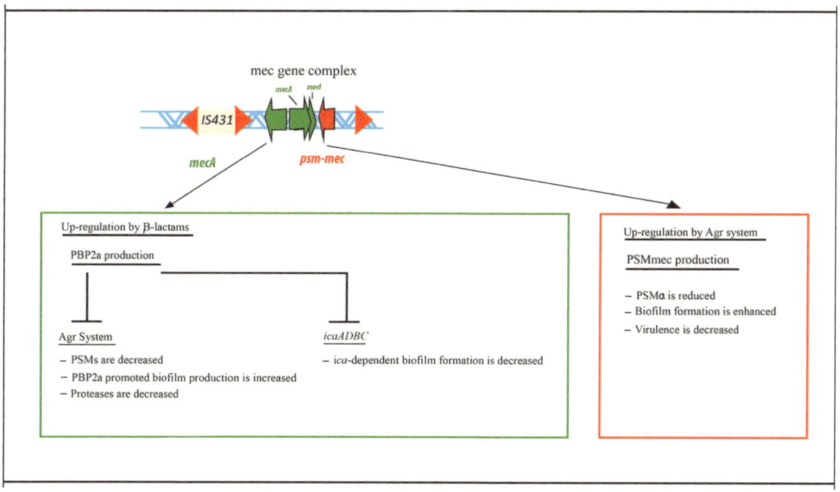

Figure 3. The effect of *mecA* and *psm-mec* induction of Staphylococcus aureus on biofilm formation and virulence.

Biofilm formation (adherence to surfaces and intercellular aggregations) of MSSA and MRSA strains is contributed by PIA in *ica*-dependent manner and surface proteins in *ica*-independent manner, respectively [4, 14]. Interestingly, in spite of the biofilm of MSSA that is formed by *ica*-independent manner is not seen or seen less prevalent, the *psm-mec* gene of type II *SCCmec* enhances expression of Atl and FnBPA in MSSA isolates [42].

5.2. mecA

Agr system is repressed by expression of PBP2a that is encoded by *mecA*, as a result of oxacillin usage [10]. PSMs are downregulated, proteases and virulence are decreased, and PBP2a promoted biofilm formation enhanced by repressed Agr regulator system. In contrary to this, *ica*-dependent biofilm formation is decreased by *ica* that is repressed by PBP2a (**Figure 3**) [42].

6. β-Lactam, methicillin, and multidrug resistance

6.1. Peptidoglycan biosynthesis of *S. aureus*

Peptidoglycan, surface proteins such as protein A, clumping factor A, fibronectin-binding protein (FnBP), collagen-binding protein, and teichoic acids construct the cell wall of *S. aureus*. Peptidoglycan is constructed by polypeptides containing L-alanine, D-glutamic acid, L-lysin and D-alanine, respectively, and glycan polysaccharide strands [5].

At the beginning of peptidoglycan synthesis, UDP-*N*-acetylmuramyl-pentapeptide (UDP-NAM-pentapeptide) and UDP-*N*-acetylglucosamine (UDP-NAG) that are nucleotide sugar-linked precursors are synthesized in cytoplasm of *S. aureus*. Pentapeptide with the sequence of L-alanine, D-glutamic acid, L-lysin, D-alanine, and D-alanine, respectively, is linked to NAM in cytoplasm. Then, bactoprenol that is a membrane-bound lipophilic acceptor transfers UDP-NAM-pentapeptide and UDP-NAG that are hydrophilic precursors from cytoplasm to the outer surface of cell membrane, respectively [5].

Then, transglycosylation and transpeptidation reactions are catalyzed by penicillin-binding proteins (PBPs) of which 4 types (PBP1, PBP2, PBP3, PBP4) are present in *S. aureus* [5]. PBPs that are DD-peptidases are bound to membrane [36]. *N*-acetylglucosamines (NAG) and *N*-acetylmuramic acids (NAM) that are bound by β(1-4) glycosidic bond catalyzed by PBPs in transglycosylation process construct glycan strands that form backbone of peptidoglycan. Transglycosylation reaction is catalyzed by PBPs, especially penicillin-binding protein 2 (PBP2) and glycosyltransferase Mtg. In transpeptidation reaction that is catalyzed by PBPs, L-lysine that is the amino acid of polypeptide linked to NAM of one glycan strand is cross-linked to D-alanine that is the amino acid of polypeptide linked to NAM of other glycan strand by pentaglycine cross bridge synthesized by family of FemABX non-ribosomal peptide. The last D-alanine of pentapeptide of UDP-NAM-pentapeptide is cleaved during transpeptidation reaction that cross-links peptidoglycan (**Figure 4**) [5].

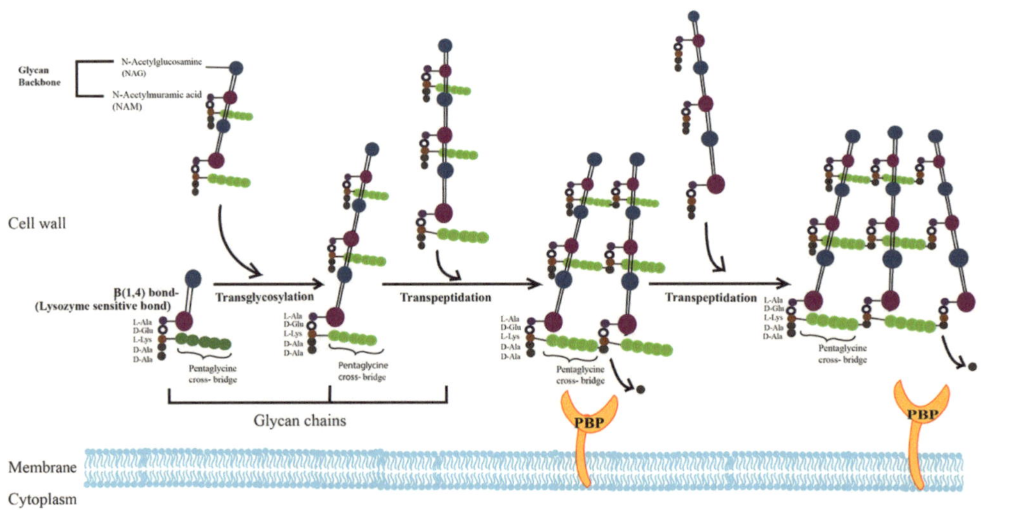

Figure 4. Biosynthesis of staphylococcal peptidoglycan. Peptidoglycan is constructed by transglycosylation and transpeptidation reactions catalyzed by penicillin-binding proteins (PBPs).

Teichoic acids that are polymers of glycerol phosphate or ribitol residues give negative feature to cell membrane and act as receptor of *S. aureus* phage [5].

6.2. Effect of β-lactam antibiotics against cell wall

Binding of β-lactams to PBPs that have high affinity to β-lactams is lethal for *Staphylococcus* [36]. Transpeptidase domain of PBPs in peptidoglycan is inactivated by β-lactam agents such as penicillins, cephalosporins, and methicillin and oxacillin that are both penicillinase-insensitive β-lactams acting as substrate of PBPs, rather than D-alanyl-D-alanine. Before enzyme substrate complex of β-lactam and PBP is formed completely, they can be dissociated by disrupting noncovalent association between them at the beginning of this complex. Later on, irreversible complex is formed by covalently binding of β-lactam that is a structural analog of D-alanyl-D-alanine substrate of PBP to active site of PBP complex that is the site for the binding of D-alanyl-D-alanine as a substrate during transpeptidation reaction (**Figure 4**). By this way, transpeptidation reaction that is the last step of peptidoglycan biosynthesis is blocked by β-lactam antibiotics that inactivate PBP. *Staphylococcus* undergoes to death due to the inhibition of peptidoglycan biosynthesis [5, 47].

6.3. Mechanism of β-lactam resistance of *Staphylococcus aureus*

β-lactamase enzymes cause resistance of cell to β-lactam antibiotics by inactivating β-lactam antibiotics. β-lactamase inactivates β-lactam antibiotics by disrupting amide bond of β-lactam ring [5].

Expression of the *bla*Z gene that is located in plasmid or transposon and encodes β-lactamase is regulated by *bla*I and *bla*RI that are own regulators. In the lack of β-lactam antibiotic, BlaI that bound to promoter-operator region repress *bla*Z gene, *bla*I-*bla*RI operon, so transcription of *bla*Z is not happen. In the usage in treatment or supplementation of β-lactam antibiotic to growth media, β-lactam binds to BlaRI that is a β-lactam-sensing signal transducer, and then, intracellular zinc metalloprotease domain of BlaRI is separated and cleaves BlaI that is already bound to operator. By this way, in the presence of β-lactam, *blaZ* is transcribed to β-lactamase that permits MRSA to grow by inactivating β-lactam (**Figure 2**) [5].

A study that showed the association between the antibiotic susceptibility patterns and the antibiotic resistance genes in staphylococcal isolates obtained from various clinical samples of patients revealed that 93.5% of *S. aureus* clinical isolates and 86.8% coagulase negative *Staphylococci* strains carry the blaZ gene [48].

6.4. Mechanism of methicillin resistance of *Staphylococcus aureus*

Resistance to methicillin, oxacillin, and nafcillin that are semisynthetic β-lactamase-insensitive β-lactams has developed by acquiring of the *mecA* gene [5]. MRSA is not only resistant to methicillin, but also resistant to all β-lactams [5, 36].

*mec*A gene expression is regulated by *mec*I and *mec*RI that are own regulators. In the lack of β-lactam antibiotic, MecI that bound to promoter-operator region repress *mecA*, and *mec*I-*mec*RI operon, so transcription of *mec*A is not happen. In the usage or supplementation of β-lactam antibiotic to growth media, β-lactam binds to MecRI that is a β-lactam-sensing signal transducer, and then, metallo-protease domain of MecRI that is placed in cytoplasmic site is separated and cleaves MecI that is already bound to operator. By this way, *mecA* is transcribed to PBP2a of which affinity is low to β-lactams [49]. Low affinity of PBP2a to β-lactams permits MRSA to grow as a result of peptidoglycan synthesis in the presence of β-lactams concentrations that can inactivate transpeptidase activity of PBPs. PBP2a that belongs to PBPs contains transpeptidase domain and non-penicillin-binding protein (**Figure 2**) [5].

Structure, function, mechanism, and molecular organization of *mec*I and *mec*RI are similar to *bla*I and *bla*RI, respectively [36]. Expression of *mecA* is regulated by both MecI and BlaI. When MecI and BlaI are both present at the same time, *mec*A is repressed even stronger; the *mec*I gene of most of the clinical MRSA isolates has deletions; due to this, expression of *mec*A is regulated by BlaI [5].

6.5. Multidrug resistance

There are eight types of *SCCmec* (I-VIII). *SCCmec* type II and III that demonstrate multi-resistance also contain additional antibiotic resistance genes such as erythromycin and tetracycline as well as methicillin. *SCCmec* type IV that is essential for community-acquired MRSA strains (CA-MRSA) that is one of the virulent strains and infect healthy person in community rather than hospital arised. The other types of *SCCmec* are rare [7].

IS*431* is mainly found in chromosome and plasmids of *Staphylococcus* and is also related to encoding various resistance factors such as tetracycline, mercury, and cadmium resistance. If other additional resistance genes such as *aadD* encoding an enzyme for tobramycin resistance are integrated within *SCCmec* cassette (IS*431mec*), multiple drug resistance is developed in methicillin-resistant *Staphylococcus* [36]. Plasmids pUB110, pI258, and pT181 integrated in *SCCmec* have additional resistance genes encoding kanamycin, tobramycin and bleomycin resistance (*ant(4')*), penicillin and heavy metal resistance, and tetracyclin resistance, respectively. Tn554 integrated in *SCCmec* have additional resistance gene *erm*A encoding inducible macrolide, lincosamide, and streptogramin resistance [49].

6.6. Homogeneous and heterogeneous resistance of MRSA

Heterogeneity is a characteristic of MRSA of which resistance level varies according to contents and ingredients of culture medium in which MRSA is grown and β-lactam antibiotic used. Most of the cells of heterogeneous methicillin resistance (HeR) strains (~99.9% or above) are susceptible to β-lactam of which concentration is low that is about 1–5 μg/mL of methicillin, whereas just a few subpopulations (such as 1 in 10^6 cfu/mL) grow in 50 μg/mL or above of methicillin by expressing high-level resistance. Homogeneous strains (HoR) are resistant to low concentration of β-lactam and can grow in higher concentrations of methicillin that is about 5 μg/mL or above [36].

Heterogeneity of MRSA is unstable and changeable according to growth conditions. HeR strains become homogeneous strains (HoR) by growth media supplemented with NaCI or sucrose for providing hypertonicity of media, or supplemented with higher concentrations of β-lactam antibiotic, or incubated at 30°C in incubator. Supplementation of growth media with EDTA or incubation at 37–43°C leads to conversion of HoR strains to HeR [36]. This conversion

http://dx.doi.org/10.5772/65452

of HeR and HoR in distinct culture conditions is due to the regulation of gene expression by Agr regulator system [42]. These conversions of MRSA can be repeated by repeated culturing in changed media that have different supplementations.

Most clinical isolates of MRSA grow as HeR in routine growth conditions, and most of them show low or moderate level of resistance, whereas a few subpopulations show high-level resistance [36].

Author details

Sahra Kırmusaoğlu

Address all correspondence to: kirmusaoglu_sahra@hotmail.com

Department of Molecular Biology and Genetics, Faculty of Arts and Sciences, T.C. Haliç University, Istanbul, Turkey

References

[1] Hall-Stoodley L and Stoodley P. Evolving concepts in biofilm infections. Cellular Microbiology. 2009;11(7):1034–1043.

[2] Stoodley P, Sauer K, Davies DG and Costerton JW. Biofilms as complex differentiated communities. Annual Review of Microbiology. 2002;56:187–209.

[3] Bjarnsholt T, Moser C, Jensen PO and Hoiby N. Biofilm Infections. New York, Dordrecht, Heidelberg, London: Springer Science Business Media, LLC, 2011;215–225.

[4] McCarthy H, Rudkin JK, Black NS, Gallagher L, O'Neill E and O'Gara JP. Methicillin resistance and the biofilm phenotype in *Staphylococcus aureus*. Frontiers in Cellular and Infection Microbiology. 2015;5(1):1–9.

[5] Plata K, Rosato AE and Wegrzyn G. *Staphylococcus aureus* as an infectious agent: overview of biochemistry and molecular genetics of its pathogenicity. Acta Biochimica Polonica. 2009;56(4):597–612.

[6] Nguyen KV, Zhang T, Thi Vu BN, Dao TT, Tran TK, Thi Nguyen DN, Thi Tran HK, Thi Nguyen CK, Fox A, Horby P and Wertheim H. *Staphylococcus aureus* nasopharyngeal carriage in rural and urban northern Vietnam. Transactions of the Royal Society of Tropical Medicine and Hygiene. 2014;108:783–790.

[7] Otto M. *Staphylococcus aureus* toxin gene hitchhikes on a transferable antibiotic resistance element. Virulence. 2010;1(1):49–51.

[8] Huang SS and Platt R. Risk of methicillin-resistant *Staphylococcus aureus* infection after previous infection or colonization. Clinical Infectious Diseases. 2003;36:281–285.

[9] Chatterjee SS, Chen L, Joo HS, Cheung GYC, Kreiswirth GYC and Otto M. Distribution and regulation of the mobile genetic element-encoded phenol-soluble modulin PSM-mec in methicillin-resistant *Staphylococcus aureus*. PLoS One. 2011;6(12):e28781.

[10] Rudkin JK, Laabel M, Edwards AM, Joo HS, Otto M, Lennon KL, O'Gara JP, Waterfield NR and Massey RC. Oxacillin alters the toxin expression profile of community associated methicillin-resistant *Staphylococcus aureus*. Antimicrobial Agents and Chemotherapy. 2014;58(2):1100–1107.

[11] Rehm SJ and Tice A. *Staphylococcus aureus*: methicillin-susceptible *S. aureus* to methicillin-resistant *S. aureus* and vancomycin-resistant *S. aureus*. Clinical Infectious Diseases. 2010;51(S2):S176–S182.

[12] Donlan RM and Costerton JW. Biofilms: survival mechanisms of clinically relevant microorganisms. Clinical Microbiology Reviews. 2002;15:167–193.

[13] Archer NK, Mazaitis MJ, Costerton JW, Leid JG, Powers ME and Shirtliff ME. *Staphylococcus aureus* biofilms properties, regulation and roles in human disease. Virulence. 2011;2(5):445–459.

[14] Kırmusaoğlu S. Staphylococcal biofilms: pathogenicity, mechanism and regulation of biofilm formation by quorum-sensing system and antibiotic resistance mechanisms of biofilm-embedded microorganisms. In: Dhanasekaran D, Thajuddin N, editors. Microbial Biofilms—Importance and Applications. Croatia: InTech; 2016. p. 189–209. doi:10.5772/61499

[15] Fitzpatrick F, Humphreys H and O'Gara JP. Evidence for icaADBC-independent biofilm development mechanism in methicillin-resistant *Staphylococcus aureus* clinical isolates. Journal of Clinical Microbiology. 2005;43:1973–1976.

[16] Houston P, Rowe SE, Pozzi C, Waters EM and O'Gara JP. Essential role for the major autolysin in the fibronectin-binding protein-mediated *Staphylococcus aureus* biofilm phenotype. Infection and Immunity. 2011;79:1153–1165.

[17] O'Neill E, Pozzi C, Houston P, Humphreys H, Robinson DA, et al. A novel *Staphylococcus aureus* biofilm phenotype mediated by the fibronectin-binding proteins, FnBPA and FnBPB. Journal of Bacteriology. 2008;190:3835–3850.

[18] McCourt J, O'Halloran DP, McCarthy H, O'Gara JP and Geoghegan JA. Fibronectin-binding proteins are required for biofilm formation by community-associated methicillin-resistant *Staphylococcus aureus* strain LAC. FEMS Microbiology Letters. 2014;353:157–164.

[19] Otto M. *Staphylococcal* infections: mechanisms of biofilm maturation. Annual Review of Medicine. 2013;64:175–188.

[20] Schwartz K, Syed AK, Stephenson RE, Rickard AH and Boles BR. Functional amyloids composed of phenol soluble modulins stabilize *Staphylococcus aureus* biofilms. PLoS Pathogens. 2012;8:e1002744.

[21] Boles BR and Horswill AR. Agr-mediated dispersal of *Staphylococcus aureus* biofilms. PLoS Pathogens. 2008;4:e1000052.

[22] Speziale P, Pietrocola G, Foster TJ, Geoghegan JA. Protein-based biofilm matrices in *Staphylococci*. Frontiers in Cellular and Infection Microbiology. 2014;4:171. doi:10.3389/fcimb.2014.00171

[23] Fitzpatrick F, Humphreys H and O'Gara JP. Environmental regulation of biofilm development in methicillin-resistant and methicillin-susceptible *Staphylococcus aureus* clinical isolates. Journal of Hospital Infection. 2006;62:120–122.

[24] O'Neill E, Pozzi C, Houston P, Smyth D, Humphreys H, Robinson DA and O'Gara JP. Association between methicillin susceptibility and biofilm regulation in *Staphylococcus aureus* isolates from device-related infections. Journal of Clinical Microbiology. 2007;45(5):1379–1388.

[25] Regassa LB, Novick RP and Betley MJ. Glucose and nonmaintained pH decrease expression of the accessory gene regulator (agr) in *Staphylococcus aureus*. Infection and Immunity. 1992;60:3381–3388.

[26] Fournier B and Hooper DC. A new two component regulatory system involved in adhesion, autolysis, and extracellular proteolytic activity of *Staphylococcus aureus*. Journal of Bacteriology. 2000;182:3955–3964.

[27] Novick RP and Subedi A. The SaPIs: mobile pathogenicity islands of *Staphylococcus*. Chemical Immunology and Allergy. 2007;93:42–57.

[28] Novick RP. Mobile genetic elements and bacterial toxinoses: the superantigen-encoding pathogenicity islands of *Staphylococcus aureus*. Plasmid. 2003;49(2):93–105.

[29] Dongsheng C, Mohammad SHH and Bernard C. Identifying pathogenicity islands in bacterial pathogenomics using computational approaches. Pathogens. 2014;3:36–56.

[30] Klug WS, Cummings MR, Spencer CA and Palladino MA. Concepts of Genetics. 11th ed. London: Pearson Education, 2015.

[31] Novick RP. *Staphylococcal* plasmids and their replication. Annual Review of Microbiology. 1989;43:537–565.

[32] Noto MJ, Kreiswirth BN, Monk AB and Archer GL. Gene acquisition at the insertion site for SCCmec the genomic island conferring methicillin resistance in *Staphylococcus aureus*. Journal of Bacteriology. 2008;190:1276–1283.

[33] Rise LB. Antimicrobial resistance in gram-positive bacteria. American Journal of Medicine. 2006;119(6):S11–S19.

[34] Hiramatsu K, Konodo N and Ito T. Genetic basis for molecular epidemiology of MRSA. Journal of Infection and Chemotheropy. 1996;2:117–129.

[35] Wu SW, de Lencastre H and Tomasz A. Recruitment of the mecA gene homologue of *Staphylococcus sciuri* into a resistance determinant and expression of the resistant phenotype in *Staphylococcus aureus*. Journal of Bacteriology. 2001;183:2417–2424.

[36] Chambers HF. Methicillin resistance in *Staphylococci*: molecular and biochemical basis and clinical implications. Clinical Microbiology Reviews. 1997;10(4):781–791.

[37] Kobayashi N, Urasawa S, Uehara N and Watanabe N. Distribution of insertion sequence-like element IS1272 and its position relative to methicillin resistance genes in clinically important *Staphylococci*. Antimicrobial Agents and Chemotheropy. 1999;43(11):2780–2782.

[38] Wielders CL, Vriens MR, Brisse S, de Graaf-Miltenburg LA, Troelstra A, Fleer A, Schmitz FJ, Verhoef J and Fluit AC. *In-vivo* transfer of mecA DNA to *Staphylococcus aureus* [corrected]. Lancet. 2001;357:1674–1675.

[39] Mempel M, Feucht H, Ziebuhr W, Endres M, Laufs R and Grüter L. Lack of mecA transcription in slime-negative phase variants of methicillin-resistant *Staphylococcus epidermidis*. Antimicrobial Agents and Chemotherapy. 1994;38(6):1251–1255.

[40] Mempel M, Muller E, Hoffmann R, Feucht H, Laufs R and Grüter L. Variable degree of slime production is linked to different levels of beta-lactam susceptibility in *Staphylococcus epidermidis* phase variants. Medical Microbiology and Immunology (Berl). 1995;184:109–113.

[41] Christensen G, Baddour LM, Madison BM, Parisi JT, Abraham SN, Hasty JH, Lowrance JA, Josephs JA and Simpson A. Colonial morphology of *Staphylococci* on Memphis agar: phase variation of slime production, resistance to beta-lactam antibiotics, and virulence. Journal of Infectious Diseases. 1990;161(6):1153–1169.

[42] Pozzi C, Waters EM, Rudkin JK, Schaeffer CR, Lohan AJ, Tong P, Loftus PJ, Pier GB, Fey PD, Massey RC and O'Gara JP. Methicillin resistance alters the biofilm phenotype and attenuates virulence in *Staphylococcus aureus* device-associated infections. PLoS Pathogens. 2012;8:e1002626.

[43] Rudkin JK, Edwards AM, Bowden MG, Brown EL, Pozzi C, Waters EM, Chan WC, Williams P, O'Gara JP and Massey RC. Methicillin resistance reduces the virulence of healthcare-associated methicillin-resistant *Staphylococcus aureus* by interfering with the agr quorum sensing system. Journal of Infectious Diseases. 2012;205(5):798–806.

[44] Queck SY, Khan BA, Wang R, Bach TH, Kretschmer D, Chen L, Kreiswirth BN, Peschel A, DeLeo FR and Otto M. Mobile genetic element-encoded cytolysin connects virulence to methicillin resistance in MRSA. PLoS Pathogens. 2009;5(7):e1000533.

[45] Kaito C, Omae Y, Matsumoto Y, Nagata M, Yamaguchi H, Aoto T, Ito T, Hiramatsu K and Sekimizu K. A novel gene, fudoh, in the SCCmec region suppresses the colony spreading ability and virulence of *Staphylococcus aureus*. PLoS One. 2008;3(12):e3921.

[46] Kaito C, Saito Y, Nagano G, Ikuo M, Omae Y, Hanada Y, Han X, Kuwahara-Arai K, Hishinuma T, Baba T, Ito T, Hiramatsu K and Sekimizu K. Transcription and translation products of the cytolysin gene psm-mec on the mobile genetic element SCCmec regulate *Staphylococcus aureus* virulence. PLoS Pathogens. 2011;7(2):e1001267.

[47] Sangappa M and Thiagarajan P. Methicillin-resistant *Staphylococcus aureus*: resistance genes and their regulation. International Journal of Pharmacy and Pharmaceutical Sciences. 2012;4:658–667.

[48] Duran N, Ozer B, Duran GG, Onlen Y and Demir C. Antibiotic resistance genes and susceptibility patterns in *Staphylococci*. Indian Journal of Medical Research. 2012;135(3): 389–396.

[49] Deurenberg RH, Vink C, Kalenic S, Friedrich AW, Bruggeman CA and Stobberingh EE. The molecular evolution of methicillin-resistant *Staphylococcus aureus*. Clinical Microbiology Infection. 2007;13:222–235.

Chapter 3

Glycopeptide Resistance in *S. aureus*

Hasan Cenk Mirza

Additional information is available at the end of the chapter

http://dx.doi.org/10.5772/65471

Abstract

The glycopeptides (particularly vancomycin) have been the recommended therapy for serious methicillin-resistant *Staphylococcus aureus* (MRSA) infections. The increased incidence of MRSA has led to the frequent use of vancomycin. Unfortunately, with the increased use of vancomycin, isolates of *S. aureus* have been discovered with reduced susceptibility to vancomycin. Several studies suggest that reduced vancomycin susceptibility is associated with vancomycin treatment failure. Various forms of glycopeptide resistance have appeared in MRSA strains, including high-level resistance, homogeneous and heterogeneous intermediate resistance. While vancomycin-resistant *S. aureus* (VRSA) strains are limited to a handful of reported cases and vancomycin-intermediate *S. aureus* (VISA) strains remain rare; heterogeneous VISA (hVISA) strains are more common. This article summarizes the current knowledge regarding the history, definition, mechanisms, detection methods, epidemiology and clinical significance of 'glycopeptide resistance in *S. aureus*' and discusses therapeutic options for the treatment of hVISA/VISA infections.

Keywords: *S. aureus*, glycopeptide resistance, vancomycin, teicoplanin, hVISA, VISA

1. Introduction

Glycopeptide group antibiotics—notably vancomycin—have traditionally been the mainstay of therapy for infections caused by methicillin-resistant *Staphylococcus aureus* (MRSA) [1]. However, the increased incidence of MRSA infections has led to increased use of vancomycin and has resulted in the emergence of *S. aureus* with reduced susceptibility to vancomycin. Both the terms vancomycin-intermediate *S. aureus* (VISA) and glycopeptide-intermediate *S. aureus* (GISA) have been used in the literature [2]. Since many VISA isolates also have been intermediate to glycopeptide teicoplanin, the term GISA may be more accurate. However, the acronym VISA is more frequently used. Various studies have associated the presence of VISA and heterogeneous VISA (hVISA) with vancomycin treatment failure.

This article focuses on the history, definition, mechanisms, detection methods, epidemiology, and clinical significance of 'glycopeptide resistance in *S. aureus*' and the therapeutic options for the treatment of hVISA/VISA infections.

2. History and definition of glycopeptide resistance

The glycopeptide vancomycin was isolated from a Gram-positive filamentous actinomycete called *Amycolatopsis orientalis* and was approved for use by the U.S. Food and Drug Administration in 1958 [2, 3]. Vancomycin acts by inhibiting proper cell wall synthesis. It binds with high affinity to D-alanyl-D-alanine (D-Ala-D-Ala) terminal end of peptidoglycan precursors and prevents cross-linking of peptidoglycan by inhibiting the action of transglycosidase and transpeptidases. Vancomycin has been in clinical use for decades and there was no notable resistance to vancomycin reported in *S. aureus* until 1996. In 1996, a MRSA strain with vancomycin MIC of 8 μg/ml (Mu50, VISA) was isolated from the surgical wound infection from a 4-month-old male infant who had undergone cardiac surgery [4]. After this case, two patients from USA and one patient from France with infections due to *S. aureus* with intermediate resistance to vancomycin were reported [5, 6]. After the emergence of VISA; a new model of vancomycin resistance (hVISA) was defined by Hiramatsu *et al.* in 1997 [7]. The first hVISA strain Mu3 was isolated from the sputum of a 64-year-old patient with MRSA pneumonia who failed vancomycin therapy. hVISA strains are susceptible to vancomycin by the standard broth microdilution reference method (vancomycin MIC ≤2 μg/ml) but contain subpopulations of cells (one in every 10^5–10^6) for which the vancomycin MIC is in the intermediate range, currently defined as 4–8 μg/ml by the Clinical and Laboratory Standards Institute (CLSI) [8]. hVISA strains are more commonly found than VISA and different rates of hVISA are reported from different countries.

In 2002, the first *S. aureus* fully resistant to vancomycin [vancomycin-resistant *S. aureus* (VRSA), vancomycin MIC ≥16 μg/ml] was reported in Michigan, United States (U.S). Fortunately, VRSA is very rare as only 14 cases of VRSA have been reported in U.S. so far [9].

3. Phenotypic changes and mechanisms of resistance

3.1. hVISA and VISA

Heterogeneous VISA appears to be the phase before the development of VISA. Vancomycin exhibits a selective pressure that leads to the growth of VISA subpopulations, eventually creating a uniform population of VISA [10].

One of the most common phenotypic changes observed in hVISA/VISA is the thickened cell wall with reduced peptidoglycan cross-linking (**Figure 1**) [2, 10, 11]. Reduced cross-linking of peptidoglycan leads to an increase in free D-Ala-D-Ala residues (binding sites for vancomycin). It is supposed that vancomycin binds to these free D-Ala-D-Ala residues in the outer layers of the thickened cell wall and is unable to reach its site of action at the cell membrane [12]. The trapped vancomycin molecules within the cell wall clog the peptidoglycan meshwork and form a physical barrier towards further incoming vancomycin molecules. Thus, collaboration of the clogging and cell wall thickening leads to glycopeptide resistance (**Figure 2**) [13, 14].

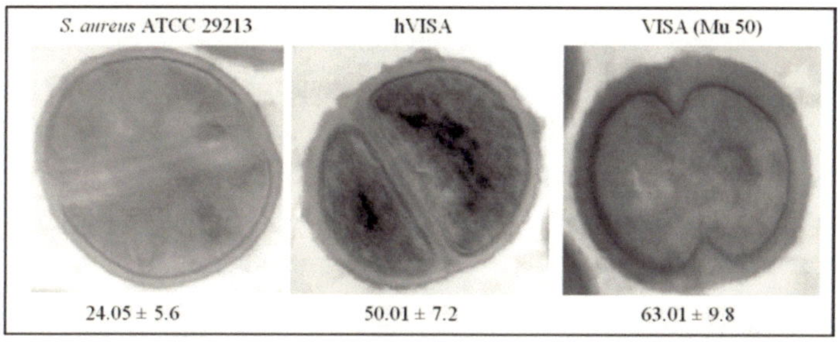

Figure 1. Comparison of the cell wall thickness of *S. aureus* ATCC 29213 [Vancomycin-susceptible *S. aureus* (VSSA)], hVISA and VISA strains by transmission electron microscopy. The cell wall thickness, in nanometers (mean ± SD), is given under each image. Magnification: × 60,000. (Adapted from Ref. [11] which was published under an open-access license agreement).

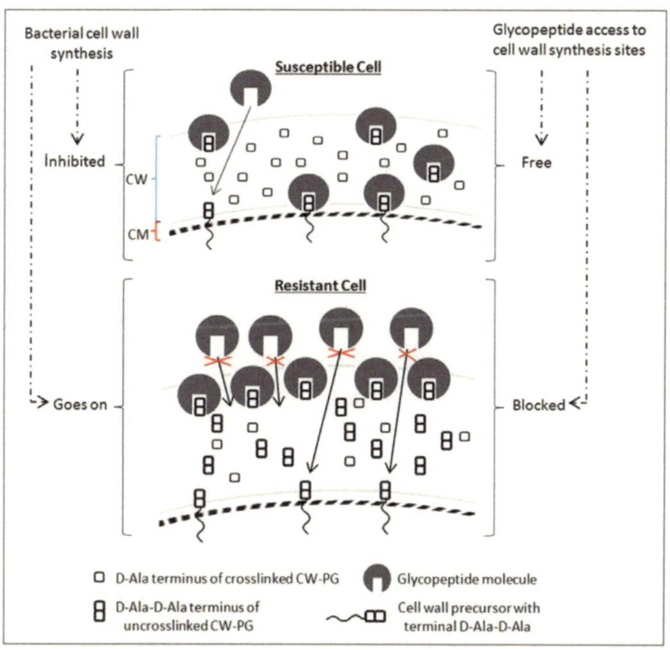

Figure 2. Model depicting the resistance mechanisms of hVISA/VISA. CW, cell wall; CM, cell membrane; PG, peptidoglycan. (Adapted with permission from Ref. [14]).

In addition to thickened cell wall, hVISA/VISA strains exhibit other phenotypic changes including reduced autolytic activity, reduced hemolytic activity and slow growth *in vitro* [10, 15].

3.1.1. Molecular mechanisms of resistance

The molecular mechanisms of glycopeptide resistance in hVISA/VISA are still not clearly understood. To date, no specific genetic determinants of hVISA/VISA have been defined. However, some of the genes whose expression has been found to be altered in VISA strains include *atl* (autolysin), *mprF* (phosphatidylglycerol lysyltransferase), *sceD* (transglycosylase), *sarA, sigB, tcaA,* and *ddh* [16]. Furthermore, mutations associated with the intermediate resistance phenotype have been identified in the two-component regulatory systems [*vraSR* (vancomycin resistance-associated sensor/regulator), *graSR* (glycopeptide resistance-associated sensor/regulator), *walKR*], and *rpoB* (RNA polymerase) gene [15].

Cellular physiology of hVISA/VISA is believed to be altered due to the cumulative effects of mutations and/or modulation of regulatory systems [17]. As a result, altered cell wall structure and metabolism resulting from multiple genetic changes appears to be responsible for intermediate resistance to glycopeptides.

3.2. VRSA

The mechanism of vancomycin resistance in VRSA strains is different from that of hVISA/VISA strains. The vanA gene complex, which confers high-level resistance to glycopeptides in enterococci, was detected in VRSA isolates.

To date, nine types of glycopeptide resistance have been described in enterococci. Eight of these types (VanA, VanB, VanD, VanE, VanG, VanL, VanM, and VanN) correspond to acquired resistance, whereas VanC is an intrinsic characteristic of *Enterococcus gallinarum* and *Enterococcus casseliflavus*. Glycopeptide resistance in enterococci results from the production of modified peptidoglycan precursors ending in D-alanyl-D-lactate (D-Ala-D-Lac) (VanA, VanB, VanD, and VanM) or D-alanyl-D-serine (D-Ala-D-Ser) (VanC, VanE, VanG, VanL, and VanN) to which vancomycin binds with low affinity and the elimination of high-affinity precursors ending in D-Ala-D-Ala [18].

Resistance in VRSA isolates is caused by the horizontal transfer of transposon Tn*1546* (carrying the *vanA* operon) from vancomycin-resistant *Enterococcus faecalis* [15, 19]. Vancomycin is known to act by binding to the terminal D-Ala-D-Ala of bacterial cell wall precursors. The *vanA gene* complex acquired by VRSA strains enables the bacteria to synthesize cell wall precursors terminating in D-Ala-D-Lac for which vancomycin has a greatly decreased affinity. In the presence of vancomycin, the novel cell wall precursors are synthesized, allowing continued peptidoglycan assembly [19, 20].

http://dx.doi.org/10.5772/65471

4. Laboratory detection of hVISA, VISA and VRSA

Laboratory detection of VISA and VRSA strains is easier than hVISA, as there are defined CLSI MIC criteria (MIC: 4–8 μg/ml for VISA and MIC ≥16 μg/ml for VRSA). These criteria have been defined using the reference broth microdilution (BMD) method. Results obtained by the use of other methods for determining the MIC should be confirmed with BMD [21]. Disk diffusion (Kirby-Bauer) is not an acceptable method for vancomycin susceptibility testing of *S.aureus* isolates.

Detection of hVISA is problematic for most clinical microbiology laboratories. The lack of a precise definition and standardized testing makes the detection of hVISA difficult [21]. hVISA strains appear susceptible to vancomycin (MIC ≤ 2 μg/ml) with conventional testing but contain subpopulations (1 per 10^5–10^6 organisms) that express reduced vancomycin susceptibility (MIC ≥4 μg/ml). Standardized methods for susceptibility testing [broth microdilution (BMD), agar dilution and standard Etest]—which use an inoculum of only 5×10^4 colony-forming unit (CFU)/well (BMD) or 1×10^4 CFU/spot (agar dilution)—fail to detect hVISA, in part due to the small inoculum, the relatively poor support of growth on Mueller-Hinton agar (MHA) plates, or a combination of both [2, 22].

The morphological features of hVISA/VISA isolates can be different from those of standard *S. aureus* cultures on agar plates. Careful observation may reveal smaller-sized colonies, "mixed" colony morphology (large and small colonies or colonies with different pigmentations in a pure culture) and reduced pigmentation. However, these changes may be subjective and are not diagnostic [2, 21].

Methods for "hVISA detection" use higher inoculum, prolonged incubation or more nutritious agar to promote the growth of subpopulations with reduced susceptibility to vancomycin. Population analysis profile-area under the curve (PAP-AUC) is considered the gold standard method for hVISA detection. However, this method is labor-intensive, time-consuming and not suitable for routine use in clinical microbiology laboratories [10, 22]. As a consequence, several screening methods have been developed for the detection of hVISA.

4.1. Screening methods for hVISA

4.1.1. Screening plates

A number of screening plates containing various concentrations of vancomycin or teicoplanin have been proposed for the detection of hVISA/VISA isolates [brain heart infusion agar (BHIA) with 3 μg/ml, 4 μg/ml or 6 μg/ml vancomycin, BHIA with 5 μg/ml teicoplanin, MHA with 5 μg/ml vancomycin or 5 μg/ml teicoplanin] [23–26]. **Figure 3** shows the growth of a hVISA strain on BHIA with 4 μg/ml vancomycin.

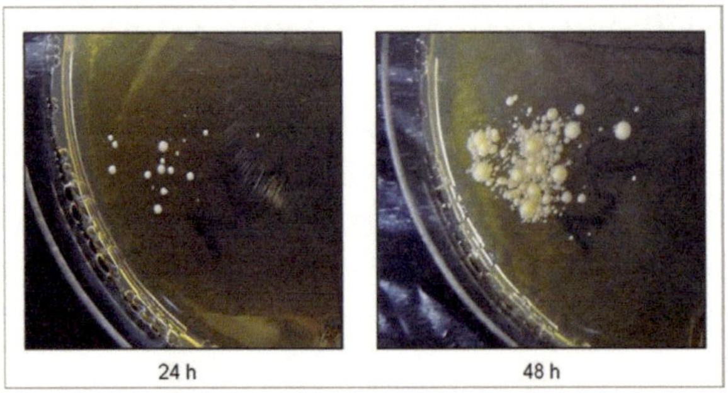

Figure 3. Photograph of a hVISA grown on BHIA with 4 μg/ml vancomycin for 24 and 48 h.

Antibiogram Committee of the French Society for Microbiology recommends the use of MHA with 5 μg/ml teicoplanin (MHA5T). This screening plate has been tested by various studies using an inoculum of 10 μl of a 2.0 McFarland standard suspension for the detection of VISA/hVISA isolates. Growth of one or more colonies is considered positive after 48 h of incubation. MHA5T has been shown to have sensitivity ranging from 65% to 79% and specificity ranging from 35 to 95% for the detection of hVISA [2].

In a study conducted by Satola *et al.*, BHIA containing 4 μg/ml vancomycin and 16 g/l pancreatic digest of casein has been shown to be 90% sensitive and 95% specific with a 0.5 McFarland inoculum and 100% sensitive and 68% specific with a 2.0 McFarland inoculum [22]. However, further studies are needed to determine the value of this screening plate.

4.1.2. Etest macromethod

Etest macromethod is performed utilizing a higher inoculum of organism (2.0 McFarland vs. 0.5 McFarland utilized in standard Etest) streaked onto BHIA. Vancomycin and teicoplanin Etest strips are applied to the dry agar surface and read after 48 h of incubation (compared to 24 h for standard Etest) at 35°C [10]. Zones must be read at complete inhibition, with care, to visualize hazy growth or microcolonies. Heteroresistance is defined as MICs for vancomycin and teicoplanin of ≥8 μg/ml or a teicoplanin MIC of ≥12 μg/ml alone. It should be noted that the result of the Etest macromethod is just a cutoff level and is not a true MIC, because this method differs from the standard MIC calculation [2, 21].

Figure 4 shows a hVISA strain (confirmed by PAP-AUC) with positive Etest macromethod result. The presence of microcolonies inside the inhibition zones reflects the heterogeneous resistant character of the strain (**Figure 5**). Subculture from a single microcolony (**Figure 5B**) done on blood agar reveals heterogeneous colony morphology (a common feature of hVISA/VISA strains) (**Figure 6**).

Various studies have evaluated the performance of Etest macromethod, using PAP-AUC as the gold standard. Etest macromethod has been shown to have sensitivity ranging from 57 to 98.5% and specificity ranging from 55 to 96% for the detection of hVISA [22, 23, 25, 27–29]. The differences in sensitivity and specificity rates may be partially explained by the use of various inoculum sizes for Etest macromethod (50, 100 or 200 μl) in different studies [27, 28, 30]. Currently, the manufacturer recommends the use of an inoculum of 100 μl [31].

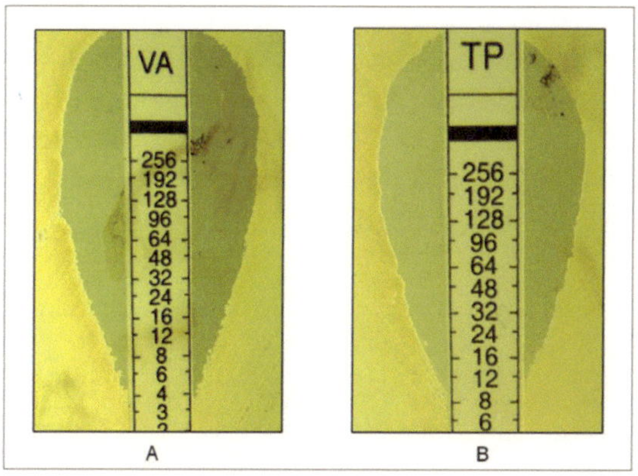

Figure 4. Positive Etest macromethod result for a hVISA strain isolated from blood culture A: Vancomycin Etest, B: Teicoplanin Etest.

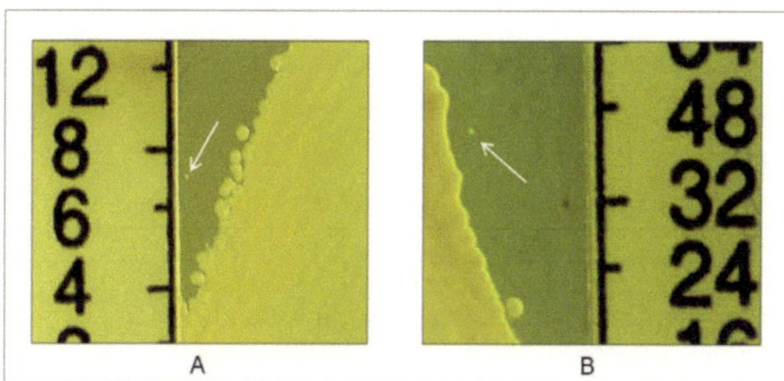

Figure 5. Magnified appearance of **Figure 4(A and B)**. The arrows indicate the presence of microcolonies growing within the zones of inhibition. A: Vancomycin Etest, B: Teicoplanin Etest.

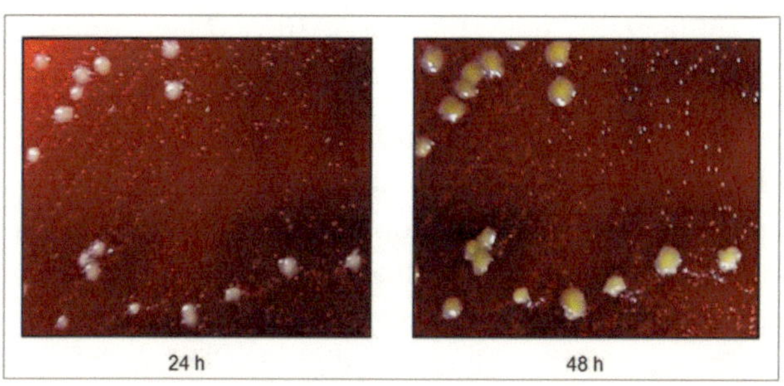

Figure 6. Subculture from a single microcolony (**Figure 5B**) on blood agar demonstrating different colony morphotypes.

4.1.3. Etest GRD

Etest glycopeptide resistance detection (GRD) is a newer Etest method for the detection of hVISA. This method involves the use of a double-ended Etest strip that contains vancomycin, teicoplanin, and a nutritional supplement to enhance the growth of hVISA. A 0.5 McFarland standard inoculum, rather than the 2 McFarland standard used for Etest macromethod, is used and inoculated onto MHA + 5% blood [2]. Etest GRD strip is applied to the agar surface and the zone of inhibition is read after 48 h of incubation at 35°C. The strain is considered positive for hVISA if the Etest GRD result is ≥8 μg/ml for either vancomycin or teicoplanin [21, 22]. **Figure 7** shows a hVISA strain with positive Etest GRD result.

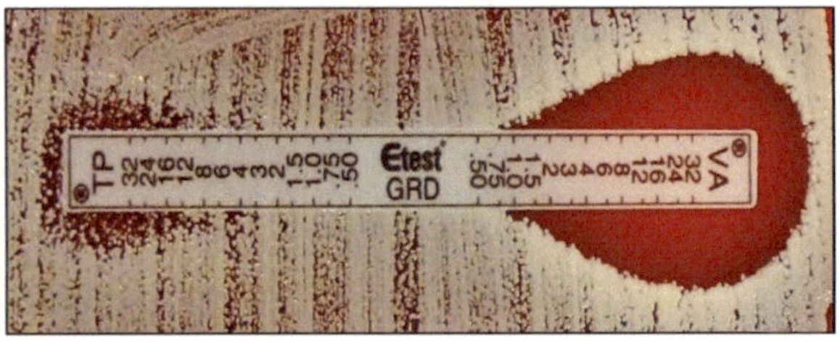

Figure 7. A hVISA strain with positive Etest GRD result. (Photograph courtesy of Dr M. Wootton).

Etest GRD has been reported to have sensitivity and specificity of 57–94% and 82–97%, respectively [22, 28, 29, 32]. Some of these differences may reflect the instability of hVISA phenotype. hVISA strains are known to be unstable, with the ability to revert to vancomycin-susceptible *S. aureus* (VSSA) under various conditions, including passage of the isolate on vancomycin-free media [29].

A possible barrier to large-scale usage of modified Etest methods is the potentially high cost to the clinical laboratory. This can be considered a disadvantage [10].

4.2. Confirmatory methods for hVISA

4.2.1. PAP-AUC

Population analysis profile-area under the curve (PAP-AUC) remains the gold standard method for detection of hVISA [10]. PAP-AUC method is performed as follows:

The isolate is incubated in tryptone soya broth (TSB) for 24 h. An undiluted culture and dilutions of $1/10^8$ and $1/10^5$ are spiral plated onto BHIA plates containing 0.5, 1, 2, 2.5, 4, and 8 μg of vancomycin per ml. After 48 h of incubation at 35°C, the colonies are counted. Log_{10} of the colony numbers (log_{10} CFU/ml) are plotted against the vancomycin concentrations. The "area under the curve (AUC)" of the isolate is calculated. The VSSA strain ATCC 29213 is used as negative control. Reference strains of hVISA (Mu3, ATCC 700698) and VISA (Mu50, ATCC 700699) are used as positive controls. A ratio is calculated by dividing the AUC of the test strain by the AUC of reference hVISA strain (Mu3). The ratios of <0.90, 0.90–1.30, and >1.30 are interpreted as VSSA, hVISA, and VISA, respectively [28, 33]. **Figure 8** shows an example of population analysis for *S. aureus* ATCC 29213 (VSSA), Mu3 (hVISA), Mu50 (VISA), a clinical hVISA isolate and a clinical VSSA isolate [11].

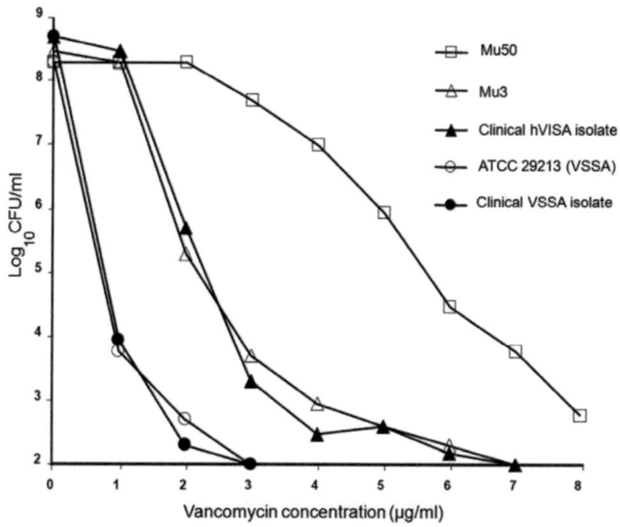

Figure 8. Example of population analysis profile curves for *S. aureus* ATCC 29213 (VSSA), Mu3 (hVISA), Mu50 (VISA), a clinical hVISA isolate and a clinical VSSA isolate. (Adapted from Ref. [11] which was published under an open-access licence agreement).

Unfortunately, PAP-AUC method is time-consuming, labor-intensive and costly which limits its use in routine clinical laboratories.

5. Epidemiology

While VRSA strains are limited to a handful of reported cases (14 total cases of VRSA in the U.S.) and VISA strains remain rare; hVISA strains are more common [9, 12, 34]. The true prevalence of hVISA is unknown, and estimates vary widely due to nonstandardized detection methods or absence of routine hVISA screening, variation in interpretation, clinical setting, geographical region, and differing patient populations [35]. Global hVISA rates among MRSA isolates have been reported to range from 0 to 73.7% [36].

In many studies, only the isolates suspected of being hVISA by screening methods (screening plates, Etest macromethod, Etest GRD) have been subjected to PAP-AUC. Some hVISA isolates may have been missed by screening methods in these studies. This may lead to an underestimation of the true prevalence [2, 27].

Although reported predominantly for MRSA; hVISA/VISA can be detected among methicillin-susceptible *S. aureus* (MSSA) strains [2, 37]. However, routine testing of MSSA isolates for the presence of hVISA/VISA for clinical purposes is not necessary and not recommended [10].

High-level resistance to vancomycin in *S. aureus* is very rare and all VRSA strains reported to date have been MRSA [9].

The proportion of *S. aureus* isolates demonstrating heteroresistance increases with increasing vancomycin MICs within the susceptible range, but heteroresistance has been reported in strains with MICs as low as 0.5 μg/ml [21, 38].

The main risk factors for hVISA and VISA infection appear to be prior MRSA colonization or infection and exposure to vancomycin. Most of hVISA/VISA infections occur in patients with serious underlying diseases such as malignancy, renal failure and diabetes, or in patients who have undergone major surgery [2, 12]. Nosocomial spread and rare outbreaks caused by VISA or hVISA have also been reported [34].

6. Clinical significance of hVISA/VISA and VRSA

The clinical significance of hVISA/VISA is difficult to determine due to differences in definitions and laboratory detection as well as the lack of well-controlled prospective studies [2, 21]. Commonly reported associations with hVISA/VISA infections include vancomycin treatment failure and high-inoculum infections such as bacteremia, endocarditis, deep abscesses, osteomyelitis, and prosthetic device infections [2, 21, 35, 36]. Some authors consider that hVISA/VISA could be responsible for treatment failure, whereas others have suggested that it has arisen as a consequence of treatment failure and prolonged vancomycin exposures [39]. It is difficult to determine, especially if it is not clear when the VISA or hVISA isolate was detected in the course of infection [21].

Interestingly, attenuated virulence of *S. aureus* with reduced susceptibility to vancomycin has been reported in some animal infection models [40, 41]. Pooled data from a meta-analysis showed similar mortality rates for hVISA and VSSA infections [36]. However, two recent studies have found a link between hVISA and higher mortality rate. Claeys *et al.* reported that patients with hVISA pneumonia experienced significantly higher inpatient mortality than those with VSSA pneumonia [42]. Hu *et al.* demonstrated that patients with hVISA bacteremia had a significantly higher in-hospital mortality than those with VSSA bacteremia [43].

The clinical significance of VRSA is unclear as only a few cases have been reported to date.

Persistent signs of infection and positive cultures for MRSA despite the administration of glycopeptide therapy, or relapse of infection after glycopeptide therapy can suggest an infection with hVISA or VISA [12]. Well-designed, large-scale prospective studies are needed to evaluate the clinical significance of these strains.

7. Therapeutic options

7.1. Role of surgery

Many patients with infections due to hVISA/VISA have high-inoculum infections (endocarditis, deep abscesses, osteomyelitis/septic arthritis and prosthetic device infections) [2, 12, 36].

Surgery is a useful adjunct to antimicrobial therapy for these patients. Main types of surgery include the drainage of abscesses or infected joints and removal of the infected prostheses [12].

7.2. Antimicrobial therapy

The emergence of hVISA/VISA clinical isolates has prompted the search for new antibiotics. While there are no guidelines regarding alternative antimicrobial therapy, there are a number of antimicrobial agents that have potential to be used in treatment of hVISA/VISA infections.

7.2.1. Daptomycin

Daptomycin is a lipopeptide antibiotic with activity against Gram-positive bacteria. In a study conducted by Wootton *et al.*, despite slightly raised MICs seen for strains with reduced susceptibility to vancomycin; daptomycin showed greater bactericidal activity than vancomycin for hVISA and VISA [44]. This indicates that, while there is a potential for cross-resistance between daptomycin and vancomycin, susceptibility to daptomycin is minimally affected by the presence of hVISA or VISA [10]. In several studies, daptomycin has been shown to have a good antimicrobial activity against the majority of hVISA isolates [27, 44, 45]. The highest rate of daptomycin nonsusceptibility was reported in a study evaluating 47 isolates of hVISA/VISA. In this study, the percentage of daptomycin nonsusceptible isolates was 15% for hVISA and 38% for VISA [35, 46]. Additionally, daptomycin has been shown to have *in vitro* activity against VRSA isolates. In a study conducted by Sievert *et al.*, one daptomycin nonsusceptible isolate was observed among 7 VRSA [47].

7.2.2. Linezolid

Linezolid is a synthetic antibacterial agent of the oxazolidinone class. Although resistance to linezolid has been reported in *S. aureus* isolates, rates of resistance remain very low. Linezolid was found to be useful for the treatment of hVISA/VISA infections [2, 48]. Also, data from a study demonstrated potent *in vitro* activity for linezolid against VRSA strains [47]. However, treatment with linezolid may be limited by toxicity. High rates of adverse reactions have been found for complex patients (seriously ill patients with multiple comorbidities) who received prolonged linezolid therapy [49]. Therefore, prolonged therapy should be used with caution in this patient group.

7.2.3. Tigecycline

Tigecycline is a glycylcycline antibiotic for intravenous infusion. In a study conducted by Sun *et al.*, 26 hVISA isolates and 1 VISA isolate were tested for tigecycline susceptibility. All isolates were found to be susceptible to tigecycline [50]. In another study, *in vitro* activity of tigecycline was evaluated against 33 VISA and 13 VRSA isolates. Tigecycline susceptibility rates were 97 and 92% for VISA and VRSA, respectively [51]. *In vitro* data have shown that tigecycline is active against hVISA/VISA as well as VRSA. Clinical studies are needed to determine the role of tigecycline in infections caused by *S. aureus* with reduced susceptibility to vancomycin.

7.2.4. New cephalosporins

New cephalosporins like ceftaroline and ceftobiprole have been shown to be active against hVISA and VISA *in vitro* and in animal studies. In rabbit models of endocarditis, these agents were superior to vancomycin against hVISA and VISA [2]. While results of *in vitro* and *in vivo* testing of these cephalosporins have been positive against hVISA/VISA, their clinical utility for infections caused by hVISA or VISA remains unknown [10].

7.2.5. Other antimicrobial agents

Other potentially active antimicrobials include lipoglycopeptides (dalbavancin, oritavancin, telavancin), quinupristin-dalfopristin, rifampin and fusidic acid. However, resistance develops rapidly with monotherapy with rifampin or fusidic acid. Therefore, these agents should be used in combination with another antistaphylococcal agent. The combination of rifampin and fusidic acid is an effective option [2]. Studies also suggest the potential for synergistic activity between vancomycin and various antimicrobials including beta-lactams and gentamicin against *S. aureus* with reduced vancomycin susceptibility [10].

Author details

Hasan Cenk Mirza

Address all correspondence to: h_cenkmirza@yahoo.com.tr

Department of Microbiology, Merzifon State Hospital, Amasya, Turkey

References

[1] Appelbaum PC. The emergence of vancomycin-intermediate and vancomycin-resistant *Staphylococcus aureus*. Clin Microbiol Infect. 2006; 12 (Suppl 1):16-23. DOI: 10.1111/j.1469-0691.2006.01344.x

[2] Howden BP, JK Davies, PD Johnson *et al.* Reduced vancomycin susceptibility in *Staphylococcus aureus*, including vancomycin-intermediate and heterogeneous vancomycin-intermediate strains: resistance mechanisms, laboratory detection, and clinical implications. Clin Microbiol Rev. 2010; 23:99-139. DOI: 10.1128/CMR.00042-09

[3] Xu L, Huang H, Wei W *et al.* Complete genome sequence and comparative genomic analyses of the vancomycin-producing *Amycolatopsis orientalis*. BMC Genomics. 2014; 15:363. DOI: 10.1186/1471-2164-15-363

[4] Hiramatsu K, Hanaki H, Ino T *et al.* Methicillin resistant *Staphylococcus aureus* clinical strain with reduced vancomycin susceptibility. J Antimicrob Chemother. 1997; 40:135-136. DOI: 10.1093/jac/40.1.135

[5] Smith TL, Pearson ML, Wilcox KR *et al.* Emergence of vancomycin resistance in *Staphylococcus aureus*. N Engl J Med. 1999; 340:493-501. DOI: 10.1056/NEJM199902183400701

[6] Ploy MC, Grelaud C, Martin C. First clinical isolate of vancomycin-intermediate *Staphylococcus aureus* in a French hospital. Lancet. 1998; 351:1212. DOI: 10.1016/S0140-6736(05)79166-2

[7] Hiramatsu K, Aritaka N, Hanaki H *et al.* Dissemination in Japanese hospitals of strains of *Staphylococcus aureus* heterogeneously resistant to vancomycin. Lancet. 1997; 350:1670-1673. DOI: 10.1016/S0140-6736(97)07324-8

[8] Tenover FC. The quest to identify heterogeneously resistant vancomycin-intermediate *Staphylococcus aureus* strains. Int J Antimicrob Agents. 2010; 36:303-306. DOI: 10.1016/j.ijantimicag.2010.06.005

[9] Walters MS, Eggers P, Albrecht V *et al.* Vancomycin-resistant *Staphylococcus aureus* – Delaware, 2015. MMWR Morb Mortal Wkly Rep. 2015; 64:1056. DOI: 10.15585/mmwr.mm6437a6.

[10] Rong SL, Leonard SN. Heterogeneous vancomycin resistance in *Staphylococcus aureus*: a review of epidemiology, diagnosis, and clinical significance. Ann Pharmacother. 2010; 44:844-850. DOI: 10.1345/aph.1M526

[11] Sola C, Lamberghini RO, Ciarlantini M *et al.* Heterogeneous vancomycin-intermediate susceptibility in a community-associated methicillin-resistant *Staphylococcus aureus* epidemic clone, in a case of Infective Endocarditis in Argentina. Ann Clin Microbiol Antimicrob. 2011; 10:15. DOI: 10.1186/1476-0711-10-15

[12] Howden BP. Recognition and management of infections caused by vancomycin-intermediate *Staphylococcus aureus* (VISA) and heterogenous VISA (hVISA). Intern Med J. 2005; 35:S136-S140. DOI: 10.1111/j.1444-0903.2005.00986.x

[13] Cui L, Iwamoto A, Lian JQ *et al.* Novel mechanism of antibiotic resistance originating in vancomycin-intermediate *Staphylococcus aureus*. Antimicrob Agents Chemother. 2006; 50:428-438. DOI: 10.1128/AAC.50.2.428-438.2006

[14] Sieradzki K, Pinho MG, Tomasz A. Inactivated pbp4 in highly glycopeptide-resistant laboratory mutants of *Staphylococcus aureus*. J Biol Chem. 1999; 274:18942-18946. DOI: 10.1074/jbc.274.27.18942

[15] Deresinski S. The multiple paths to heteroresistance and intermediate resistance to vancomycin in *Staphylococcus aureus*. J Infect Dis. 2013; 208:7-9. DOI: 10.1093/infdis/jit136

[16] Samanta D, Elasri MO. The msaABCR operon regulates resistance in vancomycin-intermediate *Staphylococcus aureus* strains. Antimicrob Agents Chemother. 2014; 58:6685-6695. DOI: 10.1128/AAC.03280-14

[17] Sakoulas G, Moellering RC Jr. Increasing antibiotic resistance among methicillin-resistant *Staphylococcus aureus* strains. Clin Infect Dis. 2008; 46 (Suppl 5):S360-S367. DOI: 10.1086/533592

[18] Garrido AM, Gálvez A, Pulido RP. Antimicrobial resistance in *Enterococci*. J Infect Dis Ther. 2014; 2:150. DOI: 10.4172/2332-0877.1000150

[19] Gardete S, Tomasz A. Mechanisms of vancomycin resistance in *Staphylococcus aureus*. J Clin Invest. 2014; 124:2836-2840. DOI: 10.1172/JCI68834

[20] Lowy FD. Antimicrobial resistance: the example of *Staphylococcus aureus*. J Clin Invest. 2003; 111:1265-1273. DOI: 10.1172/JCI200318535

[21] Holmes NE, Johnson PD, Howden BP. Relationship between vancomycin-resistant *Staphylococcus aureus*, vancomycin-intermediate *S. aureus*, high vancomycin MIC, and outcome in serious *S. aureus* infections. J Clin Microbiol. 2012; 50:2548-2552. DOI: 10.1128/JCM.00775-12

[22] Satola SW, Farley MM, Anderson KF *et al*. Comparison of detection methods for heteroresistant vancomycin-intermediate *Staphylococcus aureus*, with the population analysis profile method as the reference method. J Clin Microbiol. 2011; 49:177-183. DOI: 10.1128/JCM.01128-10

[23] Wootton M, MacGowan AP, Walsh TR *et al*. A multicenter study evaluating the current strategies for isolating *Staphylococcus aureus* strains with reduced susceptibility to glycopeptides. J Clin Microbiol. 2007; 45:329-332. DOI: 10.1128/JCM.01508-06

[24] Riederer K, Shemes S, Chase P *et al*. Detection of intermediately vancomycin-susceptible and heterogeneous *Staphylococcus aureus* isolates: comparison of Etest and Agar screening methods. J Clin Microbiol. 2011; 49:2147-2150. DOI: 10.1128/JCM.01435-10

[25] Voss A, Mouton JW, van Elzakker EP *et al*. A multi-center blinded study on the efficiency of phenotypic screening methods to detect glycopeptide intermediately susceptible *Staphylococcus aureus* (GISA) and heterogeneous GISA (h-GISA). Ann Clin Microbiol Antimicrob. 2007; 6:9. DOI: 10.1186/1476-0711-6-9

[26] Fitzgibbon MM, Rossney AS, O'Connell B. Investigation of reduced susceptibility to glycopeptides among methicillin-resistant *Staphylococcus aureus* isolates from patients in Ireland and evaluation of agar screening methods for detection of heterogeneously glycopeptide-intermediate *S. aureus*. J Clin Microbiol. 2007; 45:3263-3269. DOI: 10.1128/JCM.00836-07

[27] Mirza HC, Sancak B, Gür D. The Prevalence of vancomycin-intermediate *Staphylococcus aureus* and heterogeneous VISA among methicillin-resistant strains isolated from

pediatric population in a Turkish University Hospital. Microb Drug Resist. 2015; 21:537-544. DOI: 10.1089/mdr.2015.0048

[28] Yusof A, Engelhardt A, Karlsson A *et al.* Evaluation of a new Etest vancomycin-teicoplanin strip for detection of glycopeptide-intermediate *Staphylococcus aureus* (GISA), in particular, heterogeneous GISA. J Clin Microbiol. 2008; 46:3042-3047. DOI: 10.1128/JCM.00265-08

[29] van Hal SJ, Wehrhahn MC, Barbagiannakos T *et al.* Performance of various testing methodologies for detection of heteroresistant vancomycin-intermediate *Staphylococcus aureus* in bloodstream isolates. J Clin Microbiol. 2011; 49:1489-1494. DOI: 10.1128/JCM.02302-10

[30] Maor Y, Rahav G, Belausov N *et al.* Prevalence and characteristics of heteroresistant vancomycin-intermediate *Staphylococcus aureus* bacteremia in a tertiary care center. J Clin Microbiol. 2007; 45:1511-1514. DOI: 10.1128/JCM.01262-06

[31] Etest® Application Guide [Internet]. Available from: http://www.biomerieux-usa.com/sites/subsidiary_us/files/supplementary_inserts_-_16273_-_b_-_en_-_eag_-_etest_application_guide-3.pdf

[32] Leonard SN, Rossi KL, Newton KL *et al.* Evaluation of the Etest GRD for the detection of *Staphylococcus aureus* with reduced susceptibility to glycopeptides. J Antimicrob Chemother. 2009; 63:489-492. DOI: 10.1093/jac/dkn520

[33] Walsh TR, Bolmström A, Qwärnström A *et al.* Evaluation of current methods for detection of staphylococci with reduced susceptibility to glycopeptides. J Clin Microbiol. 2001; 39:2439-2444. DOI: 10.1128/JCM.39.7.2439–2444.2001

[34] Dhand A, Sakoulas G. Reduced vancomycin susceptibility among clinical *Staphylococcus aureus* isolates ('the MIC Creep'): implications for therapy. F1000 Med Rep. 2012; 4:4. DOI: 10.3410/M4-4

[35] Gomes DM, Ward KE, LaPlante KL. Clinical implications of vancomycin heteroresistant and intermediately susceptible *Staphylococcus aureus*. Pharmacotherapy. 2015; 35:424-432. DOI: 10.1002/phar.1577

[36] van Hal SJ, Paterson DL. Systematic review and meta-analysis of the significance of heterogeneous vancomycin-intermediate *Staphylococcus aureus* isolates. Antimicrob Agents Chemother. 2011; 55:405-510. DOI: 10.1128/AAC.01133-10

[37] Pillai SK, Wennersten C, Venkataraman L *et al.* Development of reduced vancomycin susceptibility in methicillin-susceptible *Staphylococcus aureus*. Clin Infect Dis. 2009; 49:1169-1174. DOI: 10.1086/605636

[38] Rybak MJ, Leonard SN, Rossi KL *et al.* Characterization of vancomycin-heteroresistant *Staphylococcus aureus* from the metropolitan area of Detroit, Michigan, over a 22-year period (1986 to 2007). J Clin Microbiol. 2008; 46:2950-2954. DOI: 10.1128/JCM.00582-08

[39] Di Gregorio S, Perazzi B, Ordoñez AM *et al.* Clinical, microbiological, and genetic characteristics of heteroresistant vancomycin-intermediate *Staphylococcus aureus* bacteremia in a teaching hospital. Microb Drug Resist. 2015; 21:25-34. DOI: 10.1089/mdr.2014.0190

[40] Majcherczyk PA, Barblan JL, Moreillon P *et al.* Development of glycopeptide-intermediate resistance by *Staphylococcus aureus* leads to attenuated infectivity in a rat model of endocarditis. Microb Pathog. 2008; 45:408-414. DOI: 10.1016/j.micpath.2008.09.003

[41] Peleg AY, Monga D, Pillai S *et al.* Reduced susceptibility to vancomycin influences pathogenicity in *Staphylococcus aureus* infection. J Infect Dis. 2009; 199:532-536. DOI: 10.1086/596511

[42] Claeys KC, Lagnf AM, Hallesy JA *et al.* Pneumonia caused by methicillin-resistant *Staphylococcus aureus*: does vancomycin heteroresistance matter? Antimicrob Agents Chemother. 2016; 60:1708-1716. DOI: 10.1128/AAC.02388-15

[43] Hu HC, Kao KC, Chiu LC *et al.* Clinical outcomes and molecular typing of heterogenous vancomycin-intermediate *Staphylococcus aureus* bacteremia in patients in intensive care units. BMC Infect Dis. 2015; 15:444. DOI: 10.1186/s12879-015-1215-2

[44] Wootton M, MacGowan AP, Walsh TR. Comparative bactericidal activities of daptomycin and vancomycin against glycopeptide-intermediate *Staphylococcus aureus* (GISA) and heterogeneous GISA isolates. Antimicrob Agents Chemother. 2006; 50:4195-4197. DOI: 10.1128/AAC.00678-06

[45] Leonard SN, Rybak MJ. Evaluation of vancomycin and daptomycin against methicillin-resistant *Staphylococcus aureus* and heterogeneously vancomycin-intermediate *S. aureus* in an in vitro pharmacokinetic/pharmacodynamic model with simulated endocardial vegetations. J Antimicrob Chemother. 2009; 63:155-160. DOI: 10.1093/jac/dkn439

[46] Kelley PG, Gao W, Ward PB *et al.* Daptomycin non-susceptibility in vancomycin-intermediate *Staphylococcus aureus* (VISA) and heterogeneous-VISA (hVISA): implications for therapy after vancomycin treatment failure. J Antimicrob Chemother. 2011; 66:1057-1060. DOI: 10.1093/jac/dkr066.

[47] Sievert DM, Rudrik JT, Patel JB *et al.* Vancomycin-resistant *Staphylococcus aureus* in the United States, 2002–2006. Clin Infect Dis. 2008; 46:668-674. DOI: 10.1086/527392

[48] Howden BP, Ward PB, Charles PG *et al.* Treatment outcomes for serious infections caused by methicillin-resistant *Staphylococcus aureus* with reduced vancomycin susceptibility. Clin Infect Dis. 2004; 38:521-528. DOI: 10.1086/381202

[49] Bishop E, Melvani S, Howden BP *et al.* Good clinical outcomes but high rates of adverse reactions during linezolid therapy for serious infections: a proposed protocol for monitoring therapy in complex patients. Antimicrob Agents Chemother. 2006; 50:1599-1602. DOI: 10.1128/AAC.50.4.1599-1602.2006

[50] Sun W, Chen H, Liu Y *et al*. Prevalence and characterization of heterogeneous vancomycin-intermediate *Staphylococcus aureus* isolates from 14 cities in China. Antimicrob Agents Chemother. 2009; 53:3642-3649. DOI: 10.1128/AAC.00206-09

[51] Saravolatz LD, Pawlak J, Johnson LB. In vitro susceptibilities and molecular analysis of vancomycin-intermediate and vancomycin-resistant *Staphylococcus aureus* isolates. Clin Infect Dis. 2012; 55:582-586. DOI: 10.1093/cid/cis492

Chapter 4

Mechanisms of Horizontal Gene Transfer

Fabio Cafini, Veronica Medrano Romero and
Kazuya Morikawa

Additional information is available at the end of the chapter

http://dx.doi.org/10.5772/65967

Abstract

Horizontal gene transfer plays important roles in the evolution of *S. aureus*, and indeed, a variety of virulence factors and antibiotic resistance genes are embedded in a series of mobile genetic elements. In this chapter, we review the mechanisms of horizontal gene transfer, including recent findings on the natural genetic competence. Then, we consider the transfer of two important antibiotic resistance genes: the methicillin resistance gene, *mecA* (in Staphylococcal Cassette Chromosome) and the linezolid resistance gene, *cfr* (in plasmid). In either case, distinct mechanisms driving the gene dissemination support the prominent evolutionary ability of this important human pathogen.

Keywords: Transduction, Conjugation, Transformation, staphylococcal cassette chromosome (SCC), *cfr*

1. Introduction

Staphylococcus aureus is an opportunistic pathogen responsible for diverse infectious diseases ranging from food poisoning and superficial skin abscesses to more serious infections such as pneumonia, meningitis, osteomyelitis, septicemia, endocarditis and toxic shock syndrome. The resistance to a wide variety of antibiotics [1, 2] is a global concern in clinical settings, and methicillin-resistant strains (MRSA), the most common cause of nosocomial infections, are now spreading into the community [3]. The emergence and dissemination of further resistant strains such as vancomycin-resistant *S. aureus* (VRSA) [4] and linezolid-resistant *S. aureus* (LRSA) [5, 6] are anticipated. Major parts of staphylococcal virulence and antibiotics resistance are acquired characteristics, evidenced by many of the toxin and antibiotic resistance genes embedded in mobile genetic elements such as transposons, bacteriophages, insertion sequences, pathogenicity islands and the staphylococcal cassette chromosome (SCC) [7, 8]. In this chapter, we review the current understanding about horizontal gene transfer (HGT) in *S. aureus* including the recently discovered natural transformation. We also discuss how two important mobile genetic elements (SCC and *cfr* plasmid) would be transferred from cell to cell.

2. Horizontal gene transfer mechanisms

2.1. Phage-related mechanisms

Phage-mediated horizontal gene transfer is the major driving force for *S. aureus* evolution and is well reviewed elsewhere [9]. The experimental protocols for the phage transduction are also established [10]. Staphylococcal phages can also serve as a helper phage to transfer *Staphylococcus aureus* pathogenicity islands (SaPIs) [11]. SaPI carries toxin genes including the toxic shock syndrome toxin 1 and superantigens. In addition to the conventional transduction by staphylococcal phages, atypical giant phage in environment is also capable of transduction [12].

In 1970s, a transformation-like phenomenon (now termed "pseudo-competence" or "pseudo-transformation") was described [13]. A series of studies have confirmed that it is a HGT mechanism that requires the presence of a staphylococcal phage [14]. The "competence-conferring factor" was most likely the phage tail that has lytic activity. In some old bacteriology books, pseudo-competence is regarded as competence, but the first report on genuine natural genetic competence was published on 2012 [15]. Pseudo-competence was demonstrated to be distinct from natural competence: the important competence genes encoded in the *comG* and *comE* operons were dispensable for pseudo-competence [15].

2.2. Conjugation

Bacterial conjugation has been studied in Gram-negative and Gram-positive species. Although broad-host-range plasmids able to replicate in both groups exist, the differences in terms of membrane and peptidoglycan cell wall require different conjugation systems on the basis of cell-to-cell recognition and contact.

Most of the conjugative staphylococcal plasmids studied belong to the incQ family. One of the better known staphylococcal conjugative plasmid is pGO1 [16], considered as the prototype of this type of plasmids. All the conjugative genes are located on a 14.5 kb region, and the minimal machinery necessary for conjugation includes the *oriT*, a nickase protein (*nes*) and the *tra* operon. This plasmid shows high similarities, in terms of genetic organization of the *tra* operon, with other Gram-positive conjugative plasmids such as the staphylococcal pSK41 plasmid [17], the lactococcal pMRC01 [18] and the enterococcal pRE25 [19].

Staphylococcal plasmids related to the pGO1/pSK41 family share an important homology regarding the organization of conjugative genes and, in addition, present an identical IncQ-type relaxase and a nickase gene (*nes*) responsible for the generation of the nick at the *oriT* [17]. The plasmids belonging to this family are self-conjugative, and they are able to mobilize small non-conjugative coresident plasmids. They are also associated with gentamicin (and other aminoglycosides) resistance and can be related to resistance to penicillin, trimethoprim, bleomycin, tetracycline, macrolides, lincosamide, streptogramin B and antiseptics [20]. These plasmids have contributed to the evolution of staphylococcal species in antibiotic-enriched environments, and recently, they have been reported to be related to resistance against the most important antimicrobials used in MRSA treatment: linezolid and vancomycin.

2.3. Natural transformation

Natural transformation requires the uptake of environmental DNA by the action of a set of DNA-uptake proteins that are expressed in the bacterial membrane. Once DNA is incorporated into the cytoplasm, it can be used as a source of nutrients, as a template to repair damaged genetic material or to enhance bacterial fitness by generating diversity or introducing novel traits [21].

To undergo transformation, bacteria need to develop a specific physiological state called genetic competence. Competence is achieved through the regulated expression of the genes encoding the DNA uptake machinery [22]. In general, Gram-positive DNA uptake machinery is formed by a pseudopilus (ComG proteins) that brings extracellular DNA to the cytoplasmic transport machinery, a DNA-binding protein (the receptor ComEA) and a channel (ComEC). Only a single strand enters the cytosol, while the complementary strand is degraded by an endonuclease [23].

S. aureus had been regarded as a non-transformable species until natural transformation was demonstrated in 2012 [15]. Natural transformation can transfer long DNA fragments that are too large to be transferred by bacteriophages (transduction) [22]. Indeed, the long staphylococcal cassette chromosome *mec* (SCC*mec*) type II element was successfully transferred by transformation [15], leading to the idea that the exchange of large DNA regions between distinct *S. aureus* clonal complexes may be also due to the natural transformation [24].

The regulation of competence development is a species-specific process. In *S. aureus*, the main competence regulator is the alternative sigma factor H (SigH). SigH activates the transcription of the competence machinery genes (*comG* and *comE* operons) that are essential for the development of natural transformation [15, 25]. In addition, the transcription factor ComK enhances the expression of the SigH regulon [26]. SigH is expressed in a minor population by two distinct mechanisms. The *sigH* gene can be rearranged by a "short-junction duplication," or be post-transcriptionally regulated through an inverted repeat (IR) sequence at the 5′-UTR of *sigH* mRNA. The IR is thought to hinder the ribosome-binding site to suppress the SigH expression, but the activation mechanism is not clarified yet.

Competence development is a species-specific process that requires particular environmental conditions. These conditions include nutrient access, starvation, altered growth conditions and cell density [22]. Natural transformation in *S. aureus* is detectable under specific conditions when cells are grown in the chemically defined CS2 medium [15]. Under these growth conditions, wild-type strains (N315 and its derivative) show low transformation frequencies ($<10^{-11}$), partly attributed to the subpopulation limited SigH expression. Overexpression of SigH increases the transformation frequencies up to $\sim 10^{-9}$ when purified plasmid DNA is used as donor and to $\sim 10^{-7}$ if living *S. aureus* COL cells carrying pT181 are used. Moreover, there seems to be more preferable growth conditions that facilitate transformation (Ohniwa et al., in preparation). So far, we achieved c.a. 10^{-6} level frequency in the unmodified N315 derivative strains, as well as in a part of the clinical isolates, which will be published elsewhere.

Even in SigH-expressing cells, the transformation frequencies change depending on the growth conditions, suggesting that there are additional levels of regulations for an efficient transformation. Importantly, antimicrobial agents also affect the transformation efficiencies in the SigH-expressing cells [27]. **Table 1** summarizes the effect of the antibiotics in *S. aureus* and other species. **Table 1** also includes the SOS response, because it is a complementary response in some bacteria: antibiotics that induce SOS response, such as fluoroquinolone or mitomycin C, induce competence in species lacking the SOS system [28–30] but suppress competence in species harboring the SOS system [31]. Although SOS response in *S. aureus* is limited and its accessories are simple, it does exist [32, 33]. The treatment with mitomycin C suppresses transformation in *S. aureus*. However, ciprofloxacin (fluoroquinolone) has no effect. This might indicate that the interplay between natural transformation and SOS response cannot be simplified. *S. aureus* response to β-lactam antibiotics is also linked to SOS response [34–36]. Fosfomycin and vancomycin increase natural transformation in SigH-expressing cells, but the detailed response mechanism involved is not known. Whether these inducing effects can be observed in the unmodified strains needs to be tested in a future study.

		S. aureus (+ **SigH cells)**		*S. thermophilus*		**S. p***	**L. p***	**H. p***
		TF**	**SOS**	**TF****	**SOS**	**TF****	**TF****	**TF****
	Fosfomycin	+ [27]						
	Vancomycin	+[27]				No effect [28]		
	Oxacillin	- [27]	Yes [34, 35]					
	Cefazolin	- [27]						
	Ampicillin		Yes [36]			No effect [28]	No effect [29]	No effect [30]
Quinolones	Ciprofloxacin	No effect [27]	Yes [32] [37]					+ [30]
	Norfloxacin			- [31]	Yes [31]	+ [28]	+ [29]	
	Mitomycin C	- [27]	Yes [37] [38]	- [31]	Yes [31]	+ [28]		

*S. p, L. p, H. p lack SOS system [29, 33].
**TF: transformation and/or competence gene expression.
S. p: *Streptococcus pneumoniae*, L. p: *Legionella pneumophila*, H. p: *Helicobacter pylori.*

Table 1. Effects of antibiotics on transformation and SOS response.

3. Dissemination of antibiotic resistance determinants

Since Fleming's discovery of penicillin and its application to treatment, *S. aureus* has experienced a variety of antibiotics in clinical settings. Penicillin-resistant *S. aureus* was described before the introduction of penicillin to the market in 1943. It carried a β-lactamase gene in a plasmid. Methicillin was developed as a β-lactam derivative that cannot be degraded by β-lactamase, but methicillin-resistant *S. aureus* (MRSA) was described soon after its introduction. The methicillin resistance gene is in a mobile genetic element designated staphylococcal cassette chromosome (SCC). Vancomycin is one of the effective resources for MRSA treatment, though vancomycin-resistant *S. aureus* (VRSA) has already been reported [39]. Linezolid is another promising anti-MRSA drug, but the dissemination of linezolid resistance is also anticipated. The antibiotic resistance genes and a series of reports on their transfer mechanisms are summarized in **Table 2**. Here, we focus on the dissemination mechanisms of SCC and linezolid resistance.

3.1. Dissemination of SCC

β-lactams were the first line of antibiotics against *S. aureus* infections. However, resistance has rapidly emerged. The first methicillin-resistant *S. aureus* (MRSA) strain was identified in 1961, only one year after the clinical introduction of methicillin [76]. Methicillin is a semisynthetic penicillin that resists the action of β-lactamases. It was introduced as a first choice treatment against infections caused by penicillin-resistant *S. aureus*. The methicillin resistance gene (*mecA*) encodes an alternative penicillin-binding protein (PBP2a) that has low affinity for all β-lactams. PBP2a can maintain the cell wall synthesis, while all the other PBPs are inhibited by β-lactams [77].

The *mecA* gene is carried in a variable mobile element called staphylococcal cassette chromosome *mec* (SCC*mec*). SCC*mec* is integrated in a unique orientation into a specific chromosomal attachment site (*attB*SCC) [78]. The basic structure of the SCC*mec* element consists of a cassette chromosome recombinase (*ccr*) and a *mec* complex. The *mec* complex contains the *mecA* gene and its regulatory genes (not always present) [79]. The cassette is classified according to a combination of both complexes [80]. The International Working Group on the Staphylococcal Cassette Chromosome elements reports 11 types of *SCCmec* (**http://www.sccmec.org/Pages/SCC_TypesEN.html**). SCC*mec* varies in size (from 20 to 67 kb), and it can carry other elements such as resistance genes, insertion elements, plasmids or transposons. SCC*mec* elements have only been found in staphylococci with the exception of *Macrococcus caseolyticus* [43]. This species is closely related to the staphylococci, and it was part of the *Staphylococcus* genus until 1998 when it was reclassified [81].

MRSA strains appeared in the hospital environment and spread rapidly causing serious clinical problems and several hospital outbreaks. The first MRSA strain was identified in the United Kingdom in 1961, and it carried the type I SCC*mec*. Types II and III were identified in the early 1980s in Japan and New Zealand, respectively. These types of SCC*mec* were all identified in the hospital environment; they are the largest types and can carry additional

Type	Antibiotic	Gene	Location	Origin	Reported/probable HGT mechanism	Refs.
β-lactams	Penicillin	*blaZ*	Plasmid (transposon)	*S. haemolyticus?*	Conjugation Pseudo-transformation	[40–42]
	Methicillin	*mecA*	Chromosome (SCC*mec*)	CoNS	Transduction Conjugation Transformation	[15, 43–49]
Glycopeptides	Vancomycin	*vanA*	Plasmid (transposon)	*Enterococcus* spp.	Conjugation	[50, 51]
Aminoglycosides	Gentamicin Kanamycin Tobramycin	*aacA–aphD*	Plasmid (transposon)	*Bacillus* spp.?	Conjugation Transduction	[52]
Antifolates	Trimethoprim	*dfrA*	Plasmid (transposon)	*Bacillus* spp.?	Conjugation	[53, 54]
		dfrG	Chromosome (IS)	*E. faecium?*	–	[55]
		dfrK	Plasmid Chromosome (transposon)	?	Conjugation -	[56–58]
Macrolide Lincosamide Streptogramin B		*ermB*	Plasmid (transposon)	Streptococci	Conjugation Transduction	[59–61]
		ermC	Plasmid	CoNS	Transduction	[60, 62]
		ermA	Chromosome (transposon)	CoNS	Conjugation	[60, 62, 63]
Tetracyclines	Tetracycline	*tetK tetL*	Plasmid	Streptococci Enterococci	Conjugation	[64, 65]
		tetM	Chromosome (transposon)	Streptococci *E. faecalis*	Conjugation	[61, 64]
Chloramphenicol	Chloramphenicol	*cat*	Plasmid	*S. epidermidis*	Conjugation Transduction	[8, 66, 67]
Oxazolidinones	Lynezolid	*cfr*	Plasmid	CoNS?	Conjugation Transduction	[6]
Streptogramins	Dalfopristin	*vgaA, vgaB, vatA, vatB, vatC*	Plasmid	?	Conjugation	[68, 69]
Fusidanes	Fusidic acid	*fusB*	Chromosome (SaPI) Plasmid	CoNS	Transduction	[11, 70]
		fusC	Chromosome (SCC)	CoNS	–	[7 –75]
Phosphonic acids	Fosfomycin	*fosB*	Chromosome (SaPI)	?	Transduction	[11]

Table 2. Antibiotics resistance genes.

http://dx.doi.org/10.5772/65967

resistance elements; strains that carry them are usually multi-resistant [78, 82]. During the 1990s, community-associated MRSA strains were identified, and during the early 2000s, the SCC*mec* type IV and V were described in USA and Australia, respectively. These types are smaller elements that rarely carry extra resistance elements, and they are described as community-associated SCC*mec* types [83, 84]. Types I to V are the main and widely distributed elements; since their description, new variants have been reported (SCC*mec* VI–XI).

The origin of the SCC*mec* element is not clear, but evidence indicates that it comes from coagulase negative staphylococci (CoNS). Ancestral forms have been identified in *S. sciuri, S. fleuretti, S. xylosus, S. hominis* and *M. caseolyticus* [43–45]. The source of the *mec* and *ccr* complex is unknown, but they may have assembled into *SCCmec* in CoNS where they were modified and then transferred to *S. aureus* [46]. The primary source of SCC*mec* for *S. aureus* seems to be *S. epidermidis.* SCC*mec* type IV shares high homology between both species [85]; *S. haemolyticus* and *S. hominis* appear to be reservoirs for specific classes of *mec* complex and *ccr* genes [86, 87].

The transfer mechanism of SCC*mec* is not well defined. Successful transfer via transduction, conjugation and natural transformation has been reported. Although transduction of small SCC*mec* elements (type IV, I and V) has been described [47, 48], it is unlikely that this is the predominant method. Many of the SCC*mec* are too big (up to ~60 kb) to be encapsulated by a phage. Conjugation is an alternative mechanism. Ray et al. demonstrated the transfer of a 30.8 kb element (modified from SCC*mec* II) via conjugation, the spontaneous excision from the conjugative plasmid and the insertion into the recipient chromosome of *S. aureus* and *S. epidermidis* [49]. However, these authors induced the transfer by overproducing *ccrAB*. Natural transformation can also explain the transfer of large SCC*mec* types. We have successfully transferred the SCC*mec* II [15]. However, the interspecies transfer by natural transformation has not been tested.

3.2. Dissemination of *cfr*

The *cfr* gene was identified in 2000; it was described as a new chloramphenicol/florfenicol resistance element located on the pSCFS1 plasmid [88]. This plasmid was the first multi-resistance plasmid found in a *Staphylococcus sciuri* (isolate from the nasal swab of a calf) and was associated with resistance to chloramphenicol, florfenicol, spectinomycin and MLSB (macrolide, lincosamide and streptogramin B) antibiotics. The *cfr* gene was associated with the tn558 transposon, closely related to the tn554 associated with erythromycin resistance [89].

The *cfr* gene was not associated with clinical cases until 2007, when it was demonstrated that this gene was responsible for the elevated MIC to linezolid in one clinical MRSA strain isolated in Medellin (Colombia) [90]. Linezolid is a synthetic inhibitor of protein synthesis. Its activity against Gram-positive bacteria (including MRSA and *Enterococcus* sp., even in the case of reduced vancomycin susceptibility) made this antibiotic an essential tool in the treatment of resistant pathogens [91].

Up to 2007, the only known mechanism for linezolid resistance known in staphylococci was the spontaneous mutations in ribosomal proteins [92]. This non-transmissible mechanism was associated with the previous intensive use of linezolid. The association of a potential transmissible mechanism of resistance to this antibiotic represented a global concern due to the scarce alternatives for the infections caused by these pathogens and also, due to the potential spreading of this resistance mechanism to the pathogenic bacterial pool.

When the first *cfr*-positive clinical isolate was detected, sequencing analysis showed the absence of any mutation previously associated with linezolid resistance. The strains showed an unexpected post-transcriptional modification at A2503 in the 23S rRNA. The mechanism underlying the resistance conferred by *cfr* is related to the modification of the antibiotic target site on the 23S ribosomal RNA [90]. Thus, cfr is a methyltransferase that causes a reduced ribose methylation at C2498 and the addition of an extra methylation at A2503.

In 2008, the first outbreak of linezolid-resistant MRSA strain was reported in Spain [93]. The outbreak took place in the intensive care unit (ICU) of a public hospital and lasted 3 months. A total of 15 patients infected or colonized with linezolid-resistant MRSA were detected. In this case, some isolates showed identical PFGE profiles, showing the clonal dissemination of the same linezolid-resistant strain, but other *cfr*-positive strains showed a different PFGE profile. As *cfr* prevalence was extremely low, the existence of a horizontal gene transfer event was strongly suggested, and specially, the potential existence of some undetected reservoir, capable of spreading the *cfr* gene among the pathogenic staphylococcal pool, was hypothesized. The association of a potentially transmissible mechanism of resistance to this antibiotic represented a global concern due to the scarce treatment alternatives and the potential spreading to the pathogenic bacterial pool.

In 2008, the presence of plasmid-borne *cfr* in two strains isolated in Ohio hospitals was described [94]. In this case, two staphylococci, one MRSA and one *S. epidermidis*, with linezolid MICs of 8 and 256 mg/L, respectively, were isolated from two different patients. Sequence analysis found two different plasmids on the basis of the *cfr* insertion context. The *S. epidermidis* insertion couldn't be determined, but the plasmid harbored by the *S. aureus* strain showed a pSCFS3-like genetic environment [95]. In this genetic context, the Tn558 transposon was truncated by the tandem insertion of *istAS-istBS*, potentially related to *cfr* gene mobilization. Since 2008 several studies detected the presence of this gene in livestock-associated strains belonging to different bacterial species such as *Proteus vulgaris, Enterococcus* spp., *Macrococcus caseolyticus* or *Jeotgalicoccus pinnipedialis* [96–98]. These findings showed the spread of these resistance traits among livestock-associated bacteria known as reservoir for clinical-associated strains.

In 2010, during the analysis of a collection of Panton-Valentine leukocidin (PVL)-positive MRSA isolates from Ireland, one *cfr*-positive strain was detected [99]. This strain harbored a ca. 40 kbp plasmid with *cfr* associated with the Tn558 transposon. However, this gene was located in a genetic context not previously described. In this plasmid, named pSCFS7, *cfr* gene was found inserted in the *tnpB* gene reading frame. In this case, this gene was truncated by the insertion of the terminal region of *istBS*. The detection of the pSCFS7 plasmid was especially relevant; on one hand, the *cfr*-positive MRSA strain belonged to the USA 300 genotype (ST8-MRSA-IVa), which is predominant among community-acquired MRSA

http://dx.doi.org/10.5772/65967

(CA-MRSA) in the United States [100]. And on the other hand, pSCFS7 plasmid demonstrated the capability to be transferred by conjugation to other *S. aureus* strains. Thus, this was the first report of a conjugative plasmid on *S. aureus* strain belonging to genotypes with clinical relevance.

Linezolid susceptibility among clinically significant isolates is monitored by different surveillance programs, such as Zyvox Annual Appraisal of Potency and Spectrum (ZAAPS) and the USA Linezolid Experience and Accurate Determination of Resistance (LEADER). According to the results obtained by these programs, linezolid resistance was 0.05% for *S. aureus* and 1.4% for CoNS between 2002 and 2010 [101, 102]. CoNS, not considered as true pathogens, show higher levels of resistance and could act as *cfr* reservoir for the *S. aureus* pool. In fact, the high incidence of unique clones (40%) among *cfr*-positive MRSA suggested that the transmission of the *cfr* gene by HGT could be a common phenomenon [5].

The impact of the transmission of *cfr* among potential reservoirs was determined in Spain after the *cfr*-positive MRSA outbreak in the same hospital [103]. In this study, 100 linezolid-resistant *S. epidermidis* strains obtained between 2008 and 2011 were analyzed. Authors did not recover *cfr*-positive MRSA strains, but they detected this gene in the 58% of the linezolid-resistant *S. epidermidis* isolates, again suggesting the potential role of CoNS as linezolid resistance reservoirs. In 2012, two geographically independent staphylococci harboring conjugative *cfr*-associated plasmids were detected in Spain. One of them was located on a MRSA belonging to ST125 genotype, prevalent among hospital-associated strains (HA-MRSA). This plasmid, named pERGB, showed a new genetic environment of *cfr* insertion, associated with the *istAS-istBS* tandem but not with the TN558 transposon [104]. In addition, it also showed the ability to be transferred by conjugation to the ATCC 29213 *S. aureus* strain.

The second *cfr*-associated vector detected in Spain was found on a ST22 *S. epidermidis* strain [105]. In this case, *cfr* was inserted on a genetic environment identical to the pSCFS7 vector and the plasmid also showed an *in vitro* conjugative transmission. This was the first report of pSCFS7-like plasmids in Spain associated with clinical staphylococci, followed by the finding of two more strains harboring similar vectors in 2014 [106]. Two staphylococcal strains (one *Staphylococcus haemolyticus* and one *S. aureus*) obtained from two clinical cases of septic shock were identified in the same hospital in Spain. Both strains harbored similar ca.40 kb conjugative pSCFS7-like vectors. Although plasmid restriction analysis profiles showed small differences between both strains, the emergence of unrelated *cfr*-positive *S. aureus* and CoNS and the presence of this gene in similar pSCFS7-like plasmids in Spain [105, 106] suggest the potential spread of these vectors among the staphylococcal pool in Spain.

While the observed situation suggested the spread of pSCFS7 among the staphylococci in Spain, in the USA, the situation regarding the prevalence of *cfr* vectors was different. In addition to the pSCFS3-like vector described in 2008 [94], *cfr*-positive strains carrying these plasmids were found in 2013 [107]. The study comprised 19 *S. epidermidis* and 2 *S. aureus* linezolid-resistant strains. Among the studied strains, one *S. aureus* strain did not share a similar plasmid profile. Plasmid sequence analysis demonstrated the existence of identical 39.3 kb pSCFS3-like plasmids in one *S. epidermidis* and *S. aureus* isolates [6]. As pSCFS3 plasmids were considered as non-conjugative vectors [94], this indirect demonstration of plasmid transmission questioned the nature of the HGT involved in the spread of these plasmids. In addition, an unexpected result was obtained analyzing the sequence of two *cfr* plasmids obtained in staphylococcal clinical isolates from German hospitals [108]. In this study, 6 *cfr*-positive strains were identified among 36 linezolid-resistant *S. epidermidis* isolated between January 2012 and April 2013. Sequence analysis showed the existence of pSCFS6 and pSCFS7-like plasmids. The pSCFS6-like plasmid showed substantial homology to pGO1 plasmid, meanwhile the pSCFS7, as well as pSCFS3-like plasmids, showed the most significant homology to pSK73 plasmid [107]. The presence of pSCFS7-like plasmids in clinical isolates from Germany may suggest the potential spread of these plasmids among European hospitals. Nevertheless, although pSCFS6 harbored the pGO1 *tra* and *nes* conjugative machinery, none of these genes were located in the pSCFS7 sequence, suggesting potential mobilization events of *cfr* environment onto different plasmids backbones [108].

Although conjugation alone was the recognized transmission mechanism for the *cfr* gene, the presence of identical putative non-conjugative pSCFS3 plasmids in different staphylococcal species suggested the existence of other HTG mechanisms involved in the spreading of linezolid resistance [107]. Our group answered this question demonstrating an alternative mechanism for *cfr* spread based on phage transduction among MRSA [6]. By using a *S. aureus* N315 derivate strain harboring a pSCFS7-like vector obtained by conjugation from one clinical *S. epidermidis* strain, we transferred this gene to other MRSA strains by conjugation as well as transduction. In addition, this transmission allowed transductant MRSA *cfr*-positive strains to retain the conjugative capability, suggesting the complete transmission of this vector, or at least all the necessary genes to allow conjugative transmission.

4. Conclusion

The prominent evolutionary ability of *Staphylococcus aureus* partly relies on the gene transfer mechanisms ranging from the conventional phage transduction and conjugation to the unique staphylococcal mechanisms such as SaPI-helper phage. Recently found staphylococcal natural transformation further explains the ability to transfer larger genetic elements. The surveillance for antibiotics resistance (especially for the last resort antibiotics such as linezolid and vancomycin) is critical, and the test of emerging resistant pathogens in terms of their ability to use these distinct gene dissemination pathways might help to control the evolution of this important human pathogen.

Acknowledgements

We thank Ms. Nguyen Thi Le Thuy for her help. We acknowledge the supports from Pfizer Academic Contributions and Takeda Science Foundation.

http://dx.doi.org/10.5772/65967

Author details

Fabio Cafini[1,†], Veronica Medrano Romero[2,†] and Kazuya Morikawa[3*]

*Address all correspondence to: morikawa.kazuya.ga@u.tsukuba.ac.jp

1 Universidad Europea de Madrid, Department of Basic Biomedical Science, Madrid, Spain

2 Graduate School of Comprehensive Human Sciences, University of Tsukuba, Tsukuba, Japan

3 Division of Biomedical Science, Faculty of Medicine, University of Tsukuba, Tsukuba, Japan

† These authors contributed equally

References

[1] Lowy, F.D., Antimicrobial resistance: the example of Staphylococcus aureus. J Clin Invest, 2003. **111**(9): p. 1265–73.

[2] Ito, T., et al., Insights on antibiotic resistance of Staphylococcus aureus from its whole genome: genomic island SCC. Drug Resist Updat, 2003. **6**(1): p. 41–52.

[3] Chambers, H.F. and F.R. Deleo, Waves of resistance: Staphylococcus aureus in the antibiotic era. Nat Rev Microbiol, 2009. **7**(9): p. 629–41.

[4] Mongodin, E., et al., Microarray transcription analysis of clinical Staphylococcus aureus isolates resistant to vancomycin. J Bacteriol, 2003. **185**(15): p. 4638–4643.

[5] Gu, B., et al., The emerging problem of linezolid-resistant Staphylococcus. J Antimicrob Chemother, 2013. **68**(1): p. 4–11.

[6] Cafini, F., et al., Horizontal gene transmission of the cfr gene to MRSA and Enterococcus: role of Staphylococcus epidermidis as a reservoir and alternative pathway for the spread of linezolid resistance. J Antimicrob Chemother, 2016. **71**(3): p. 587–92.

[7] Lindsay, J.A., Genomic variation and evolution of Staphylococcus aureus. Int J Med Microbiol, 2010. **300**(2–3): p. 98–103.

[8] Malachowa, N. and F.R. DeLeo, Mobile genetic elements of Staphylococcus aureus. Cell Mol Life Sci, 2010. **67**(18): p. 3057–71.

[9] Deghorain, M. and L. Van Melderen, The Staphylococci phages family: an overview. Viruses, 2012. **4**(12): p. 3316–35.

[10] McNamara, P.J., Genetic manipulation of Staphylococcus aureus, in Staphylococcus molecular genetics, J.A. Lindsay, Editor. 2008, Caister Academic Press: Norfolk, UK. p. 89–130.

[11] Novick, R.P., G.E. Christie, and J.R. Penades, The phage-related chromosomal islands of Gram-positive bacteria. Nat Rev Microbiol, 2010. **8**(8): p. 541–51.

[12] Uchiyama, J., et al., Intragenus generalized transduction in Staphylococcus spp. by a novel giant phage. ISME J, 2014. **8**(9): p. 1949–52.

[13] Pattee, P.A. and D.S. Neveln, Transformation analysis of three linkage groups in Staphylococcus aureus. J Bacteriol, 1975. **124**(1): p. 201–11.

[14] Birmingham, V.A. and P.A. Pattee, Genetic transformation in Staphylococcus aureus: isolation and characterization of a competence-conferring factor from bacteriophage 80 alpha lysates. J Bacteriol, 1981. **148**(1): p. 301–7.

[15] Morikawa, K., et al., Expression of a cryptic secondary sigma factor gene unveils natural competence for DNA transformation in Staphylococcus aureus. PLoS Pathog, 2012. **8**(11): p. e1003003.

[16] Thomas, W.D., Jr. and G.L. Archer, Identification and cloning of the conjugative transfer region of Staphylococcus aureus plasmid pGO1. J Bacteriol, 1989. **171**(2): p. 684–91.

[17] Berg, T., et al., Complete nucleotide sequence of pSK41: evolution of staphylococcal conjugative multiresistance plasmids. J Bacteriol, 1998. **180**(17): p. 4350–9.

[18] Dougherty, B.A., et al., Sequence and analysis of the 60 kb conjugative, bacteriocin-producing plasmid pMRC01 from Lactococcus lactis DPC3147. Mol Microbiol, 1998. **29**(4): p. 1029–38.

[19] Schwarz, F.V., V. Perreten, and M. Teuber, Sequence of the 50-kb conjugative multiresistance plasmid pRE25 from Enterococcus faecalis RE25. Plasmid, 2001. **46**(3): p. 170–87.

[20] Ramsay, J.P., S.M. Kwong, Murphy, R.J.T., Eto, K.Y., Price, K.J., Nguyen, Q.T., O'Brien, F.G., Grubb, W.B., Coombs, G.W. Neville Firth An updated view of plasmid conjugation and mobilization in Staphylococcus. Mob Genet Elements, 2016. **6**(4): p. 1–11.

[21] Chen, I., The ins and outs of DNA transfer in bacteria. Science, 2005. **310**(5753): p. 1456–60.

[22] Thomas, C.M. and K.M. Nielsen, Mechanisms of, and barriers to, horizontal gene transfer between bacteria. Nat Rev Microbiol, 2005. **3**(9): p. 711–21.

[23] Chen, I. and D. Dubnau, DNA uptake during bacterial transformation. Nat Rev Microbiol, 2004. **2**(3): p. 241–9.

[24] Lindsay, J.A., Staphylococcus aureus genomics and the impact of horizontal gene transfer. Int J Med Microbiol, 2014. **304**(2): p. 103–9.

[25] Morikawa, K., et al., A new staphylococcal sigma factor in the conserved gene cassette: functional significance and implication for the evolutionary processes. Genes Cells, 2003. **8**(8): p. 699–712.

[26] Fagerlund, A., P.E. Granum, and L.S. Havarstein, Staphylococcus aureus competence genes: mapping of the SigH, ComK1 and ComK2 regulons by transcriptome sequencing. Mol Microbiol, 2014. **94**(3): p. 557–79.

[27] Thi, Le T.N., V.M. Romero, and K. Morikawa, Cell wall-affecting antibiotics modulate natural transformation in SigH-expressing Staphylococcus aureus. J Antibiot (Tokyo), 2016. **69**(6): p. 464–6.

[28] Prudhomme, M., et al., Antibiotic stress induces genetic transformability in the human pathogen Streptococcus pneumoniae. Science (New York, N.Y.), 2006. **313**(5783): p. 89–92.

[29] Charpentier, X., et al., Antibiotics and UV radiation induce competence for natural transformation in Legionella pneumophila. J Bacteriol, 2011. **193**(5): p. 1114–21.

[30] Dorer, M.S., J. Fero, and N.R. Salama, DNA damage triggers genetic exchange in Helicobacter pylori. PLoS Pathog, 2010. **6**(7): p. e1001026.

[31] Boutry, C., et al., SOS response activation and competence development are antagonistic mechanisms in Streptococcus thermophilus. J Bacteriol, 2013. **195**(4): p. 696–707.

[32] Cirz, R.T., et al., Complete and SOS-mediated response of Staphylococcus aureus to the antibiotic ciprofloxacin. J Bacteriol, 2007. **189**(2): p. 531–9.

[33] Ambur, O.H., et al., Genome dynamics in major bacterial pathogens. FEMS Microbiol Rev, 2009. **33**(3): p. 453–70.

[34] Plata, K.B., et al., Targeting of PBP1 by beta-lactams determines recA/SOS response activation in heterogeneous MRSA clinical strains. PLoS One, 2013. **8**(4): p. e61083.

[35] Cuirolo, A., K. Plata, and A.E. Rosato, Development of homogeneous expression of resistance in methicillin-resistant Staphylococcus aureus clinical strains is functionally associated with a beta-lactam-mediated SOS response. J Antimicrob Chemother, 2009. **64**(1): p. 37–45.

[36] Maiques, E., et al., beta-lactam antibiotics induce the SOS response and horizontal transfer of virulence factors in Staphylococcus aureus. J Bacteriol, 2006. **188**(7): p. 2726–9.

[37] Mesak, L.R., V. Miao, and J. Davies, Effects of subinhibitory concentrations of antibiotics on SOS and DNA repair gene expression in Staphylococcus aureus. Antimicrob Agents Chemother, 2008. **52**(9): p. 3394–7.

[38] Anderson, K.L., et al., Characterization of the Staphylococcus aureus heat shock, cold shock, stringent, and SOS responses and their effects on log-phase mRNA turnover. J Bacteriol, 2006. **188**(19): p. 6739–56.

[39] Kali, A., Antibiotics and bioactive natural products in treatment of methicillin resistant Staphylococcus aureus: a brief review. Pharmacogn Rev, 2015. **9**(17): p. 29–34.

[40] Anthonisen, I.L., et al., Organization of the antiseptic resistance gene qacA and Tn552-related β-lactamase genes in multidrug-resistant Staphylococcus haemolyticus strains of animal and human origins. Antimicrob Agents Chemother, 2002. **46**(11): p. 3606–3612.

[41] Novick, R.P., Genetic systems in staphylococci. Methods Enzymol, 1991. **204**: p. 587–636.

[42] Lindberg, M., Sjostrom, J., Johansson, T., Transformation of chromosomal and plasmid characters in Staphylococcus aureus. J Bacteriol, 1972. **109**(2): p. 844–847.

[43] Tsukubakishita, S., Kuwahara-Arai, K., Baba, T., Hiramatsu, K., Staphylococcal cassette chromosome mec-like element in Macrococcus caseolyticus. Antimicrob Agents Chemother, 2010. **54**(4): p. 1469–75.

[44] Tsukubakishita, S., Kuwahara-Arai, K., Sasaki, T., Hiramatsu, K., Origin and molecular evolution of the determinant of methicillin resistance in staphylococci. Antimicrob Agents Chemother, 2010. **54**(10): p. 4352–9.

[45] Wu, S., Piscitelli, C., de Lencastre, H., Tomasz, A., Tracking the evolutionary origin of the methicillin resistance gene: cloning and sequencing of a homologue of mecA from a methicillin susceptible strain of Staphylococcus sciuri. Microb Drug Resist, 1996. **2**: p. 435–41.

[46] Otto, M., Coagulase-negative staphylococci as reservoirs of genes facilitating MRSA infection. Bioassays, 2013. **35**(1): p. 4–11.

[47] Scharn, C., Tenover, F.C., Goering, R.V., Transduction of staphylococcal cassette chromosome mec elements between strains of Staphylococcus aureus. Antimicrob Agents Chemother, 2013. **57**(11): p. 5233–8.

[48] Chlebowicz, M., Maslanova, I., Kuntova, L., Grundmann, H., Pantucek, R., Doskar, J., van Dijl, J.M, The Staphylococcal Cassette Chromosome mec type V from Staphylococcus aureus ST398 is packaged into bacteriophage capsids. Int J Med Microbiol, 2014. **304**(5–6): p. 764–74.

[49] Ray, M., Boundy, S., Archer, G.L., Transfer of the methicillin resistance genomic island among staphylococci by conjugation. Mol Microbiol, 2016. **100**(4): p. 675–85.

[50] Noble, W.C., Virani, Z., Cree R.G.A., Co-transfer of vancomycin and other resistance genes from Enterococcus faecalis NCTC 12201 to Staphylococcus aureus. FEMS Microbiol Lett, 1992. **93**: p. 195–8.

[51] Sievert, D.M., M.L. Boulton, G. Stolman, D. Johnson, M.G. Stobierski, F.P. Downes, P.A. Somsel, J.T. Rudrik, W. Brown, W. Hafeez, T. Lundstrom, E. Flanagan, R. Johnson, J. Mitchel, S. Chang, Staphylococcus aureus resistant to vancomycin. MMWR Morb Mortal Wkly Rep, 2002. **51**: p. 565–7.

[52] Rouch, D.A., Byrne, M.E., Kong, Y.C., Skurray, R.A., The aacA-aphD gentamicin and kanamycin resistance determinant of TN4001 from Staphylococcus aureus: expression and nucleotide sequence analysis. J Gen Microbiol, 1987. **133**: p. 3039–52.

[53] Rouch, D.A., Messerotti, L.J., Loo, L.S.L., Jackson, C.A., Skurray, R.A., Trimethroprim resistance transposon Tn4003 from Staphylococcus aureus encodes genes for a dihydrofolate reductase and thymidylate synthetase flanked by three copies of IS257. Mol Microbiol, 1989. **3**(2): p. 161–75.

[54] Archer, G.L., Coughter, J.P., Johnston J.L, Plasmid-encoded trimethoprim resistance in Staphylococci. Antimicrob Agents Chemother, 1986. **29**(5): p. 733–40.

[55] Sekiguchi, J., et al., Cloning and characterization of a novel trimethoprim-resistant dihydrofolate reductase from a nosocomial isolate of Staphylococcus aureus CM.S2 (IMCJ1454). Antimicrob Agents Chemother, 2005. **49**(9): p. 3948–51.

[56] Kadlec, K. and S. Schwarz, Identification of a novel trimethoprim resistance gene, dfrK, in a methicillin-resistant Staphylococcus aureus ST398 strain and its physical linkage to the tetracycline resistance gene tet(L). Antimicrob Agents Chemother, 2009. **53**(2): p. 776–8.

[57] Kadlec, K., et al., Unusual small plasmids carrying the novel resistance genes dfrK or apmA isolated from methicillin-resistant or -susceptible staphylococci. J Antimicrob Chemother, 2012. **67**(10): p. 2342–5.

[58] Schwarz, S., et al., Plasmid-mediated antimicrobial resistance in staphylococci and other firmicutes. Microbiol Spectr, 2014. **2**(6):PLAS-0020-2014.doi:10.1128/microbiolspec. PLAS-0020-2014

[59] Khan, S.A., Novick R., Terminal nucleotide sequences of Tn551, a transposon specifying erythromycin resistance in Staphylococcus aureus: homology with Tn3. Plasmid, 1980. **4**: p. 148–54.

[60] Leclercq, R., Courvalin, P., Bacterial resistance to macrolide, lincosamide, and streptogramin antibiotics by target modification. Antimicrob Agents Chemother, 1991. **35**(7): p. 1267–72.

[61] Trieu-Cuot P, Poyart-Salmeron C, Carlier C, Courvalin P. Molecular dissection of the transposition mechanism of conjugative transposons from Gram-positive cocci. In: Dunny G M, Patrick P, Cleary L L, editors. Genetics and molecular biology of streptococci, lactococci, and enterococci. Washington, D.C: American Society for Microbiology; 1991. pp. 21–27.

[62] Thakker-Varia, S., Jenssen, W.D., Moon-Mcdermott, L., Weinstein, M.P., Dubin, D.T., Molecular epidemiology of Macrolides-Lincosamides-Streptogramin B resistance in Staphylococcus aureus and Coagulase-Negative Staphylococci. Antimicrob Agents Chemother, 1987. **31**(5): p. 735–43.

[63] Murphy, E., Nucleotide Sequence of ermA, a macrolide-lincosamide-streptogramin B determinant in Staphylococcus aureus. J Bacteriol, 1985. **162**(2): p. 633–40.

[64] Chopra, I. and M. Roberts, Tetracycline antibiotics: mode of action, applications, molecular biology, and epidemiology of bacterial resistance. Microbiol Mol Biol Rev, 2001. **65**(2): p. 232–60.

[65] Bismuth, R., Zilhao, R., Sakamoto, H., Guesdon, J., Courvalin, P, Gene heterogeneity for tetracycline resistance in Staphylococcus spp. Antimicrob Agents Chemother, 1990. **34**(8): p. 1611–14.

[66] Lyon, B.R., Skurray, R., Antimicrobial resistance of Staphylococcus aureus: genetic basis. Microbiol Rev, 1987. **51**(1): p. 88–134.

[67] Tennent, J.M., May, J.W., Skurray, R.A., Characterisation of chloramphenicol resistance plasmids of Staphylococcus aureus and S. epidermidis by restriction enzyme mapping techniques. J Med Microbiol, 1986. **22**: p. 79–84.

[68] Hershberger, E., Donabedian, S., Konstantinou, K., Zervos, M.J., Quinupristin-Dalfopristin resistance in Gram-Positive bacteria: mechanism of resistance and epidemiology. Clin Infect Dis, 2004. **38**(92–98).

[69] Allignet, J., El Solh, N., Comparative analysis of staphylococcal plasmids carrying three streptogramin-resistance genes: vat-vgb-vga. Plasmid, 1999. **42**: p. 134–138.

[70] Yazdankhah, S.P., et al., Fusidic acid resistance, mediated by fusB, in bovine coagulase-negative staphylococci. J Antimicrob Chemother, 2006. **58**(6): p. 1254–1256.

[71] Hung, W.C., et al., Skin commensal staphylococci may act as reservoir for fusidic acid resistance genes. PLoS One, 2015. **10**(11): p. e0143106.

[72] Lin, Y.T., et al., A novel staphylococcal cassette chromosomal element, SCCfusC, carrying fusC and speG in fusidic acid-resistant methicillin-resistant Staphylococcus aureus. Antimicrob Agents Chemother, 2014. **58**(2): p. 1224–7.

[73] Holden, M.T., et al., Complete genomes of two clinical Staphylococcus aureus strains: evidence for the rapid evolution of virulence and drug resistance. Proc Natl Acad Sci U S A, 2004. **101**(26): p. 9786–91.

[74] Ender, M., B. Berger-Bachi, and N. McCallum, Variability in SCCmecN1 spreading among injection drug users in Zurich, Switzerland. BMC Microbiol, 2007. **7**: p. 62.

[75] Kinnevey, P.M., et al., Emergence of sequence type 779 methicillin-resistant Staphylococcus aureus harboring a novel pseudo staphylococcal cassette chromosome mec (SCCmec)-SCC-SCCCRISPR composite element in Irish hospitals. Antimicrob Agents Chemother, 2013. **57**(1): p. 524–31.

[76] Jevons, M., "Celbenin"-resistant staphylococci. Br Med J, 1961. **124**: p. 124–5.

[77] Peacock, S., Paterson, GK., Mechanisms of methicillin resistance in Staphylococcus aureus. Annu Rev Biochem, 2015. **84**: p. 577–601.

[78] Ito, T., Y. Katayama, and K. Hiramatsu, Cloning and nucleotide sequence determination of the entire mec DNA of pre-methicillin-resistant Staphylococcus aureus N315. Antimicrob Agents Chemother, 1999. **43**(6): p. 1449–58.

[79] Katayama, Y., T. Ito, and K. Hiramatsu, A new class of genetic element, staphylococcus cassette chromosome mec, encodes methicillin resistance in Staphylococcus aureus. Antimicrob Agents Chemother, 2000. **44**(6): p. 1549–55.

[80] (IWG-SCC), I.W.G.o.t.C.o.S.C.C.E., Classification of staphylococcal cassette chromosome mec (SCCmec): guidelines for reporting novel SCCmec elements. Antimicrob Agents Chemother, 2009. **53**(12): p. 4961–7.

[81] Kloos, W.E., Ballard, D.N., George, C.G., Webster, J.A., Hubner, R.J., Ludwig, W., Schleifer, K.H. Fiedler, F. and Schubert, K., Delimiting the genus Staphylococcus through description of Macrococcus caseolyticus gen. nov., comb. nov. and Macrococcus equipercicus sp. nov., and Macrococcus bovicus sp. nov. and Macrococcus carouselicus sp. nov. J Syst Bacteriol, 1998. **48**: p. 859–77.

[82] Ito, T., Katayama, Y., Asada, K., Mori, N., Tsutsumimoto, K., Tiensasitorn, C., Hiramatsu, K., Structural Comparison of Three Types of Staphylococcal Cassette Chromosome mec Integrated in the Chromosome in Methicillin-Resistant Staphylococcus aureus. Antimicrob Agents Chemother, 2001. **45**(5): p. 1323–36.

[83] Ito, T., Ma, XX., Takekuchi, F., Okuma, K., Yuzawa, H., Hiramatsu, K., Novel type V staphylococcal cassette chromosome mec driven by a novel cassette chromosome recombinase, ccrC. Antimicrob Agents Chemother, 2004. **48**(7): p. 2637–51.

[84] Ma, X., Ito, T., Tiensasitorn, C., Jamklnag, M., Chongtrakool, P., Boyle-Vavra, S., Daum, R.S., Hiramatsu, K., Novel type of staphylococcal cassette chromosome mec identified in community-acquired methicillin-resistant Staphylococcus aureus strains. Antimicrob Agents Chemother, 2002. **46**(4): p. 1147–52.

[85] Barbier, F., Ruppe, E., Hernandez, D., Lebaux, D., Methicillin-resistant coagulase-negative staphylococci in the community: high homology of SCCmec IVa between Staphylococcus epidermidis and major clones of methicillin-resistant Staphylococcus aureus. J Infect Dis, 2010. **202**: p. 270–281.

[86] Bouchami, O., Ben Hassen, A., Lencastre, H., Miragaia, M., Molecular epidemiology of methicillin-resistant Staphylococcus hominis (MRSHo): low clonality and reservoirs of SCCmec structural elements. PLoS One, 2011. **6**(7): p. e21940.

[87] Bouchami, O., Ben Hassen, A., Lencastre, H., Miragaia, M., High prevalence of mec complex C and ccrC is independent of SCCmec type V in Staphylococcus haemolyticus. Eur J Clin Microbiol Infect Dis, 2011. **31**(4): p. 605–14.

[88] Schwarz, S., C. Werckenthin, and C. Kehrenberg, Identification of a plasmid-borne chloramphenicol-florfenicol resistance gene in Staphylococcus sciuri. Antimicrob Agents Chemother, 2000. **44**(9): p. 2530–3.

[89] Murphy, E., L. Huwyler, and C. de Freire Bastos Mdo, Transposon Tn554: complete nucleotide sequence and isolation of transposition-defective and antibiotic-sensitive mutants. EMBO J, 1985. **4**(12): p. 3357–65.

[90] Toh, S.M., et al., Acquisition of a natural resistance gene renders a clinical strain of methicillin-resistant Staphylococcus aureus resistant to the synthetic antibiotic linezolid. Mol Microbiol, 2007. **64**(6): p. 1506–14.

[91] Livermore, D.M., Linezolid in vitro: mechanism and antibacterial spectrum. J Antimicrob Chemother, 2003. **51**(Suppl 2): p. ii9–16.

[92] Locke, J.B., M. Hilgers, and K.J. Shaw, Mutations in ribosomal protein L3 are associated with oxazolidinone resistance in staphylococci of clinical origin. Antimicrob Agents Chemother, 2009. **53**(12): p. 5275–8.

[93] Sanchez Garcia, M., et al., Clinical outbreak of linezolid-resistant Staphylococcus aureus in an intensive care unit. JAMA, 2010. **303**(22): p. 2260–4.

[94] Mendes, R.E., et al., First report of cfr-mediated resistance to linezolid in human staphylococcal clinical isolates recovered in the United States. Antimicrob Agents Chemother, 2008. **52**(6): p. 2244–6.

[95] Kehrenberg, C. and S. Schwarz, Distribution of florfenicol resistance genes fexA and cfr among chloramphenicol-resistant Staphylococcus isolates. Antimicrob Agents Chemother, 2006. **50**(4): p. 1156–63.

[96] Wang, Y., et al., Detection of the staphylococcal multiresistance gene cfr in Proteus vulgaris of food animal origin. J Antimicrob Chemother, 2011. **66**(11): p. 2521–6.

[97] Wang, Y., et al., Detection of the staphylococcal multiresistance gene cfr in Macrococcus caseolyticus and Jeotgalicoccus pinnipedialis. J Antimicrob Chemother, 2012. **67**(8): p. 1824–7.

[98] Liu, Y., et al., Transferable multiresistance plasmids carrying cfr in Enterococcus spp. from swine and farm environment. Antimicrob Agents Chemother, 2013. **57**(1): p. 42–8.

[99] Shore, A.C., et al., Identification and characterization of the multidrug resistance gene cfr in a Panton-Valentine leukocidin-positive sequence type 8 methicillin-resistant Staphylococcus aureus IVa (USA300) isolate. Antimicrob Agents Chemother, 2010. **54**(12): p. 4978–84.

[100] Klevens, R.M., et al., Invasive methicillin-resistant Staphylococcus aureus infections in the United States. JAMA, 2007. **298**(15): p. 1763–71.

[101] Flamm, R.K., et al., An international activity and spectrum analysis of linezolid: ZAAPS Program results for 2011. Diagn Microbiol Infect Dis, 2013. **76**(2): p. 206–13.

[102] Flamm, R.K., et al., Linezolid surveillance results for the United States: LEADER surveillance program 2011. Antimicrob Agents Chemother, 2013. **57**(2): p. 1077–81.

[103] Baos, E., et al., Characterization and monitoring of linezolid-resistant clinical isolates of Staphylococcus epidermidis in an intensive care unit 4 years after an outbreak of infection by cfr-mediated linezolid-resistant Staphylococcus aureus. Diagn Microbiol Infect Dis, 2013. **76**(3): p. 325–9.

[104] Gopegui, E.R., et al., Transferable multidrug resistance plasmid carrying cfr associated with tet(L), ant(4')-Ia, and dfrK genes from a clinical methicillin-resistant Staphylococcus aureus ST125 strain. Antimicrob Agents Chemother, 2012. **56**(4): p. 2139–42.

[105] Lozano, C., et al., Characterization of a cfr-positive methicillin-resistant Staphylococcus epidermidis strain of the lineage ST22 implicated in a life-threatening human infection. Diagn Microbiol Infect Dis, 2012. **73**(4): p. 380–2.

[106] Fessler, A.T., et al., Cfr-mediated linezolid resistance in methicillin-resistant Staphylococcus aureus and Staphylococcus haemolyticus associated with clinical infections in humans: two case reports. J Antimicrob Chemother, 2014. **69**(1): p. 268–70.

[107] Mendes, R.E., et al., Dissemination of a pSCFS3-like cfr-carrying plasmid in Staphylococcus aureus and Staphylococcus epidermidis clinical isolates recovered from hospitals in Ohio. Antimicrob Agents Chemother, 2013. **57**(7): p. 2923–8.

[108] Bender, J., et al., Linezolid resistance in clinical isolates of Staphylococcus epidermidis from German hospitals and characterization of two cfr-carrying plasmids. J Antimicrob Chemother, 2015. **70**(6): p. 1630–8.

Chapter 5

Effects of Alterations in *Staphylococcus aureus* Cell Membrane and Cell Wall in Antimicrobial Resistance

Andrea de Souza Monteiro,
Wallace Ribeiro Nunes Neto,
Aleff Ricardo Santos Mendes,
Bruna Lorrana dos Santos Pinto,
Luís Cláudio Nascimento da Silva and
Gabriella Freitas Ferreira

Additional information is available at the end of the chapter

http://dx.doi.org/10.5772/66954

Abstract

Staphylococcus aureus is one of the most successful opportunistic pathogen able to cause serious infections due to its ability to produce virulence factors and acquire antimicrobial resistance. Recent reports indicate that the phenotypic changes in the cell wall and cell membrane are essential mechanisms related to the resistance to several antibacterial drugs (such as daptomycin and vancomycin). These alterations involve changes in cell wall composition and chemical modifications of some components (point mutation leading to modification in phosphatidylglycerol molecule, in the production of the aberrations in peptidoglycan structure and decrease in autolytic activity of the components of the cell envelope), leading to changes in electric charge of the cell surface, cell membrane fluidity and cell morphology. In fact, *S. aureus* develops several multifactorial and strain-specific adaptive mechanisms to survival in host. The study of such mechanisms is very important. The aim of this chapter is to review the phenotypic mechanisms related to drug resistance in *S. aureus*.

Keywords: *Staphylococcus aureus*, daptomycin, vancomycin, heteroresistance, stress stimulon response

1. Introduction

The lipopeptide and glycopeptide antibiotics are very effective against infections caused by Gram-positive cocci, showing good efficacy against *Staphylococcus aureus*. The mechanism of action of these antibiotics is linked with their ability to block cell wall bacterial synthesis. As examples of the most used drugs to treat *S. aureus* infection, we have daptomycin (DAP) and vancomycin. However, currently, the indiscriminate use of these antimicrobials has decreased their effectiveness against *S. aureus* strains [1].

Daptomycin (DAP) is a cyclic lipopeptide antibiotic obtained from *Streptomyces roseosporus* with activity against the most Gram-positive bacteria, including vancomycin-resistant enterococci (VRE) and methicillin-resistant *S. aureus* (MRSA) [2–4]. DAP appears to have multiple effects on the Gram-positive bacterial cell membrane (BCM) [5]. The mechanism of action proposed is the aggregation between DAP and BMC, which alters the architecture of cell membrane and forms pores, leading to ion loss. This new arrangement leads to a rapid depolarization, resulting in a loss of membrane potential that culminates in bacterial cell death. Regarding the interaction mechanisms with the formation of cell wall and surface, a special mention should be given to the interference in peptidoglycan and lipoteichoic biosynthesis [6–8].

The glycopeptide antibiotics were introduced in therapy against infections caused by *S. aureus* in 1955 [9]. The vancomycin is glycopeptide produced by *Amycolatopsis orientalis* (actinomycete) and is the representative of this class of antibiotic widely used in medical practice today, especially after the appearance of resistant strains of *S. aureus* to methicillin [10]. However, the emergence of molecular mechanisms of resistance to vancomycin and the appearance of phenotypic resistance profiles in heterogeneous subpopulations of *S. aureus* as described susceptible have hindered the use of glycopeptide as first choice agent in antibiotic therapy [11]. Some reduced susceptibility phenotypes are classified in some profiles as vancomycin-intermediate *S. aureus* (VISA) and vancomycin-resistant *S. aureus* (VRSA) [11]. Subpopulations of heterogeneous *S. aureus* with heterogeneous resistance to vancomycin and notoriously sensitive to vancomycin are classified as heteroresistant vancomycin-intermediate *S. aureus* (hVISA) [1].

Heteroresistance is defined as resistance to antibiotics expressed by a subset of a microbial population that initially is considered susceptible to these antibiotics. These resistant subpopulations are able to adapt to increasing drug concentrations in a stepwise manner [12]. This phenomenon has been described in a wide range of bacteria and fungi, but attention has been directed toward *S. aureus* [13]. For the *S. aureus* hVISA strains containing subpopulations of vancomycin-intermediate daughter cells, the minimal inhibitory concentrations (MICs) for the parent strains of these daughter cells fall within the susceptible range of 1–4 μg/mL. However, if the lineage is exposed to increasing concentrations of vancomycin, a new generation of cells with reduced susceptibility profiles will be favored. This exhibition creates a selective pressure that favors the outgrowth of rare vancomycin-resistant clones leading to hVISA clones. Eventually, the continued exposure to vancomycin culminates in a uniform population of VISA phenotypes [14]. Evidence in clinical case studies which monitored *S. aureus* infections in 250 patients showed that the hVISA phenotype is closely related with significantly prolonged bacteremia events and associated with increased rates of endocarditis and osteomyelitis, compared with *methicillin-resistant Staphylococcus aureus* (MRSA) bacteremia [15].

VISA and hVISA have an increased D-Ala-D-Ala moieties in their thickness cell wall that form false targets that sequester vancomycin, with reduced autolytic activity and slow growth in vitro ([14]. This phenomenon is believed to "trap" vancomycin and this, together with the thickened cell wall, may act as a barrier to the diffusion of large molecules, like daptomycin (as cited below) [16, 17]. In this way, the emergence of these bacterial phenotypes cited above has put into question the effectiveness of these antibiotics against *S. aureus* [1, 18, 19]. These changes in susceptibility seem to be related to the difficulty of resolving cases of *S. aureus* infection, leading to increased mortality of patients [20]. Altered host-pathogen interaction due to hVISA strains may change the course of the infection to worst prognostic for the patient. In a macrophage model of infection, hVISA/VISA strains showed increased capsule and reduced protein A (SpA, a protein surface cell), associated with reduced NF-κB activation and reduced TNF-α and IL-1β expression [21]. The persistent infections associated with hVISA/VISA strains can be a result of changes in host-pathogen interactions that culminate in attenuated host immune response [14].

2. Mechanisms for daptomycin resistance associated to modifications in cell membrane of the *Staphylococcus aureus*

A few years ago, antibiotic therapy using DAP to treat MRSA infections appeared to be a good choice; however, there are reports in the literature about bacterial strains with resistance to daptomycin (DAP-R) and with intermediary resistance (DAP-I) [19, 22]. *S. aureus* DAP-R infection has been associated with endocarditis and abscesses; it is characterized by high concentration of microorganisms in infected area with oral administration of low doses of DAP (i.e., ≤ 6 mg/kg/day) [23, 24]. In addition, it was observed the emergence of DAP non-susceptible *S. aureus* phenotypes in a patient with persistent VISA bacteremia [1]. The resistant phenotypes of VISA strains have developed an increased DAP resistance during therapy [25, 26]. Besides, it could be associated with the previous use of vancomycin [27]. DAP-I mechanisms in *S. aureus* have not yet been elucidated completely, but a possible predominant phenomenon for the appearance of this phenotype would be an increase repulsion of DAP molecules of the surface cell. This modification is generally associated with an overall net charge change on the cell surface (for a more positive charge) [23].

The lysyl-phosphatidylglycerol (Lys-PG) is an important membrane lipid in bacteria, more common in Gram-positive cells [28]. The Lys-PG is incorporated into the microbial cell membrane by the activity *of the* multiple peptide resistance factor (MprF) *gene* product (encoded by the *mprF*/*fmtC* gene). The MprF is a bifunctional protein composed by C-terminal part responsible by synthesize of the Lys-PG and the N-terminal hydrophobic protein domain is essential for efficient translocation of Lys-PG from the inner to the outer leaflet of the cytoplasmic membrane bacteria [28, 29].

The MprF protein catalyzes the modification of the negatively charged in phosphatidylglycerol (PG) with l-lysine and translocation of Lys-PG from the inside to the outside of the cell membrane leaflet [30]. MprF proteins in *S. aureus* encompass a lysyl-phosphatidylglycerol synthase and a Lys-PG flippase domain, responsible for aiding the movement of phospholipid molecules between the two leaflets in cell membrane ("flip-flop" transition). Moreover, in *S. aureus* the Lys-PG flippase and synthase in the MprF can understand two different proteins fused with distinct functional subunits [29].

The neutralization of the cell membrane surface leads to MprF triggered by bacterial resistance to cationic antimicrobial peptides (CAMPs) [31]. MprF was first described as a virulence factor of *S. aureus* by Peschel et al. [32], analyzing a mutant strain observed for MprF gene, which was unable to modify phosphatidylglycerol with L-lysine, was considerably faster killed by human neutrophils and exhibited an attenuated virulence in mice. This study indicated a key role of MprF for the resistance to defensins and cathelicidins (secreted peptides in host mucosal) and implied a higher pathogenicity of *S. aureus*. Interestingly, MprF is involved in the development of DAP-R in *S. aureus* [33]. These observations related to cells with DAP-R prolife take into account several factors. Among these are mechanisms that can interfere with the balance in incorporation of the PG into membrane. Also, it was verified that the co-expression of the alanyl-PG (Ala-PG) synthase with flippase domains of Lys-PG synthesizing MprF proteins led to a wild-type level of daptomycin susceptibility, indicating that Ala-PG can also protect bacterial membrane against DAP [33]. Moreover, the incorporation of the point mutations leading to amino acid exchanges in the MprF proteins of *S. aureus* strains leads to a decreased susceptibility to daptomycin [34].

Several hypotheses have been raised about the interference mechanisms of a mutant gene for the MprF protein in the dynamics of PG synthesis in *S. aureus*. It is considered that the biophysicist repulsion process of DAP molecules from the bacterial surface would be assigned to an increased PG incorporation by Δ*mprF* strain with singly point-mutated *mprF* gene ($mprF_{S295L}$ or $mprF_{T345A}$) [35]. More recently, it was noted that the decrease in susceptibility to DAP in some mutant strains for the MprF gene was the result of the critical effects caused by PG poor incorporation, resulting in failures in the oligomerization in the cell membrane, which compromise its antibacterial activity [23]. In addition, the possibility of antibiotic repulsion (such as DAP) triggered by the increase in positive charge can be seen in some *S. aureus* strains with a significant increase in cell wall thickness. These strains exhibit increased MICs for drug antibiotic and VISA-DAP-R phenotype [1].

3. Mechanisms for vancomycin resistance associated to modifications in cell envelope of the *Staphylococcus aureus*

The resistance mechanisms for both VISA and hVISA appear to have common features. However, it is always observed in patterns that distinguish them from vancomycin-susceptible *Staphylococcus aureus* (VSSA). Although the gene expression of hVISA or VISA during exposure to vancomycin denotes some patterns, subtle differences in the contribution of transcripts of these two phenotypes are found. One basic evidence regarding decrease in susceptibility is related to the cell wall thickening in bacterial cells. This process seems to initiate with the acquisition of a reduced autolysis caused by downregulation of autolysin genes, such as *atl*/*lyt*M [1]. A thickened cell wall has been highlighted as a characteristic phenotype commonly found in clinical VISA. This feature is intimately associated with peptidoglycan-clogging theory that explains vancomycin resistance by passage delay of antibiotic molecules across the thickened peptidoglycan layers [18]. Punctual mutations by genetic manipulation in *S. aureus* strains that could lead to cell wall thickening were investigated thoroughly. However, these studies did not conclude that active point mutations involving genes of regulatory systems, autolysins and major catalytic enzymes could be involved in the appearance of VISA phenotypes [36, 37].

Studies conducted on gene transcription analysis showed that after exposure of DAP, the cells exhibit a regulation of the cell wall "stimulon," similar to that observed in response to vancomycin [1, 38]. Comparison of DAP-I and DAP-*S. aureus* strain pairs, which are located in the genes that have been associated with VISA phenotype, indicated that the genes involved in the synthesis and/or homeostasis of the cell wall play an important role in the resistance to vancomycin observed to DAP strains [39].

Signal transduction mediated by two-component systems (TCSs)*YycFG* or sensor histidine kinase *WalK* (also called *WalRK*) is a regulatory system of two essential components of cell wall synthesis and homeostasis, which has also been implicated in DAP-R and VISA/VSSA cell phenotypes [1, 40]. Members of the two-component regulatory system *WalK/WalR* that regulate genes are involved in autolysis, biofilm formation and cell wall metabolism [1]. *WalK* functions as a sensor protein kinase, which is autophosphorylated at a histidine residue and transfers its phosphate group to *walk* [40]. The impacts of the single substitutions in either *WalR* or *WalK*, dramatically change the bacterial cell physiology, with significant reductions in autolytic activity and increases in cell wall thickness linked to the insertion of *WalR* or *WalK* alleles from the VISA strain into vancomycin-susceptible *S. aureus* (VSSA).

The impacts of the single substitutions in either *WalR* or *WalK* dramatic changes the cell bacterial physiology, with significant reductions in autolytic activity and increases in cell wall thickness linked to the introduction of the *walR* or *walk* allele from the VISA strain into the room fully vancomycin-susceptible *S. aureus* (VSSA). Vancomycin-intermediate *S. aureus* (VISA) is generated from vancomycin *S. aureus* sensible by multiple spontaneous mutations in two-component regulatory systems as standing for vancomycin resistance-associated sensor/regulator (V*raSR*) and inducible by cationic antimicrobial peptides (CAMPs), which could be important for bacterial cells in resisting the harmful effects of CAMPs and possibly other antimicrobial agents [41].

The assessment of the effects of mutations directed at specific targets, which are responsible for the metabolism of the cell wall in *S. aureus*, indicated that the synergistic mutations (double mutation) might have a more significant effect on the appearance of the VISA phenotype. Recently, it was observed that a deletion mutation in genes of the two-component regulatory system *walRK* (synonyms: *vicRK and yycFG*) might result in an increased resistance to vancomycin and appearance of VISA phenotype from the *S. aureus* LR5P1-V3 strain. On the other hand, LR5P1 strain with double mutation (*walK**clpP**) exhibited a thickened cell wall, slow growth and decreased autolytic activity [37]. Similarly, Hu et al. [42], also studying the participation of point mutation in *WalK* (G223D) gene in *S. aureus* MW2 (community-acquired methicillin-resistant), reported a decreased expression of genes associated with the cell wall metabolism, decreased autolytic activity and a reduced vancomycin susceptibility. In addition, the electrophoretic mobility shift assay (EMSA) indicated that *WalK* (G223D)-phosphorylated *WalR* had a reduced capacity to bind the *atlA* promoter. The *atlA* promoter is one of the component potential members of the *WalK/WalR* regulon and is involved in cell wall metabolism in *S. aureus*.

The ATP-dependent Clp protease (ClpP) consists of two heptameric rings and belongs to the family of serine peptidases [43]. ClpP plays an essential role in the degradation of pathogen cell wall but also in the regulation of their virulence [44]. The ClpP components in *S. aureus* are responsible for initiating physiological adaptive responses against different external pressures, including extreme changes in temperature, osmolarity and oxidative stress [45]. In addition, the ClpP protease presented chaperone-like functions, recognizing and refolding misfolded proteins accumulated or aggregated proteins in the cell, consequently participates in the cell envelope turnover in microbial cells [46, 47].

In various pathogenic microorganisms, such as *Listeria monocytogenes, Streptococcus pneumoniae* and *S. aureus, ClpP* proteases have been identified in in vivo expression studies as an important virulence factor [44, 48, 49]. Knockout studies of the *clpP* ATP-dependent gene in *S. aureus,* followed by global transcriptional analysis using DNA microarray technology, showed that the loss of *clpP* leads to complete derepression of transcription of the *CtsR* gene (or *yacG,* a polypeptide transcriptional regulator). The ClpP proteins are regulated by the *CtsR* heat-shock repressor controlled by HRCA (heat-inducible chaperone, a heat-shock regulon) and a partial derepression of genes involved in response to oxidative stress and DNA repair system SOS response pathway. Moreover, the expression of genes whose products are involved in autolysis of microbial cells was unregulated. This culminated in a dramatic increase in autolysis processes in *S. aureus* Δ*clpP* mutant [46]. In addition, other observations on the effect of the mutation identified in *clpP* system in *S. aureus* LR5P1-V3 strain indicated that deregulation is a new mechanism, which can lead to resistance to vancomycin. It was observed that the LR5P1-V3 mutant, derived from N315LR5P1, exhibited increased resistance to vancomycin, as MIC values rose from 1 to 8 μg/mL [37].

Recently, a genetic evaluation of vancomycin-intermediate *S. aureus* (VISA) isolated from the same patient at different times tightly corroborates an association of this phenotype with evidence mutations in the novel class of genes, encoding LPXTG motif-containing cell wall-anchoring proteins. These proteins contain an LPXTG sequence motif at their C-terminus, which is a cleavage signal that leads to the covalent binding of the proteins to the cell wall [50]. The presence of covalently bound LPXTG proteins has been shown to contribute to the regular cross-linked structure of the cell wall and anchoring of surface proteins to the peptidoglycan layer [51]. It is hypothesized that the origin of the VISA phenotype may be also related to mutations in the genes encoding LPXTG-associated proteins, leading to an aberrant peptidoglycan structure [50]. This new architecture would provide false binding sites for vancomycin, thus reducing the permeation of this antibiotic in to the cell wall [50]. Mutations evidenced in the anchor domain LPXTG family proteins indicate that the phenotype VISA can have a reduced susceptibility to vancomycin in vivo resulting from spontaneous or induced mutations of little-known character [52].

4. Mechanisms resistant to β-lactam antibiotics associated to penicillin-binding protein in *Staphylococcus aureus*

With regard to β-lactam antibiotics, one mechanism-conditioned resistance to these antibiotics, mainly to methicillin and others related drugs, is the expression of penicillin-binding protein modified (PBP2s). The PBP2 is a bifunctional protein produced by *S. aureus* and has binding specificity to β-lactam antibiotics. This protein presented a functional transpeptidase domain and carboxypeptidase domain; it is directly linked to the cell wall metabolism in bacteria [53]. In *S. aureus*, both PBPs and (PBP2) are membrane-associated proteins that catalyze the final step of peptidoglycan biosynthesis. The transpeptidase and carboxypeptidase activities of PBPs occur at the D-Ala-D-Ala terminus of a peptidoglycan precursor containing N-acetylglucosamine and N-acetyl-muramic acid L-Ala-D-Glu-L-Lys-D-Ala-D-Ala (pentapeptide chain) [53].

The β-lactam antibiotics inhibit PBPs by competing with the precursor [undecaprenyl-pyrophosphoryl-MurNAc-(pentapeptide)] for binding to the active site of the enzyme. PBP2s enzymes are associated with decreased bacterial susceptibility to oral cephalosporins and recently, they have been implicated in the emergence of the "MRSA superbugs" [54]. One of the most worrisome evidence on MRSA is related to high mortality rates among infected patients. It is estimated that for MRSA patients, the mortality rate is two to three times higher than for patients infected with *S. aureus* susceptibly strains [55].

In methicillin-resistant *S. aureus* strains (MRSA), the enzymatic function can be replaced by PBP2 and PBP2s, proteins encoded by the *mecA* gene, which act as substitutes for the transpeptidase [56]. The *mecA* gene is present on the staphylococcal cassette chromosome (*SCC mec*), a genomic island in staphylococci and other Gram-positive bacteria that encode methicillin resistance. Its mobile nature allows it to become widespread among microorganisms [57]. Generally, in susceptible *S. aureus* cells, the vancomycin molecules bind on the C-terminal D-Ala-D-Ala, thereby inhibiting the catalytic reactions of the transglycosylation and transpeptidation, mediated by PBPs. Moreover, PBP2 also plays an important role in the resistance in MRSA; it is related to expression of high-level resistance to vancomycin [58]. This resistance profile is an associated expression of *VanA* operon, one complex genic in *S. aureus* and *Enterococcus* species designated as vancomycin-resistant enterococci (VRE) [59]. The *vanA* operon was acquired by VRSA from serving of the transposon *Tn*1546 residing on a conjugal plasmid; possibly, its origin is related to a transfer of the genetic element by association with *Enterococcus faecalis* in the same niche located in the host [60].

5. The cell-wall-stress stimulon response in *Staphylococcus aureus*

Some antibiotics related to cell wall biogenesis and its stability can influence gene expression and produce a cell-wall-stress stimulon (CWSS) in the *S. aureus* cells. The oxacillin antibiotics, widely used until recently against *S. aureus* infections, appear to interfere in transcription of genes required for the synthesis of peptidoglycan in the bacterial cells. Analysis of the dynamics of gene expression and proteomic studies using GeneChipsTM approach hypothesized on an upregulation for some proteins and transcription factors involved in cell wall metabolism and response to stress. The same experimental approach that indicated the main influence of amoxicillin during cell exposure is related to increased expression of genes encoding involved in cell wall metabolism, including *pbpB*, *Vras* and *Murz* genes. This pattern of transcriptional response can represent the signature of a stimulon cell wall induced in response to antibiotics, which interfere with the synthesis and structure of the cell wall [61].

Recently, by using a reporter gene system based on a highly sensitive luciferase fused with *tcaA* and *sa0908* genes, it was demonstrated that gene expression in *S. aureus* occurs in different kinetic patterns [62]. The *tcaA* and *sa0908* genes relate to encoding a membrane protein related to signature resistance to glycopeptide antibiotics and encoding protein for the cell envelope (member of the LytR-CpsA-Psr family), respectively. These patterns were determined from observations of the fluorescence intensity during growth of *S. aureus* (susceptible strain BB255) in the presence of various antibiotics at subinhibitory and inhibitory concentrations. From their results, it was possible to establish that all drugs tested induced the CWSS and that the induction patterns varied according to the drug. One of the hypotheses raised in this study would be that the standard kinetics observed could perhaps be related to the specificity or antibiotic mechanism action. These findings are based on fluorescence results obtained for different drug groups such as tunicamycin, flavomycin, oxacillin and fosfomycin, which presented high levels of maximal induction (RLU > 40,000); and daptomycin and lysostaphin exhibiting fluorescence indices below 10,000. Moreover, some antibiotics such as fosfomycin and D-cycloserine showed a lag-phase induction for all tested concentrations of about 30 and 10 min, respectively. Possibly, these antibiotics act in the early stages of peptidoglycan synthesis, which could be linked to delays in the induction CWSS in the *S. aureus*.

6. Conclusion

Multiple mechanisms contribute to the increased antimicrobial resistance in S. aureus, culminating in a more robust cellular adaptation against antibiotics that act on the synthesis of components of the cell envelope. These multiple mechanisms of adaptation in *S. aureus* include heteroresistance or mutational events, make the bacteria to evolve from a susceptible strain in to a resistant clone; thus significantly interfering with the bacterial response to antibiotics. Finally, further knowledge of these mechanisms may considerably impact the development of new drugs designed to specific targets in the microbial cell.

Author details

Andrea de Souza Monteiro[1]*, Wallace Ribeiro Nunes Neto[1], Aleff Ricardo Santos Mendes[1], Bruna Lorrana dos Santos Pinto[1], Luís Cláudio Nascimento da Silva[2] and Gabriella Freitas Ferreira[3]

*Address all correspondence to: andreasmont@gmail.com

1 Laboratório de Microbiologia, Universidade CEUMA, São Luis, Maranhão, Brazil

2 Laboratório de Prospecção Molecular, Universidade CEUMA, São Luis, Maranhão, Brazil

3 Departamento de Farmácia, Universidade Federal de Juiz de Fora, Governador Valadares, Brazil

References

[1] V. Cafiso, et al. Modulating activity of vancomycin and daptomycin on the expression of autolysis cell-wall turnover and membrane charge genes in hVISA and VISA strains. PLoS One. 2012;**7**(1):e29573. DOI: 10.1371/journal.pone.0029573.

[2] S.D. Taylor, M. Palmer. The action mechanism of daptomycin. Bioorganic & Medicinal Chemistry. 2016; **24** (24):6253-6268. DOI: 10.1016/j.bmc.2016.05.052.

[3] C.L. Moore, et al. Daptomycin versus vancomycin for bloodstream infections due to methicillin-resistant *Staphylococcus aureus* with a high vancomycin minimum inhibitory concentration: a case-control study. Clinical Infectious Diseases. 2012;**54**(1):51–58. DOI: 10.1093/cid/cir764.

[4] F.P Tally, et al. Daptomycin: a novel agent for gram-positive infections. Expert Opinion on Investigational Drugs. 1999;**8**(8):1223–1238. DOI: 10.1517/13543784.8.8.1223.

[5] J.K. Hobbs, et al. Consequences of daptomycin-mediated membrane damage in *Staphylococcus aureus*. Journal of Antimicrobial Chemotherapy. 2008;**62**(5):1003–1008. DOI: 10.1093/jac/dkn321.

[6] P. Canepari, et al. Lipoteichoic acid as a new target for activity of antibiotics: mode of action of daptomycin (LY146032). Antimicrobial Agents and Chemotherapy. 1990;**34**(6):1220–1226. DOI: 10.1128/AAC.34.6.1220.

[7] N.E. Allen, J.N. Hobbs, W.E. Alborn Jr. Inhibition of peptidoglycan biosynthesis in gram-positive bacteria by LY146032. Antimicrobial Agents and Chemotherapy. 1987;**31**(7):1093–1099. DOI: 10.1128/AAC.31.7.1093.

[8] J.K. Muraiha, et al. Oligomerization of daptomycin on membranes. Biochimica et Biophysica Acta (BBA)—Biomembranes. 2011;**1808**(4):1154–1160. DOI: 10.1016/j.bbamem.2011.01.001.

[9] R.D. Süssmuth, W. Wohlleben. The biosynthesis of glycopeptide antibiotics—a model for complex, non-ribosomally synthesized, peptidic secondary metabolites. Applied Microbiology and Biotechnology. 2004;**63**(4):344–350. DOI: 10.1007/s00253-003-1443-z.

[10] H. Jeong, et al. Genome sequence of the vancomycin-producing amycolatopsis orientalis subsp. orientalis strain KCTC 9412T. Genome Announcements. 2013;**1**(3):e00408–e00413. DOI: 10.1128/genomeA.00408-13.

[11] S.T. Micek. Alternatives to vancomycin for the treatment of methicillin-resistant *Staphylococcus aureus* infections. Clinical Infectious Diseases. 2007;**45**(3):S184–S190. DOI: 10.1086/519471.

[12] G.F. Ferreira, et al. Heteroresistance to itraconazole alters the morphology and increases the virulence of cryptococcus gattii. Antimicrobial Agents and Chemotherapy. 2015;**59**(8):4600–4609. DOI: 10.1128/AAC.00466-15.

[13] S. Deresinski. Vancomycin heteroresistance and methicillin-resistant *Staphylococcus aureus*. The Journal of Infectious Diseases. 2009;**199**(5):605–609. DOI: 10.1086/596630.

[14] C. Liu, H.F. Chambers. *Staphylococcus aureus* with heterogeneous resistance to vancomycin: epidemiology, clinical significance and critical assessment of diagnostic methods. Antimicrobial Agents and Chemotherapy. 2003;**47**(10):3040–3045. DOI: 10.1128/AAC.47.10.3040-3045.2003.

[15] Y. Maor, et al. Clinical features of heteroresistant vancomycin-intermediate *Staphylococcus aureus* bacteremia versus those of methicillin-resistant *S. aureus* bacteremia. The Journal of Infectious Diseases. 2009;**199**(5):619–624. DOI: 10.1086/596629.

[16] G. Sakoulas, et al. Adaptation of methicillin-resistant *Staphylococcus aureus* in the face of vancomycin therapy. Clinical Infectious Diseases. 2006;**42**(1):S40–S50. DOI: 10.1086/491713.

[17] L. Cui, et al. Novel mechanism of antibiotic resistance originating in vancomycin-intermediate *Staphylococcus aureus*. Antimicrobial Agents and Chemotherapy. 2006;**50**(2):428–438. DOI: 10.1128/AAC.50.2.428-438.2006.

[18] F. Bert, et al. Prevalence, molecular epidemiology and clinical significance of heterogeneous glycopeptide-intermediate *Staphylococcus aureus* in liver transplant recipients. Journal of Clinical Microbiology. 2003;**41**(11):5147–5152. DOI: 10.1128/JCM.41.11.5147-5152.2003.

[19] A. Capone, et al. *In vivo* development of daptomycin resistance in vancomycin-susceptible methicillin-resistant *Staphylococcus aureus* severe infections previously treated with glycopeptides. European Journal of Clinical Microbiology & Infectious Diseases. 2016;**35**(4):625–631. DOI: 10.1007/s10096-016-2581-4.

[20] G. Sakoulas, et al. Human cathelicidin LL-37 resistance and increased daptomycin MIC in methicillin-resistant *Staphylococcus aureus* strain USA600 (ST45) are associated with increased mortality in a hospital setting. Journal of Clinical Microbiology. 2014;**52**(6):2172–2174. DOI: 10.1128/JCM.00189-14.

[21] B.P. Howden, et al. Reduced vancomycin susceptibility in *Staphylococcus aureus*, including vancomycin-intermediate and heterogeneous vancomycin-intermediate strains: resistance mechanisms, laboratory detection and clinical implications. Clinical Microbiology Reviews. 2010;**23**(1):99–139. DOI: 10.1128/CMR.00042-09.

[22] N.N. Mishra, et al. *In vitro* cross-resistance to daptomycin and host defense cationic antimicrobial peptides in clinical methicillin-resistant *Staphylococcus aureus* isolates. Antimicrobial Agents and Chemotherapy. 2011;**55**(9):4012–4018. DOI: 10.1128/AAC.00223-11.

[23] T.T. Tran, et al. Mechanisms of drug resistance: daptomycin resistance. Annals the New York Academy of Sciences. 2015;**1354**:32–53. DOI: 10.1111/nyas.12948.

[24] L. Dortet, et al. *In vivo* acquired daptomycin resistance during treatment of methicillin-resistant *Staphylococcus aureus* endocarditis. International Journal of Infectious Diseases. 2013;**17**(11):e1076–e1077. DOI: 10.1016/j.ijid.2013.02.019.

[25] K. Julian, et al. Characterization of a daptomycin-nonsusceptible vancomycin-intermediate *Staphylococcus aureus* strain in a patient with endocarditis. Antimicrobial Agents and Chemotherapy. 2007;**51**(9):3445–3448. DOI: 10.1128/AAC.00559-07.

[26] S.J. van Hal, et al. Emergence of daptomycin resistance following vancomycin-unresponsive *Staphylococcus aureus* bacteraemia in a daptomycin-naïve patient—a review of the literature. European Journal of Clinical Microbiology & Infectious Diseases. 2011;**30**(5):603–610. DOI: 10.1007/s10096-010-1128-3.

[27] J.B. Patel, et al. An association between reduced susceptibility to daptomycin and reduced susceptibility to vancomycin in *Staphylococcus aureus*. Clinical Infectious Diseases. 2006;**42**(11):1652–1653. DOI: 10.1086/504084.

[28] Y. Oku, et al. Characterization of the *Staphylococcus aureus* mprF gene, involved in lysinylation of phosphatidylglycerol. Microbiology. 2004;**150**(1):45–51. DOI: 10.1099/mic.0.26706-0.

[29] C.M. Ernst, et al. The lipid-modifying multiple peptide resistance factor is an oligomer consisting of distinct interacting synthase and flippase subunits. MBio. 2015;**6**(1):e02340–e02414. DOI: 10.1128/mBio.02340-14.

[30] J. Andrä, et al. Multiple peptide resistance factor (MprF)-mediated resistance of *Staphylococcus aureus* against antimicrobial peptides coincides with a modulated peptide interaction with artificial membranes comprising Lysyl-phosphatidylglycerol. The Journal of Biological Chemistry. 2011;**286**:18692–18700. DOI: 10.1074/jbc.M111.226886.

[31] C.M. Ernst, et al. The bacterial defensin resistance protein MprF consists of separable domains for lipid lysinylation and antimicrobial peptide repulsion. PLoS Pathogens. 2009;**5**(11):e1000660. DOI: 10.1371/journal.ppat.1000660.

[32] A. Peschel, et al. *Staphylococcus aureus* resistance to human defensins and evasion of neutrophil killing via the novel virulence factor mprf is based on modification of membrane lipids with L-lysine. JEM. 2001;**193**(9):1067. DOI: 10.1084/jem.193.9.1067.

[33] C.J. Slavetinsky, A. Peschel, C.M. Ernst. Alanyl-phosphatidylglycerol and lysyl-phosphatidylglycerol are translocated by the same MprF flippases and have similar capacities to protect against the antibiotic daptomycin in *Staphylococcus aureus*. Antimicrobial Agents and Chemotherapy. 2012;**56**(7):3492–3497. DOI: 10.1128/AAC.00370-12.

[34] R.H Baltz. Daptomycin: mechanisms of action and resistance and biosynthetic engineering. Current Opinion in Chemical Biology. 2009;**13**(2):144–151. DOI: 10.1016/j.cbpa.2009.02.031.

[35] S.J. Yang, et al. Causal role of single nucleotide polymorphisms within the mprF gene of *Staphylococcus aureus* in daptomycin resistance. Antimicrobial Agents and Chemotherapy. 2013;**57**(11):5658–5664. DOI: 10.1128/AAC.01184-13.

[36] A. Jansen, et al. Role of insertion elements and yycFG in the development of decreased susceptibility to vancomycin in *Staphylococcus aureus*. International Journal of Medical Microbiology. 2007;**297**(4):205–215. DOI: 10.1016/j.ijmm.2007.02.002.

[37] M. Shoji, et al. WalK and clpP mutations confer reduced vancomycin susceptibility in *Staphylococcus aureus*. Antimicrobial Agents Chemotherapy. 2011;**55**(8):3870–3881. DOI: 10.1128/AAC.01563-10.

[38] A. Muthaiyan, et al. Transcriptional profiling reveals that daptomycin induces the *Staphylococcus aureus* cell wall stress stimulon and genes responsive to membrane depolarization. Antimicrobial Agents and Chemotherapy. 2008;**52**(3):980–990. DOI: 10.1128/AAC.01121-07.

[39] A. Fischer, et al. Daptomycin resistance mechanisms in clinically derived *Staphylococcus aureus* strains assessed by a combined transcriptomics and proteomics approach. Journal of Antimicrobial Chemotherapy. 2011;**66**(8):1696–1711. DOI: 10.1093/jac/dkr195.

[40] Q. Ji, et al. Structure and mechanism of the essential two-component signal-transduction system WalKR in *Staphylococcus aureus*. Nature Communications. 2016;7(11000). DOI: 10.1038/ncomms11000.

[41] S. Dubrac, T. Msadek. Identification of genes controlled by the essential YycG/YycF two-component system of *Staphylococcus aureus*. Journal of Bacteriology. 2004;**186**(4):1175–1181. DOI: 10.1128/JB.186.4.1175-1181.2004.

[42] J. Hu, et al. Mechanism of reduced vancomycin susceptibility conferred by walk mutation in community-acquired methicillin-resistant *Staphylococcus aureus* strain MW2. Antimicrobial Agents and Chemotherapy. 2014;**59**(2):1352–1355. DOI: 10.1128/AAC.04290-14.

[43] M.R. Maurizi. Clp P represents a unique family of serine proteases. The Journal of Biological Chemistry. 1990;**265**(21):12546–12552. http://www.jbc.org/content/265/21/12546.long.

[44] A.J. Farrand, et al. Regulation of host hemoglobin binding by the *Staphylococcus aureus* Clp proteolytic system. Journal of Bacteriology. 2013;**195**(22):5041–5050. DOI: 10.1128/JB.00505-13.

[45] D. Frees, et al. Alternative roles of ClpX and ClpP in *Staphylococcus aureus* stress tolerance and virulence. Molecular Microbiology. 2003;**48**(6):1565–1578. DOI: 10.1046/j.1365-2958.2003.03524.x.

[46] A. Michel, et al. Global regulatory impact of ClpP protease of *Staphylococcus aureus* on regulons involved in virulence, oxidative stress response, autolysis and DNA repair. Journal of Bacteriology. 2006;**188**(16):5783–5796. DOI: 10.1128/JB.00074-06.

[47] A. Wawrzynow, et al. The ClpX heat-shock protein of *Escherichia coli*, the ATP-dependent substrate specificity component of the ClpP-ClpX protease, is a novel molecular chaperone. The EMBO Journal. 1995;**14**(9):1867–1877. http://www.ncbi.nlm.nih.gov/pmc/articles/PMC398286/.

[48] G.T. Robertson, et al. Global transcriptional analysis of clpP mutations of type 2 *Streptococcus pneumoniae* and their effects on physiology and virulence. Journal of Bacteriology. 2002;**184**(13):3508–3520. DOI: 10.1128/JB.184.13.3508-3520.2002.

[49] O. Gaillot, et al. The ClpP serine protease is essential for the intracellular parasitism and virulence of *Listeria monocytogenes*. Molecular Microbiology. 2000;**35**(6):1286–1294. DOI: 10.1046/j.1365-2958.2000.01773.x.

[50] L. Rishishwar, C.S. Kraft, I. King Jordan. Population genomics of reduced vancomycin susceptibility in *Staphylococcus aureus*. mSphere. 2016;**1**(4):e00094–e00116. DOI: 10.1128/mSphere.00094-16.

[51] S.K. Mazmanian, et al. *Staphylococcus aureus* sortase, an enzyme that anchors surface proteins to the cell wall. Science. 1999;**285**(5428):760–763. DOI: 10.1126/science.285.5428.760.

[52] H. Ton-That, O. Schneewind. Anchor structure of *Staphylococcal* surface proteins. The Journal of Biological Chemistry. 1999;**274**(34):24316–24320. http://www.jbc.org/content/274/34/24316.full.pdf.

[53] V. Navratna, et al. Molecular basis for the role of *Staphylococcus aureus* penicillin binding protein 4 in antimicrobial resistance. Journal of Bacteriology. 2010;**192**(1):134–144. DOI: 10.1128/JB.00822-09.

[54] A. Ojha Kshetry, et al. Minimum inhibitory concentration of vancomycin to methicillin resistant Staphylococcus aureus isolated from different clinical samples at a tertiary care hospital in Nepal. Antimicrobial Resistance Infection Control. 2016;5(27). DOI: 10.1186/s13756-016-0126-3.

[55] R. Köck, et al. Methicillin-resistant Staphylococcus aureus (MRSA): burden of disease and control challenges in Europe. European Surveillance. 2010;15(41):):pii=19688. http://www.eurosurveillance.org/images/dynamic/ee/v15n41/art19688.pdf.

[56] K. Hiramatsu, et al. The emergence and evolution of methicillin-resistant *Staphylococcus aureus*. Trends in Microbiology. 2001;**9**(10):486–493. DOI: 10.1016/S0966-842X(01)02175-8.

[57] Y. Katayama, et al. PBP 2a mutations producing very-high-level resistance to beta-lactams. Antimicrobial Agents and Chemotherapy. 2004;**48**(2):453–459. DOI: 10.1128/AAC.48.2.453-459.2004.

[58] B.J. Werth, et al. Novel combinations of vancomycin plus ceftaroline or oxacillin against methicillin-resistant vancomycin-intermediate *Staphylococcus aureus* (VISA) and heterogeneous VISA. Antimicrobial Agents and Chemotherapy. 2013;**57**(5):2376–2379. DOI: 10.1128/AAC.02354-12.

[59] B. Périchon, P. Courvalin. VanA-type vancomycin-resistant *Staphylococcus aureus*. Antimicrobial Agents and Chemotherapy. 2009;**53**(11):4580–4587. DOI: 10.1128/AAC.00346-09.

[60] L.M. Weigel, et al. Genetic analysis of a high-level vancomycin-resistant isolate of *Staphylococcus aureus*. Science. 2003;**302**(5650):1569–1571. DOI: 10.1126/science.1090956.

[61] S. Utaida, et al. Genome-wide transcriptional profiling of the response of *Staphylococcus aureus* to cell-wall-active antibiotics reveals a cell-wall-stress stimulon. Microbiology. 2003;**149**(10):2719–2732. DOI: 10.1099/mic.0.26426-0.

[62] V. Dengler, et al. Induction kinetics of the Staphylococcus aureus cell wall stress stimulon in response to different cell wall active antibiotics. BMC Microbiology. 2011;11(16). DOI: 10.1186/1471-2180-11-16.

Chapter 6

SOS Response and *Staphylococcus aureus*: Implications for Drug Development

Luís Cláudio Nascimento da Silva,
Roseane Costa Diniz,
Isana Maria de Souza Feitosa Lima,
Camilla Itapary dos Santos, Matheus Silva Alves,
Larissa Isabela Oliveira de Souza and
Andrea de Souza Monteiro

Additional information is available at the end of the chapter

http://dx.doi.org/10.5772/65960

Abstract

Damage in genetic material is induced through the action of several drugs (directly or indirectly). Specially, antimicrobials from quinolone class (such as ciprofloxacin) induce DNA damage that promotes the formation of the RecA filament leading to auto-cleavage of LexA and allows the expression of SOS genes, including the error-prone polymerase (like *umu*C). The SOS pathway plays a critical role in the acquisition of mutations that lead to the emergence of antibiotic-resistant bacteria and the spread of virulence factors. This chapter provides a comprehensive review about the SOS response of *Staphylococcus aureus* and the modulatory effects of new compounds (natural or synthetics) on this pathway. The effects of some SOS inhibitors are highlighted such as baicalein and aminocoumarins. Compounds able to prevent SOS response are extremely important to develop new combinatory approaches to inhibit *S. aureus* mutagenesis. The study of new SOS inductors could reveal new insights into the pathways used by *S. aureus* to acquire drug resistance; examples of these compounds are the lysine-peptoid hybrid LP5, cyclic peptide inhibitors, etc. These studies can impact the development of new drugs. In conclusion, we hope to provide essential information about the effects of compounds on SOS response from *S. aureus*.

Keywords: DNA damage, mutagenesis, virulence factors, small colony variants

1. Introduction

Drug resistance is a well-known problem involved in the treatment of bacterial infections and its incidence is escalating in an alarming rate [1–3]. As a result, microbial diseases are still among the most serious problems to public health system, especially in developing countries where infectious diseases still represent a major cause of human mortality. Especially alarming is the rapid global spread of multiresistant bacteria that cause common infections and that resist treatment with existing antimicrobial medicines [4, 5]. The classical paradigm suggests that antibiotic resistance emerges by selection of preexisting mutants in the bacterial population exposed to antibiotics [1]. In contrast, recent data suggested that mutations evolve after cells encounter antibiotic therapy. This kind of mutation is known as adaptive mutation, which is activated by the SOS DNA repair and mutagenesis pathways [6, 7].

The SOS system is the bacterial DNA damage response that is activated by DNA damage or stalled DNA replication caused by the exposure of bacteria to stressful conditions [8] such as antibiotic treatment [9], starvation [10], and oxidative stress [11]. Repair of damaged DNA is critical for bacterial survival, and during this process, some mutations may be introduced into the genome, which may result in bacterial drug resistance [12, 13]. Accumulation of single-stranded DNA (ss-DNA) is the signal that induces the SOS response by promoting the formation of the RecA filament, which in turn activates the auto-cleavage activity of LexA and allows expression of several genes [8]. The SOS response is a very orchestrated pathway by which the bacterial cell improves its capacity to inhibit cell division, repair DNA, and express error-prone DNA polymerases to replicate noninstructive DNA lesions [14]. This pathway has been widely studied in *Escherichia coli* where more than 40 genes are involved [15]. The first stage of SOS response is the expression of genes related to nucleotide excision repair mechanisms (*uvrA, uvrB, uvrD, polB, ruvA, ruvB,* and *dinI*). If the damaged is not repaired the genes responsible for recombination repair mechanisms (*recA* and *recN*) are expressed. Finally, if the SOS response is not successful, then the *sulA* and *umuDC* genes are expressed. SulA inhibits cell division and the *umuDC* operon encodes the error-prone DNA polV crucial in translesion error-prone DNA synthesis. When *sulA* is expressed in the late stage of the SOS gene expression, it arrests cell division by binding FtsZ and provides extra time for the mutagenic error-prone polymerases to acquire mutations that allow cells to escape from the metabolic and genomic stress [8, 16–18].

Some difference may be found in the SOS response for each species. For example, this process in *Bacillus subtilis* is mediated by a similar number of genes than in *E. coli*, however, only seven genes are common for these two bacteria [19]. In the case of *Staphylococcus aureus*, only sixteen genes have been identified under the control of LexA, between them one error-prone polymerase is designated here as *umuC* (SACOL1400) [9, 20]. The SOS pathway plays a critical role in several processes related to pathogenesis of *S. aureus*, such as emergence of antibiotic resistant strains [21], dissemination of virulence factors [22], and increase of the frequency of small colony variants (SCVs) [23]. In this sense, this chapter aims to provide a comprehensive review about the modulatory effects of compounds (natural or synthetics) on SOS response of *S. aureus*.

2. Overview of SOS response in *Staphylococcus aureus*

Since DNA damage may occur as a result of environmental agents and drugs, the role of SOS pathway in different conditions has been studied in *S. aureus* [21–23]. Most of these studies have focused on the effects of clinical relevant antibiotics, especially those from fluoroquinolone class, such as ciprofloxacin. The induction of SOS response in this pathogen has been associated with mutagenesis, spread of virulence factors, and formation of small colony variants [22–27]. We discuss some of the papers related to these subjects in the following topics.

2.1. SOS response affects the expression of virulence factors in *Staphylococcus aureus*

To prove this concept, the effects of SOS response in the dissemination of pathogenicity island-encoded virulence factors in staphylococci was evaluated [22]. *S. aureus* pathogenicity island (SaPI) comprises a large family of highly mobile phage-related chromosomal islands, which carry a range of virulence genes, for example, TSST1 (toxic shock syndrome toxin), SEB (staphylococcal enterotoxin B), and other superantigens [28]. SaPI are widely distributed among Gram-positive bacteria and they are considered as prototypes for the understanding of the mobile mechanisms of pathogenicity islands, since horizontal gene transfer has an extremely important role in bacterial evolution [29]. It was demonstrated that SOS induction (by ciprofloxacin) induced SaPI excision and replication with participation of at least three different temperate phages (80, 11, and 147). SOS pathway also regulates the replication and high-frequency transfer of this element, as well as of SaPI1. Theses finds suggested that SOS activation by antibiotics may lead to the spread of staphylococcal virulence genes, an unintended consequence [22].

The influence of subinhibitory concentrations (Sub-MIC) of others antibiotics in the induction of SOS response and horizontal transfer of virulence factors in *S. aureus* was also evaluated [24]. The authors used antibiotics with different action mechanisms such as lactams (ampicillin, penicillin, ceftriaxone, and cloxacillin), macrolide-β lincosamide-streptogramin B antibiotics (erythromycin), aminoglycosides (kanamycin), chloramphenicol, and tetracycline. From these drugs, only β-lactams induced replication of SOS- inducible prophages 80α and 11ϕ, resulting in SaPIbov1 transfer. The effects of ciprofloxacin and trimethoprim (a folic acid inhibitor from sulfonamide class) on phage induction and expression of phage-encoded virulence factors were evaluated using *S. aureus* strains isolates from patients with cystic fibrosis [25]. This study analyzed the integration of phages into the chromosomal gene coding for β-hemolysin (*hlb*), these phages encode for accessory virulence determinants such as staphylokinase (*sak*; a plasminogen activator essential for bacteria dissemination from clots and abscesses and resistance against human defensins) and enterotoxins [30, 31]. Sub-MIC of both drugs resulted in delysogenization of strains and replication of *hlb*-converting phages in a dose-dependent manner. The involvement of SOS response in phage mobilization was demonstrated by increase of *recA* expression. In addition, induction of 13 was directly associated with phage-encoded virulence gene *sak* [25].

In another study, the expression of type 5 capsular polysaccharide (CP5) in *S. aureus* was shown to be linked to SOS response [32]. CP5 is one virulence factor that is important for protection against phagocytes [33] and it is an attractive candidate for the development of immunotherapies [34]. The production of CP5 is influenced by various environmental agents (carbon dioxide, iron concentration, and specific nutrients) and controlled by a complex regulatory genetic network [35]. Using a transposon-mediated mutagenesis assay, seven genes were identified affecting the production of CP5, including *sbcD* and *sbcC* genes [35]. These genes are adjacent forming the *sbcDC* locus that negatively affects capsule production. Sub-MIC of SOS inducers (ciprofloxacin or mitomycin C) promoted the transcription of *sbcDC* locus and consequently repressed the CP5 production [32]. The authors suggested that this effect of SOS response in capsule expression could be related to (i) energy saving (the energy needed to capsule biosynthesis would be used for DNA reparation); (ii) improvement of adhesion capability (capsule absence would unmask the adhesion proteins present in cell membrane, promoting bacterial infection and thereby avoiding DNA-damaging agents). These results corroborate with previous study which showed that ciprofloxacin increased the expression of fibronectin-binding proteins (FnBPs) in fluoroquinolone-resistant *S. aureus* strains [36].

2.2. SOS response and mutagenesis in *Staphylococcus aureus*

Apart from its capacity to express virulence factors, *S. aureus* is extremely able to acquire resistance to virtually any antibiotic. For example, methicillin-resistant *S. aureus* (MRSA) strains are important etiologic agents of both nosocomial and community infections. It has been shown that Sub-MIC of fluoroquinolone drugs enhances methicillin resistance in community or nosocomial MRSA isolates [26, 37]. Community-associated MRSA isolates (CA-MRSA) grown in tryptic soy broth containing sub-MIC of fluoroquinolone (ciprofloxacin or levofloxacin) showed increased resistance in nafcillin agar, and this effect was dose-dependent. Through microarray analysis it was possible to conclude that alterations-induced fluoroquinolone drugs were mediated by SOS response [26]. In the same context, a later study evaluated the effects of Sub-MIC of ciprofloxacin in the development of rifampin resistance in methicillin-susceptible *S. aureus* (MSSA) and MRSA strains. Ciprofloxacin induced higher frequencies of rifampin-resistant mutants. A significant proportion of these mutants exhibited in-frame deletions or insertions in the *rpoB* gene at several positions, while those mutants from ciprofloxacin-free cultures essentially showed single-amino-acid substitutions [27].

2.3. Induction of SOS increases the frequency of small colony variants in *Staphylococcus aureus*

Recently, the activation of SOS response was linked with the enhanced incidence of small colony variants (SCVs) in *S. aureus* [11, 23]. *S. aureus* SCVs are marked by small colony with slow growth phenotype, which is associated with intracellular persistence and reduced antimicrobial susceptibility [38]. *S. aureus* switch to SCVs phenotype under the pressure of stress elicitors such as oxidative stress [11], cold stress [39], and drug treatment [23]. SCVs are frequently associated with latent or chronic infections, including device-associated infections, bone and tissue infections, and airway infections of cystic fibrosis patients [40].

S. aureus SCVs present mutations in one or few genes related to metabolic pathways resulting in atypical biochemical characteristics [41]. The nature of these mutations is directly related to the antibiotic resistance profile exhibited by the SCVs. Resistance to trimethoprim-sulfamethoxazole has been associated to alteration on *thyA* gene, which encodes thymidylate synthase [42, 43]. This enzyme is essential for DNA biosynthesis as it converts deoxyuridine monophosphate (dUMP) to deoxythymidine monophosphate (dTMP). Diminished concentrations of intracellular dTMP lead to thymidine-dependent SCVs phenotypes (TD-SCVs), which is associated to trimethoprim-sulfamethoxazole resistance and hypermutability [44, 45].

On the other hand, mutations in genes related to menadione or hemin synthesis result in electron transport-defective strains as bacteria are unable to produce menaquinone and cytochromes, respectively [46, 47]. SCVs auxotrophic for menadione or hemin are resistance to aminoglycosides (such as gentamicin) due to a decrease in drug uptake [48]. Fluoroquinolones and mitomycin C Sub-MIC increased the generation of gentamicin-resistant SCVs with an increased mutation rate through activation of the SOS response [23]. The SOS response is also essential for the adaptation of *S. aureus* to oxidative stress, in this case by producing hydrogen peroxide–resistant SCVs [11].

3. New compounds able to modulate the SOS response in *Staphylococcus aureus*

Given the role of SOS response in *S. aureus* survival and pathogenesis, the effects of new antimicrobial candidates on SOS genes have become more frequently evaluated, especially those which target DNA structure or DNA replication machinery [49, 50]. Gottschalk et al. [49] reported an easy and inexpensive agar-based assay to detect the expression of *recA* induced by a compound. In this assay, a *S. aureus* 8325-4 derivative strain carrying the *recA* gene fused with the reporter gene *lacZ* (which encodes for β-galactosidase) is incorporated in agar plates containing X-Gal (5-bromo-4-β chloro-3-indolyl-D-galactopyranoside). X-gal is a chromogenic substrate for β-galactosidase that produces a rich blue color that can easily be detected visually. The compound to be tested should be added in wells in these agar plates and the expression of *recA* is monitored as a blue ring at the point of bacterial growth. Using this assay, the ability of some compound to active SOS response was revealed, such as the lysine-peptoid hybrid LP5 [49], some cyclic peptide inhibitors of the β-sliding clamp [50], and the amphibian peptide fallaxin analogue FL9 [51]. The induction of SOS response was also related to the anti–*S. aureus* action of new synthetic bis-indole antibiotics [52]. All these compounds inhibit the DNA replication of *S. aureus*.

Special attention has been given to the use of SOS inhibitors as therapeutic adjuvants in combating bacterial infections. These approaches involve inhibiting the SOS-mediated mutagenesis induced by drugs and thus improving their long-term viability. In these cases, LexA and RecA represent potential targets [53, 54]. In fact, the number of SOS inhibitors is still limited and most of the studies use *E. coli* as model [55, 56]. Regarding the suppression of SOS response in *S. aureus*, a study showed baicalein as a potential compound. Baicalein is the main component of the Chinese herb Scutellaria baicalensis Georgi (Labiatae), which shows anti–*S. aureus* and antioxidant activities [57, 58]. Baicalein inhibited the expression of some SOS genes (*recA*, *lexA*, and LexA-regulated DNA polymerase SACOL1400) and the rifampin-resistant mutation ratio induced by Sub-MIC of ciprofloxacin. The authors correlated these effects in SOS response with a decrease in the formation of intracellular reactive oxygen species and ATP level after baicalein treatment [59].

In a later study, the effects of novobiocin in the SOS response induced by ciprofloxacin were evaluated. Novobiocin is an aminocoumarin, a class of antibiotics that interferes with ATPase activity of the gyrase subunit B and the topoisomerase IV subunit ParE without inducing double-strand breaks [60–62]. Differently from quinolones, aminocoumarin treatment does not activate SOS response. In fact, novobiocin inhibited the *recA* expression in a LexA-independent manner. Novobiocin was also able to suppress the SOS response induced by ciprofloxacin: it inhibited *recA* expression and partially reduced the induction of the error-prone polymerase *umuC* (regulated by LexA). These effects resulted in a reduction in the frequency of recombination, mutation, and the formation of nonhemolytic variants [20].

The concept that SOS response is a potential target was additionally explored using antimicrobial photoinactivation. Antimicrobial photodynamic therapy (aPDT) is a promising strategy for the treatment of localized infections, such as acne inflammation [63], periodontal, and peri-implant diseases [64]. aPDT consists in the use of three elements (photosensitizer agent, visible light, and oxygen), where the damage of different bacterial structures (cell envelopes, lipids, proteins, and DNA) would avoid the development of resistance [65]. The role of DNA damage and SOS response during photoinactivation was recently established. Different exogenous photosensitizers induced DNA damage and consequently the expression of *recA*. The repression of *recA* by novobiocin or gene deletion resulted in additional susceptibility of *S. aureus* toward photoinactivation through increase of DNA damage. These results suggested that the combination of *recA* inhibitors and photoinactivation could have a clinical relevance [66].

SOS response in *E. coli* has been shown to be regulated by ribonuclease E (RNase E), an enzyme involved in RNA metabolism (global mRNA degradation, maturation of rRNA, and small regulatory RNA) [67]. RNase E deficient strains exhibit a reduction in SOS activation, revealing that RNase E inhibitors could be possibly used as drug adjuvants [68]. Although RNase E orthologs have been identified in a range of other bacteria and in bacteria and chloroplasts [69, 70], RNA turnover is not regulated by an RNase E ortholog protein in *S. aureus* [70]. Instead, *S. aureus* has an mRNA degradosome complex formed by diverse proteins, including RNase enzymes (RNase J1, RNase J2, RNase Y, and RnpA), enolase, phosphofructokinase, polynucleotide phosphorylase (PNPase), and DEAD box RNA helicase. RnpA, a component of this complex, has been reported as a target to inhibit bacterial survival and pathogenesis [70, 71]. However, the role of mRNA degradosome complex in SOS response regulation remains to be elucidated in this pathogen.

4. Conclusion

The SOS response is an essential pathway for *S. aureus* survival and pathogenesis. This mechanism is activated by different stress situations (such as environmental alteration, drug, and toxins treatment), which lead to mutagenesis, phenotypical alterations, and spread of virulence factors. All these consequences of SOS activation are important to pathogen dissemination and treatment failure. SOS proteins are potential target for therapies, especially those using quinolones and RecA/LexA inhibitors. These studies have shown that SOS inhibitors are able to decrease drug-induced mutagenesis in *S. aureus*. We hope that more researches will be performed in the future to identify more compounds that are able to modulate SOS response, as well as deeper *in vivo* studies to establish the clinical relevance of them.

Author details

Luís Cláudio Nascimento da Silva[1, *], Roseane Costa Diniz[1], Isana Maria de Souza Feitosa Lima[1], Camilla Itapary dos Santos[1], Matheus Silva Alves[1], Larissa Isabela Oliveira de Souza[2] and Andrea de Souza Monteiro[1]

*Address all correspondence to: luisclaudionsilva@yahoo.com.br

1 Ceuma University, São Luís, MA, Brazil

2 Research Center Aggeu Magalhães, Recife, PE, Brazil

References

[1] Jessica MAB, Mark AW, Alison JB, David OO, Laura JVP. Molecular mechanisms of antibiotic resistance. Nature Reviews Microbiology. 2015;**13**(1):42—51. DOI: 10.1038/nrmicro3380

[2] Damien R, et al. Fitness cost of antibiotic susceptibility during bacterial infection. Science Translational Medicine. 2015;**7**(297):297ra114. DOI: 10.1126/scitranslmed.aab1621

[3] Asher B, Ofer F, Orit G, Nathalie QB. Distinguishing between resistance, tolerance and persistence to antibiotic treatment. Nature Reviews Microbiology. 2016;**14**(5):320–330. DOI: 10.1038/nrmicro.2016.34

[4] World Health Organization. Antimicrobial resistance: global report on surveillance. World Health Organization; Geneva, Switzerland, 2014. 257 p. DOI: http://www.who.int/drugresistance/documents/surveillancereport/en/

[5] Oliver W, et al. Colonisation with multidrug-resistant bacteria is associated with increased mortality in patients with cirrhosis. Gut. 2015;**64**(7):1183–1184. DOI: 10.1136/gutjnl-2014-309104

[6] Antoine G, et al. Costs and benefits of high mutation rates: adaptive evolution of bacteria in the mouse gut. Science. 2001;**291**(5513):2606–2608. DOI: 10.1126/science.1056421

[7] Clara Torres-Barceló, et al. The SOS response increases bacterial fitness, but not evolvability, under a sublethal dose of antibiotic. Proceedings of the Royal Society Biological Sciences. 2015;**282**:1816. DOI: 10.1098/rspb.2015.0885

[8] Zeynep B, Didier M. SOS, the formidable strategy of bacteria against aggressions. FEMS Microbiology Reviews. 2014;**38**(6):1126–1145. DOI: http://dx.doi.org/10.1111/1574-6976.12077

[9] Ryan TC, et al. Complete and SOS-mediated response of *Staphylococcus aureus* to the antibiotic ciprofloxacin. Journal of Bacteriology. 2007;**189**(2):531–539. DOI: 10.1128/JB.01464-06

[10] Steve PB, et al. Starvation, together with the SOS response, mediates high biofilm-specific tolerance to the fluoroquinoloneofloxacin. PLoS Genetics. 2013;**9**(1):e1003144. DOI: 10.1371/journal.pgen.1003144

[11] Kimberley LP, et al. *Staphylococcus aureus* adapts to oxidative stress by producing H_2O_2-resistant small-colony variants via the SOS response. Infection and Immunity. 2015;**83**(5):1830–1844. DOI: 10.1128/IAI.03016-14

[12] Didier H, et al. Evidence for induction of integron-based antibiotic resistance by the SOS response in a clinical setting. PLoS Pathogens. 2012;**8**(6):e1002778. DOI: 10.1371/journal.ppat.1002778

[13] Hongan L, et al. Antibiotic treatment enhances the genome-wide mutation rate of target cells. Proceedings of the National Academy of Sciences. 2016;**113**(18):E2498–E2505. DOI: 10.1073/pnas.1601208113

[14] Kelsi LA, et al. Characterization of the *Staphylococcus aureus*heat shock, cold shock, stringent, and sos responses and their effects on log-phase mRNA turnover. Journal of Bacteriology. 2006;**188**(19):6739–6756. DOI: 10.1128/JB.00609-06

[15] Justin C, et al. Comparative gene expression profiles following UV exposure in wild-type and SOS-deficient *Escherichia coli*. Genetics. 2001;**158**(1):41–64. DOI: http://www.genetics.org/content/158/1/41.long

[16] Bénédicte M. After 30 years of study, the bacterial SOS response still surprises us. PLoS Biology. 2005;**3**(7):e255. DOI: 10.1371/journal.pbio.0030255

[17] Katharina S, Phuong P, Michael MC, Myron F. Goodman. Roles of DNA polymerase V and RecA protein in SOS damage-induced mutation. Chemical Reviews. 2006;**106**(2):406–419. DOI: 10.1021/cr0404951

[18] Celina J. Inducible SOS response system of DNA repair and mutagenesis in *Escherichia coli*. International Journal of Biological Sciences. 2008;**4**(6):338–344. DOI: 10.7150/ijbs.4.338

[19] Alexi IG, et al. Characterization of the global transcriptional responses to different types of DNA damage and disruption of replication in *Bacillus subtilis*. Journal of Bacteriology. 2006;**188**(15):5595–5605. DOI: 10.1128/JB.00342-06

[20] Wiebke S, Christiane G, Christiane W. Opposing effects of aminocoumarins and fluoroquinolones on the SOS response and adaptability in *Staphylococcus aureus*. Journal of Antimicrobial Chemotherapy. 2013;**68**(3):529–538. DOI: 10.1093/jac/dks456

[21] Arabela C, Konrad P, Adriana ER. Development of homogeneous expression of resistance in methicillin-resistant *Staphylococcus aureus* clinical strains is functionally associated with a β-lactam-mediated SOS response. Journal of Antimicrobial Chemotherapy. 2009;**64**(1):37–45. DOI: 10.1093/jac/dkp164

[22] Úbeda C, Maiques E, Knecht, E, Lasa Í, Novick RP, Penadés JR. Antibiotic-induced SOS response promotes horizontal dissemination of pathogenicity island-encoded virulence factors in staphylococci. Molecular Microbiology. 2005;**56**(3):836–844. DOI: 10.1111/j.1365-2958.2005.04584.x

[23] Martin V, Wilhelm P, Hanne I. Activation of the SOS response increases the frequency of small colony variants. BMC Research Notes. 2015;**8**(749):1. DOI: 10.1186/s13104-015-1735-2

[24] Elisa M, et al. β-Lactam antibiotics induce the sos response and horizontal transfer of virulence factors in *Staphylococcus aureus*. Journal of Bacteriology. 2006;**188**(7):2726–2729. DOI: 10.1128/JB.188.7.2726-2729.2006

[25] Christiane G, Johanna K, Christiane W. Ciprofloxacin and trimethoprim cause phage induction and virulence modulation in *Staphylococcus aureus*. Antimicrobial Agents and Chemotherapy. 2006;**50**(1):171–177. DOI: 10.1128/AAC.50.1.171-177.2006

[26] Pierre T, Li B, Henry FC . Subinhibitory fluoroquinolone exposure selects for reduced beta-lactam susceptibility in methicillin-resistant *Staphylococcus aureus* and alterations in the SOS-mediated response. Research in Microbiology. 2009;**160**(3):187–192. DOI: 10.1016/j.resmic.2009.03.003

[27] Jean-Philippe D, et al. Impact of ciprofloxacin exposure on *Staphylococcus aureus*genomic alterations linked with emergence of rifampin resistance. Antimicrobial Agents and Chemotherapy. 2011;**55**(5):1946–1952. DOI: 10.1128/AAC.01407-10

[28] Richard PN, Gail EC, Jose RP. The phage-related chromosomal islands of Gram-positive bacteria. Nature Reviews Microbiology. 2010;**8**:541–551. DOI: 10.1038/nrmicro2393

[29] Carles U, María ÁT-M, José RP, Richard PN. Structure–function analysis of the SaPIbov1 replication origin in *Staphylococcus aureus*. Plasmid. 2012;**67**(2):183–190. DOI: 10.1016/j.plasmid.2012.01.006

[30] Douglas RD, Bryan U, Vincent AFi. Uncovering novel mobile genetic elements and their dynamics through an extra-chromosomal sequencing approach. Mobile Genetics Elements. 2016;**6**(4):e1189987 . DOI: 10.1080/2159256X.2016.1189987

[31] Lena T, Olaf S, Dominique M. Pathogenesis of *Staphylococcus aureus* blood stream infections. Annual Review of Pathology: Mechanisms of Disease. 2016;**11**:343–364 . DOI: 10.1146/annurev-pathol-012615-044351

[32] Zhongyi C, Thanh TL, Chia YL. The sbcDC locus mediates repression of type 5 capsule production as part of the SOS response in *Staphylococcus aureus*. Journal of bacteriology. 2007;**189**:343–7350. DOI: 1 0.1128/JB.01079-07

[33] Chia Y L, Jean CL. Staphylococcal Capsule. In: Vicent AF, et al., editor. Gram-Positive Pathogens. 2nd ed. Washington, DC: American Society for Microbiology; 2006. pp. 456–457. DOI: 10.1128/9781555816513.ch37

[34] Ivan AG, et al. Synthesis of *Staphylococcus aureus* type 5 trisaccharide repeating unit: solving the problem of lactamization. Organic Letters. 2015;**17**(4):928–931. DOI: 10.1021/acs.orglett.5b00031

[35] Thanh TL, Chia YL. The arl locus positively regulates *Staphylococcus aureus* type 5 capsule via an mgrA-dependent pathway. Microbiology. 2006;**152**(10):3123–3131. DOI: 10.1099/mic.0.29177-0

[36] Carmelo B, et al. Induction of fibronectin-binding proteins and increased adhesion of quinolone-resistant *Staphylococcus aureus* by subinhibitory levels of ciprofloxacin. Antimicrobial Agents and Chemotherapy. 2000;**44**(6):1428–1437. DOI: 10.1128/AAC.44.6.1428-1437.2000

[37] Richard AV, et al. Selection of high-level oxacillin resistance in heteroresistant *Staphylococcus aureus* by fluoroquinolone exposure. Journal of Antimicrobial Chemotherapy. 2001;**48**(3):375–381. DOI: 10.1093/jac/48.3.375

[38] Richard AP, et al. Small colony variants: a pathogenic form of bacteria that facilitates persistent and recurrent infections. Nature Reviews Microbiology. 2006;**4**:295–305. DOI: 10.1038/nrmicro1384

[39] Mousa MA, et al. Metabolomic and proteomic responses of *Staphylococcus aureus* to prolonged cold stress. Journal of Proteomics. 2015;**121**:44–55. DOI: 10.1016/j.jprot.2015.03.010

[40] Kahl BC, Becker K, Löffler B. Clinical significance and pathogenesis of staphylococcal small colony variants in persistent infections. Clinical Microbiology Reviews. 2016;**29**(2):401–427. DOI: 10.1128/CMR.00069-15

[41] Kahl BC. Small colony variants (SCVs) of *Staphylococcus aureus*—a bacterial survival strategy. Infection, Genetics and Evolution. 2014;**21**:515–522. DOI: 10.1016/j.meegid.2013.05.016

[42] Besier S, Ludwig A, Ohlsen K, Brade V, Wichelhaus TA. Molecular analysis of the thymidine-auxotrophic small colony variant phenotype of *Staphylococcus aureus*. International Journal of Medical Microbiology. 2007;**297**:217–225. DOI: 10.1016/j.ijmm.2007.02.003

[43] Chatterjee I, Kriegeskorte A, Fischer A, Deiwick S, Theimann N, Proctor RA, Peters G, Herrmann M, Kahl BC. In vivo mutations of thymidylate synthase (thyA) are responsible for thymidine dependency in clinical small-colony variants of *Staphylococcus aureus*. Journal of Bacteriology. 2008;**190**:834–842. DOI: 10.1128/JB.00912-07

[44] Zander J, Besier S, Saum SH, Dehghani F, Loitsch S, Brade V, Wichelhaus TA. Influence of dTMP on the phenotypic appearance and intracellular persistence of *Staphylococcus aureus*. Infection and Immunity. 2008;**76**:1333–1339. DOI: 10.1128/IAI.01075-07

[45] Besier S, Zander J, Kahl BC, Kraiczy P, Brade V, Wichelhaus TA. The thymidine-dependent small-colony-variant phenotype is associated with hypermutability and antibiotic resistance in clinical *Staphylococcus aureus* isolates. Antimicrobial Agents and Chemotherapy. 2008;**52**:2183–2189. DOI: 10.1128/AAC.01395-07

[46] McNamara PJ, Proctor RA. *Staphylococcus aureus* small colony variants, electron transport and persistent infections. International Journal of Antimicrobial Agents. 2000;**14**:117–122.

[47] Lannergård J, von Eiff C, Sander G, Cordes T, Seggewiss J, Peters G, Proctor RA, Becker K, Hughes D. Identification of the genetic basis for clinical menadione-auxotrophic small-colony variant isolates of *Staphylococcus aureus*. Antimicrobial Agents and Chemotherapy. 2008;**52**:4017–4022. DOI: 10.1128/AAC.00668-08.

[48] Dean MA, Olsen RJ, Long SW, Rosato AE, Musser JM. Identification of point mutations in clinical *Staphylococcus aureus*strains that produce small-colony variants auxotrophic for menadione. Infection and Immunity. 2014;**82**:1600–1605. DOI: 10.1128/IAI.01487-1.

[49] Gottschalk S, Ifrah D, Lerche S, Gottlieb CT, Cohn MT, Hiasa H, Hansen PR, Gram L, Ingmer H, Thomsen LE. The antimicrobial lysine-peptoid hybrid LP5 inhibits DNA replication and induces the SOS response in *Staphylococcus aureus*. BMC Microbiology. 2013;**13**(192):1–8. DOI: 10.1186/1471-2180-13-192

[50] Kjelstrup S, Hansen PM, Thomsen LE, Hansen PR, Løbner-Olesen A. Cyclic peptide inhibitors of the β-sliding clamp in *Staphylococcus aureus*. PLoS One. 2013;**8**(9):e72273. DOI: 10.1371/journal.pone.0072273

[51] Gottschalk S, Gottlieb CT, Vestergaard M, Hansen PR, Gram L, Ingmer H, Thomsen LE. Amphibian antimicrobial peptide fallaxin analogue FL9 affects virulence gene expression and DNA replication in *Staphylococcus aureus*. Journal of Medical Microbiology. 2015;**64**:1504–1513. DOI: 10.1099/jmm.0.000177

[52] Opperman TJ, Kwasny SM, Li JB, Lewis MA, Aiello D, Williams JD, Peet NP, Moir DT, Bowlin TL, Long EC. DNA targeting as a likely mechanism underlying the antibacterial activity of synthetic Bis-indole Antibiotics. Antimicrobial Agents and Chemotherapy. 2016; DOI: 10.1128/AAC.00309-16

[53] Culyba MJ, Mo CY, Kohli RM. Targets for combating the evolution of acquired antibiotic resistance. Biochemistry. 2015;**54**(23):3573–3582. DOI: 10.1021/acs.biochem.5b00109

[54] Mo CY, Manning SA, Roggiani M, Culyba MJ, Samuels AN, Sniegowski PD, Goulian M, Kohli RM. Systematically altering bacterial SOS activity under stress reveals therapeutic strategies for potentiating antibiotics. mSphere. 2016;**1**(4). DOI: 10.1128/mSphere.00163-16

[55] Sexton JZ, Wigle TJ, He Q, Hughes MA, Smith GR, Singleton SF, Williams AL, Yeh LA. Novel inhibitors of *E. coli* RecA ATPase activity. Current Chemical Genomics and Translational Medicine. 2010;**4**:34–42. DOI: 10.2174/1875397301004010034

[56] Peterson EJ, Janzen WP, Kireev D. Singleton SF high-throughput screening for RecA inhibitors using a transcreener adenosine 5′-O-diphosphate assay. ASSAY and Drug Development Technologies. 2012;**10**(3):260–268. DOI: 10.1089/adt.2011.0409

[57] Fujita M, Shiota S, Kuroda T, Hatano T, Yoshida T, Mizushima T, Tsuchiya T. Remarkable synergies between baicalein and tetracycline, and baicalein and β-lactams against methicillin-resistant *Staphylococcus aureus*. Microbiology and Immunology. 2005;**49**(4):391–396. DOI: 10.1111/j.1348-0421.2005.tb03732.x

[58] Sahu BD, Kumar JM, Kuncha M, Borkar RM, Srinivas R, Sistla R. Baicalein alleviates doxorubicin-induced cardiotoxicity via suppression of myocardial oxidative stress and apoptosis in mice. Life Sciences. 2016;**144**(1):8–18. DOI: 10.1016/j.lfs.2015.11.018

[59] Peng Q, Zhou S, Yao F, Hou B, Huang Y, Hua D, Zheng Y, Qian Y. Baicalein suppresses the SOS response system of *Staphylococcus aureus* induced by ciprofloxacin. Cellular Physiology and Biochemistry. 2011;**28**(5):1045–1050 . DOI: 10.1159/000335791

[60] Alt S, Mitchenall LA, Maxwell A, Heide L. Inhibition of DNA gyrase and DNA topoisomerase IV of *Staphylococcus aureus* and *Escherichia coli* by aminocoumarin antibiotics. Journal of Antimicrobial Chemotherapy. 2011;**66**(9):2061–2069. DOI: 10.1093/jac/dkr247

[61] Schröder W, Bernhardt J, Marincola G, Klein-Hitpass L, Herbig A, Krupp G, Nieselt K, Wolz C. Altering gene expression by aminocoumarins: the role of DNA supercoiling in *Staphylococcus aureus*. BMC Genomics. 2014;**15**;291. DOI:10.1186/1471-2164-15-291

[62] Heide L. New aminocoumarin antibiotics as gyrase inhibitors. International Journal of Medical Microbiology. 2014;**304**(1):31–36. DOI: 10.1016/j.ijmm.2013.08.013

[63] Jeon YM, Lee HS, Jeong D, Oh HK, Ra KH, Lee MY. Antimicrobial photodynamic therapy using chlorin e6 with halogen light for acne bacteria-induced inflammation. Life Sciences. 2015;**124**:56–63. DOI: 10.1016/j.lfs.2014.12.029

[64] Al Habashneh R, Asa'ad FA, Khader Y. Photodynamic therapy in periodontal and peri-implant diseases. Quintessence International. 2015;**46**:677–690. DOI: 10.3290/j.qi.a34078.

[65] Almeida A, Faustino MA, Tomé JP. Photodynamic inactivation of bacteria: finding the effective targets. Future Medicinal Chemistry. 2015;**7**(10):1221–1224. DOI: 10.4155/fmc.15.59

[66] Grinholc M, Rodziewicz A, Forys K, Rapacka-Zdonczyk A, Kawiak A, Domachowska A, Golunski G, Wolz C, Mesak L, Becker K, Bielawski KP. Fine-tuning recA expression in *Staphylococcus aureus* for antimicrobial photoinactivation: importance of photo-induced DNA damage in the photoinactivation mechanism. Applied Microbiology and Biotechnology. 2015;**99**(21):9161–9176. DOI: 10.1007/s00253-015-6863-z

[67] Mildenhall KB, Wiese N, Chung D, Maples VF, Mohanty BK, Kushner SR. RNase E-based degradosome modulates polyadenylation of mRNAs after Rho-independent transcription terminators in *Escherichia coli*. Molecular Microbiology. 2016;**101**(4):645–655. DOI: 10.1111/mmi.13413.

[68] Manasherob R, Miller C, Kim KS, Cohen SN. Ribonuclease E modulation of the bacterial SOS response. Plos One. 2012;**7**(6):e38426. DOI: 10.1371/journal.pone.0038426.

[69] Aït-Bara S, Carpousis AJ. RNA degradosomes in bacteria and chloroplasts: classification, distribution and evolution of RNase E homologs. Molecular Microbiology. 2015;**97**(6):1021–1135. DOI: 10.1111/mmi.13095

[70] Eidem TM, Lounsbury N, Emery JF, Bulger J, Smith A, Abou-Gharbia M, Childers W, Dunman PM. Small-molecule inhibitors of *Staphylococcus aureus*RnpA-mediated RNA turnover and tRNA processing. Antimicrobial Agents and Chemotherapy. 2015;**59**(4):2016–2028. DOI: 10.1128/AAC.04352-14

[71] Olson PD, Kuechenmeister LJ, Anderson KL, Daily S, Beenken KE, Roux CM, Reniere ML, Lewis TL, Weiss WJ, Pulse M, Nguyen P, Simecka JW, Morrison JM, Sayood K, Asojo OA, Smeltzer MS, Skaar EP, Dunman PM. Small molecule inhibitors of *Staphylococcus aureus* RnpA alter cellular mRNA turnover, exhibit antimicrobial activity, and attenuate pathogenesis. PLoS Pathogens. 2011;**7**(2): e1001287. DOI: 10.1371/journal.ppat.1001287.

Chapter 7

Antimicrobial Activity of Chitosan Membranes against *Staphylococcus aureus* of Clinical Origin

Ana A. Escárcega-Galaz, Jaime López-Cervantes,
Dalia I. Sánchez-Machado, Olga R. Brito-Zurita and
Olga N. Campas-Baypoli

Additional information is available at the end of the chapter

http://dx.doi.org/10.5772/65980

Abstract

Healthy human skin has beneficial microflora and many pathogens causing infections. *Staphylococcus aureus* is the most prevalent and can have multiresistance to antibiotics. Chitosan is a polysaccharide composed of glucosamine and N-acetyl-D-glucosamine, which is biodegradable and has antimicrobial activity. As part of a national scientific research project for the development and application of biomaterials, we decided to study the effect of different membranes based on chitosan against strains of *S. aureus* isolated from infected ulcers. The study found that seven of nine strains of *S. aureus* are sensitive to rifampin and the least eight of nine strains were multiresistant to more than ten antibiotics. All chitosan-based membranes confirm its antimicrobial effect on direct contact with an increase in its diameter. The contact area of the membranes is increased according to the concentration of chitosan. The highest average area increase was the chitosan membranes with honey and glycerin, 88.32%. Chitosan membranes have shown their effectiveness against *S. aureus* strains of clinical origin. Thus, these materials can be applied for the treatment of chronic ulcers without toxic hazards and resistance caused by antibiotics.

Keywords: chitosan, antimicrobial membranes, ulcer, biomaterials, pathogens

1. Introduction

Staphylococcus aureus is an infectious microorganism that can be both community- and hospital-acquired. Among the microorganisms causing nosocomial infections, it is second in prevalence (10.6%) of infection in surgical areas, intensive care, and pediatric areas [1, 2]. Similarly, this Gram-positive pathogen is the infectious agent in a broad spectrum of diseases from skin abscesses, dermatitis, surgical wounds, bacteremia, and osteomyelitis. The antimicrobial treatment of *S. aureus* infections has become more complicated by the increase of a broad spectrum of antibiotics and the development of resistant strains.

Chitosan is a cationic linear polysaccharide composed of glucosamine and N-acetyl glucosamine units linked by β (1-4) glucoside bonds [3]. This polymer is biodegradable and has antimicrobial activity against *S. aureus, Escherichia coli, Salmonella typhimurium,* and fungi [4]. The antimicrobial effect of chitosan is attributed to positive charges of the polymer chain. Thus, by increasing the amount of amino groups protonated, antimicrobial activity is enhanced by affecting the permeability of the bacterial cell wall. Due to its antimicrobial activity, it has been used in food preservation as antimicrobial coating of bread, fruit, vegetables, eggs, and various meat products. Because of their lack of toxicity and allergenicity, chitosan is a biomaterial with pharmaceutical and medical applications. Thus, chitosan has been used in health care products such as curing agent, dressings, skin grafts [3], hemostat, and drug carrier [5]. These biomaterials can be prepared in the form of hydrogels, membranes, and sponges.

The skin surface is characterized by a slightly acidic pH that favors the development of some bacteria [6]. However, in an open wound, within the first 24–48 h can be found *Streptococcus, S. aureus,* and *Pseudomonas aeruginosa* and then, between days 5 and 7, the bacteria found were *Klebsiella* and *Escherichia coli* [7].

Skin infections affect the epidermis, subcutaneous tissue, and muscle. Some of them require hospital admission for antimicrobial or surgical treatment. Depending on their severity, they have been associated with increased hospital stays and medical costs because traditional antibiotic treatments require long periods [8]. An alternative to antibiotics is curing materials with bioactive components. These dressings should ideally maintain a moist environment, act as antimicrobials to prevent secondary infections, remove exudate, and promote tissue regeneration [9, 10] One group evaluated the antimicrobial action of cotton textile impregnated with chitosan against bacteria isolated from the skin and found that chitosans of low- and high-molecular weight showed effective inhibition of *S. aureus* [11]. Another studied the effect of chitosan in antimicrobial ultrastructural organization of clinical *S. aureus* strains and found changes in its cell and cytoplasmic membrane. Similarly, Woo et al. [12] developed a bilayer scaffold from chitosan with TiO_2 that showed high reduction in viable *S. aureus*. To our knowledge, there are no studies on the application of chitosan membranes against *S. aureus* isolated from infected ulcers of the patients hospitalized. This chapter deals with the preparation and evaluation of the effect of different membranes based on chitosan against *S. aureus* strains of clinical origin. All chitosan membranes were prepared by solvent evaporation and the antimicrobial activity was evaluated by the agar diffusion technique.

http://dx.doi.org/10.5772/65980

2. Experimentation

2.1. Chitosan

Chitosan was obtained by thermo-alkaline hydrolysis of chitin, which was recovered by lactic fermentation of shrimp waste. The chitin was demineralized (0.1 M HCl at 25°C for 4 h) and deproteinized (4.5% NaOH at 65°C for 4 h). Afterward, purified chitin was deacetylated (40% NaOH at 110°C for 2 h) to obtain chitosan, according to reported methodologies [13]. Chitosan was washed until a neutral pH was reached and dried at 50°C. The purity of the chitosan was verified based on its moisture and ash content by method given in reference [14].

Degree of deacetylation of chitosan was determined by a spectrophotometric method reported by Liu et al. [15]. Briefly, two standard solutions were prepared; D-glucosamine (7.49 mM) and N-acetylglucosamine (0.49 mM), from these, working solutions were prepared to obtain a 12-point line of different concentrations. The absorbance of the standard solutions and samples were read at 201 nm in a UV-Vis spectrophotometer (Genesys 10 UV, Madison, IA, USA). Finally, the degree of deacetylation was calculated with the following equation, $\%DD = (161.1 \times A \times V - 0.0218m)/(3.361m - 42.1 \times A \times V)$, where, A is the absorbance of the sample, V is the volume of dilution, and m is the amount of sample in mg.

The molecular weight of chitosan was determined as proposed by Solis et al. [16], based on the intrinsic viscosity, according to Mark-Houwink's equation $n = KM_v^a$. Where, the reported values of K and a for chitosan in HAc 0.3 M and NaAc 0.2 M at 30°C are 0.074 and 0.76 mg, respectively. An Ubbelohde capillary viscometer immersed in water bath at 30 ± 0.01°C was used. The falling time of solvent (t_0) and of five polymer solutions of known concentrations (t_i) was measured.

Chitosan was identified by Fourier Transform Infrared Spectroscopy (FTIR) according to the methodology given in reference [17], with some modifications. The spectral resolution was of 4 cm^{-1} with 64 scans in a range of 600–4000 cm^{-1} using a Thermo Scientific (Nicolet5s, Madison, IA, USA) infrared spectrometer.

2.2. Chitosan membranes

Six chitosan based formulations using 1% acetic acid were prepared. Three pure chitosan solutions (1, 2, and 3%), another of 2% chitosan with glycerin (five drops per 100 ml) and two more solutions of 2% chitosan using honey (95:5, v/v) with and without glycerin. For the last two solutions, honey was diluted in distilled water (80:20, v/v) and homogenized by stirring.

All chitosan membranes were prepared by solvent evaporation. For this, solutions of each formulation were poured into polypropylene plates (10 ml in each mold) and dried at 40°C for 24 h in an oven (Felisa, Zapopan, Jalisco, Mexico). Lastly, the films were removed from the mold and stored in sterile plastic bags until use.

2.3. Collection and conservation of the sample

Between June and December 2015, a descriptive and cross-sectional study was conducted in order to evaluate the effect of chitosan membranes against *S. aureus* strains isolated from skin ulcers. Patients and involved personnel confirmed their participation by giving their consent.

The samples were obtained from the center of the ulcer by a medical epidemiologist. For this, a Stuart medium swab collection system (COPAN Transystem, Brescia, Italy) was used. The labeled samples were transported in a container to a certified microbiology laboratory for processing within the same hour.

2.4. Phenotypic identification and sensitivity tests

For microbial isolation and identification, the samples were inoculated by cross-streaking on MacConkey agar for Gram-negative bacterium and trypticase soy agar (TSA) for culture collection. Mannitol salt agar was used for Gram-positive bacterium and Biggy agar for fungi inoculated by streaking. Next, the plates were incubated at 37°C for bacteria and 30°C for fungi for 24 h. Later, macroscopic characteristics of colony-forming units (CFU) were analyzed.

For the identification of microorganisms, a broth microdilution method was used, with an inoculation Prompt™ system precision wand. Isolated colonies were emulsified in Prompt™ innoculation bottles for an equivalent concentration of 0.08 with the McFarland standard. Next, 100 μl per well were deposited in the SIEMENS microplates from a MicroScan RENOK panel which was incubated at 37°C for 24 h. Specifically, type 33 plates (B1017-211) were used for Gram-positive bacteria and type 44 (B1017-305) for Gram-negative bacteria. Later, each plate was read for the identification of studied microorganisms using a LabPro Command Center software. Antibiotic sensitivity was performed simultaneously with phenotypic identification using a RENOK MicroScan panel. The MIC (Minimum Inhibitory Concentration) was determined according to the CLSI (Clinical and Laboratory Standards Institute) criteria for each antibiotic. The studied antibiotics were oxacillin, gentamicin, tetracycline, daptomycin, ampicillin, erythromycin, penicillin, nitrofurantoin, vancomycin, levofloxacin, moxifloxacin, ciprofloxacin, linezolid, ceftriaxone, Sinercid, clindamycin, rifampin, amoxicillin/clavulanate k, trimethoprim/sulfamethoxazole, and ampicillin/sulbactam.

2.5. Sensitivity tests with chitosan membranes

The sensitivity test for *S. aureus* was performed by Kirby-Bauer's agar diffusion method [18]. From each of the identified bacterial isolates a micro-dilution was prepared in Prompt™ inoculation bottle. Afterward, plates with Muller Hinton agar were inoculated with a sterile swab and dispersed by streaking.

Chitosan based membranes were cut into 16 mm diameter discs and placed in triplicate on the inoculated agar with sterile forceps, ensuring direct contact between both surfaces. Each agar also included two blank controls that consisted of Whatman # 1 paper; one was impregnated with 1% acetic acid and the other with 0.9% sodium chloride. Plates were incubated at 37°C for 24 h. Lastly, the antimicrobial effect of chitosan was evident by observing the existence of inhibition zones below the membranes and inhibition halos around each membrane.

3. Results and discussion

3.1. Chitosan characterization

The ash content of chitosan is an indication of its purity. For chitosan with 9.42 ± 0.07% moisture, the average ash contents are 0.37 ± 0.02%. The range of ash content is 0.08% for langoustine obtained chitosan [19] and 4.0% to crab obtained chitosan [20], whereas for chitosan obtained from shrimp, the range is from 0.070 [21] to 0.832% [22]. Variations in ash content are due to the location of origin, as well as the purification and thermos-alkaline hydrolysis of chitin.

The molecular weight of chitosan determines its functional properties and its antimicrobial activity. This study found that the average molecular weight of chitosan was 119.48 kDa, estimated based on the intrinsic viscosity. With this value, chitosan can be classified as a low molecular weight (50–190 kDa) material. Therefore, the molecular weight is a reflection of the process conditions used to obtain chitosan from the purification and thermo-alkaline deacetylation of chitin. Other investigations have reported molecular weights for shrimp obtained chitosan of 136 [23], 180 [24], and 1260 kDa [25]. While the values reported for chitosan obtained from crab shells vary from 1240 [26] to 483 kDa [27]. For fungal chitosan, reports show low molecular weight, from 41 [24] to 110–150 kDa [25]. Davoodbasha et al. [28] conducted antimicrobial tests with commercial chitosan 100–300 kDa. Hernández-Ochoa et al. [29] also studied the antimicrobial activity of commercial chitosan with different molecular weight (low: 50–190 kDa, medium: 190–310 kDa and high: 310–375 kDa) finding satisfactory results with the lower molecular weight.

For the degree of deacetylation of chitosan, an average value of 84.59 ± 0.87% ($n = 6$) was found, similar to that reported in other studies; 85 [30], 82 [31], 83 [20], and 73.52% [32] varying depending on the source of chitin and the deacetylation conditions. To determine the degree of deacetylation, a variety of methods have been employed; however, among the most repetitive are the spectrophotometric and potentiometric methods and FTIR [27]. The degree of deacetylation has a strong impact on the antimicrobial activity of chitosan, mostly because its increase raises its solubility. Therefore, a greater number of amino groups with positive charge can be obtained, which are responsible for interacting with the cell wall charge of microorganisms [33].

The FTIR technique made it possible to identify the functional groups in the chitosan molecule (**Figure 1**). At 881.96 cm^{-1}, a characteristic band of the stretching of the glycosidic bond can be observed; also at 1055.62 and 1028.60 cm^{-1} the stretching of C—O can be seen. It is possible to observe the bending band N—H of the primary amide formed during deacetylation at 1545.72 cm^{-1} and the amine group at 1626.76 cm^{-1}. At the position of 2884.84 cm^{-1} the stretching of C—H and at 2962.02 cm^{-1} the tense vibration from group C—H can be observed. Ultimately, OH and N—H were identified at 3274.61 and 3359.51 cm^{-1}, respectively. These results are similar to those reports given by references [32, 34]. As reported by Shigemasa et al. [35], errors in band intensity can occurred at positions 1640 and 3450 cm^{-1} due to the effect of water absorption.

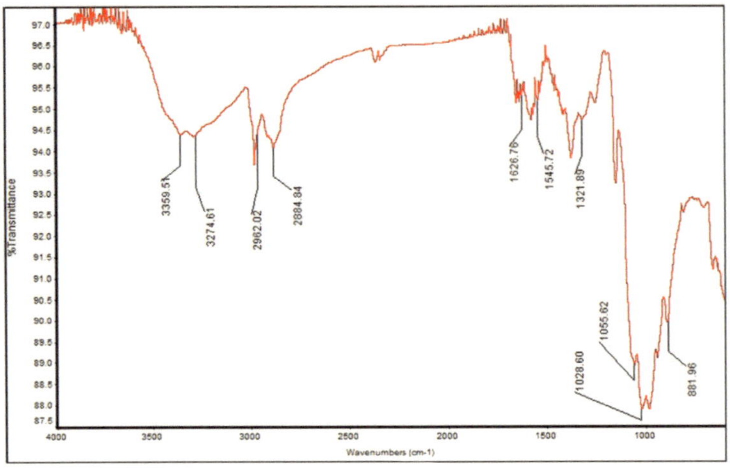

Figure 1. FTIR spectra of powdered chitosan.

3.2. Preparation of chitosan membranes

Dissolved chitosan is capable of forming a membrane due to the evaporation of the solvent, as well as forming intra and intermolecular hydrogen bonds between the chitosan polymer chains [36]. Chitosan membranes were prepared using pure chitosan and a mix of chitosan with glycerin or honey. All membranes were transparent, uniform, and smooth at the surface and with hard texture when chitosan concentration was increased. Pure chitosan membranes show a very pale yellow color and membranes containing honey show a brown tone. All membranes were easily removed from the polyethylene plates with 9.5 cm in diameter, and thickness depending on the concentration of chitosan, found in the range of 0.0131 ± 0.0021 and 0.0339 ± 0.0034 mm for 1 % and 3 %, respectively.

3.3. Phenotypic identification of microorganisms

From patients hospitalized for various reasons in a regional hospital located in northwestern Mexico, 23 infected skin ulcers derived from toes, sacral parts, coccyx, arm, and leg stumps were analyzed. The age range of the patients was from 43 to 96 years. Among the isolated and identified strains were *S. aureus*, *Proteus mirabilis*, *Candida albicans*, *E. coli*, *Enterobacter aerogenes*, *Morganella morganii*, *P. aeruginosa*, and *Klebsiella pneumoniae*. From all identified strains nine (29.03%) were *S. aureus*. The incidence of *S. aureus* in ulcers with mild type infection is 80–90% and in moderate to severe infections, it is 66% [37]. According to Barberán and Fariñas [38], *S. aureus* has been the cause of 40% of infections in skin and soft tissue [8]. Mention that the microorganisms with higher incidence in skin lesions and that increase resistance to antibiotics are *E. coli*, *K. pneumoniae*, *P. mirabilis*, *Enterobacter cloacae*, *Serratia marcescens*, *M. morganii*, *Acinetobacter baumannii*, and *P. aeruginosa*. Barberán and Fariñas [38], report that *Propionibacterium acnes* and *S. aureus* are some of the most common skin pathogens. **Figure 2**, left, shows the development of *S. aureus* on mannitol salt agar, medium that enables the growth of Gram-

http://dx.doi.org/10.5772/65980

positive bacteria and inhibits the growth of Gram-negative. **Figure 2**, right, presents a microplate which includes the identification phase and the antibiogram phase with dilutions of the antibiotics.

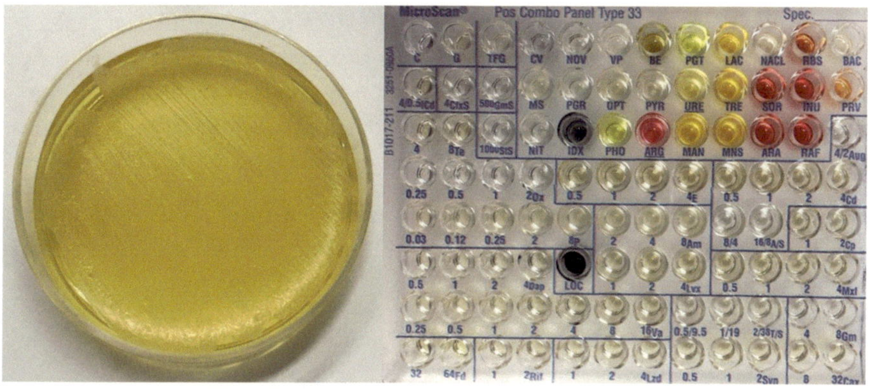

Figure 2. *S. aureus* growth in mannitol salt agar and microplate for identification with antibiogram.

Antibiogram	UD-001	UD-002	UD-020	UD-021	UD-023	UD-024	UD-025	UD-029	UD-030
Oxacillin	R >2	S < 0.25	S < 0.25	R > 2	R > 2	R > 2	R > 2	R > 2	R > 2
Gentamicin	S < 4	S < 4	S < 4	R > 8	R > 8	S < 4	R > 8	S < 4	S < 4
Tetracycline	S < 4	S < 4	S < 4	R > 8	R > 8	R > 8	S < 4	S < 4	S < 4
Daptomycin	R > 4	R >4	R >4	R > 4	R > 4	R > 4	S < 0.5	R > 4	S < 0.5
Ampicillin	R > 8	R > 8	S < 2	R > 8	R > 8	R > 8	R > 8	R > 8	R > 8
Erythromycin	R > 4	R >4	R >4	R > 4	R > 4	R > 4	R > 4	R > 4	R > 4
Penicillin	S < 0.03	R > 8	R > 8	R > 8	R > 8	R > 8	R > 8	R > 8	R > 8
Nitrofurantoin	R > 64	S < 32	S < 32	S< 32	R > 64	R > 64	S < 32	S < 32	S < 32
Vancomycin	S < 0.25	S < 0.25	R > 16	S < 0.25	S < 32	R > 16	R > 16	R > 16	R > 16
Levofloxacin	R > 4	S < 1	R > 4	R > 4	R > 4	R > 4	R > 4	R > 4	R > 4
Moxifloxacin	R > 4	S < 0.5	R > 4	R > 4	R > 4	R > 4	R > 4	R > 4	R > 4
Ciprofloxacin	R > 2	S < 1	R > 4	R > 2	R > 2	R > 2	R > 2	R > 2	R > 2
Linezolid	S < 1	S < 1	R > 4	R > 4	R > 4	S < 1	S < 1	R > 4	R > 4
Ceftriaxone	R > 32	S < 8	S < 8	S < 8	R > 32	R > 32	R > 32	S < 8	R > 32
Synercid	S < 0.5	S < 0.5	R > 2	R > 2	R > 2	S < 0.5	S < 0.5	S < 0.5	S < 0.5
Clindamycin	R > 4	S < 0.5	S < 0.5	R > 4	R > 4	R > 4	R > 4	R > 4	R > 4
Rifampin	S < 1	S < 1	S < 1	R > 2	R > 2	S < 1	S < 1	S < 1	S < 1
Amoxicillin/K clauvulanato	R > 4/2	S < 4/2	R > 4/2	R > 4/2	R > 4/2	R > 4/2	R > 4/2	R > 4/2	R > 4/2
Trimethoprim/ sulfamethoxazole	S < 0.5/9.5	S < 0.5/9.5	R > 2/38	R > 2/38	R > 2/38	S < 0.5/9.5	R > 2/38	R > 2/38	S < 0.5/9.5
Ampicillin/ sulbactam	R > 16/8	R > 16/8	S < 8/4	R > 16/8	R > 16/8	S < 8/4	S < 8/4	S < 8/4	S < 8/4

R, resistant; S, sensitive.

Table 1. Antibiogram of chronic ulcers from *S. aureus* isolates.

3.4. *S. aureus* sensitivity to antibiotics

Table 1 shows the minimum inhibitory "*in vitro*" amount of twenty antibiotics against nine strains of *S. aureus* studied with a RENOK MicroScan panel. Specifically, seven of the nine *S. aureus* strains are sensitive to rifampin (MIC < 1 μ/ml), while the least effective antibiotics were ampicillin (MIC > 8 μ/ml), erythromycin (MIC > 4 μ/ml), penicillin (MIC > 8 μ/ml), levofloxacin (MIC > 4 μ/ml), moxifloxacin (MIC > 4 μ/ml), ciprofloxacin (MIC > 2 μ/ml), and clavulanate amoxycillin (MIC > 4/2 μ/ml). In addition, eight of the nine strains were detected to be multiresistant to more than ten antibiotics. Additionally, one isolated showed sensitivity to vancomycin, while another was sensitive to 15 of the 20 studied antibiotics.

Figure 3 shows that most strains are resistant to the most commonly used antibiotics. All isolates were resistant to erythromycin. Only one of the nine strains showed sensitivity toward ampicillin, penicillin, levofloxacin, ciprofloxacin, and amoxicillin.

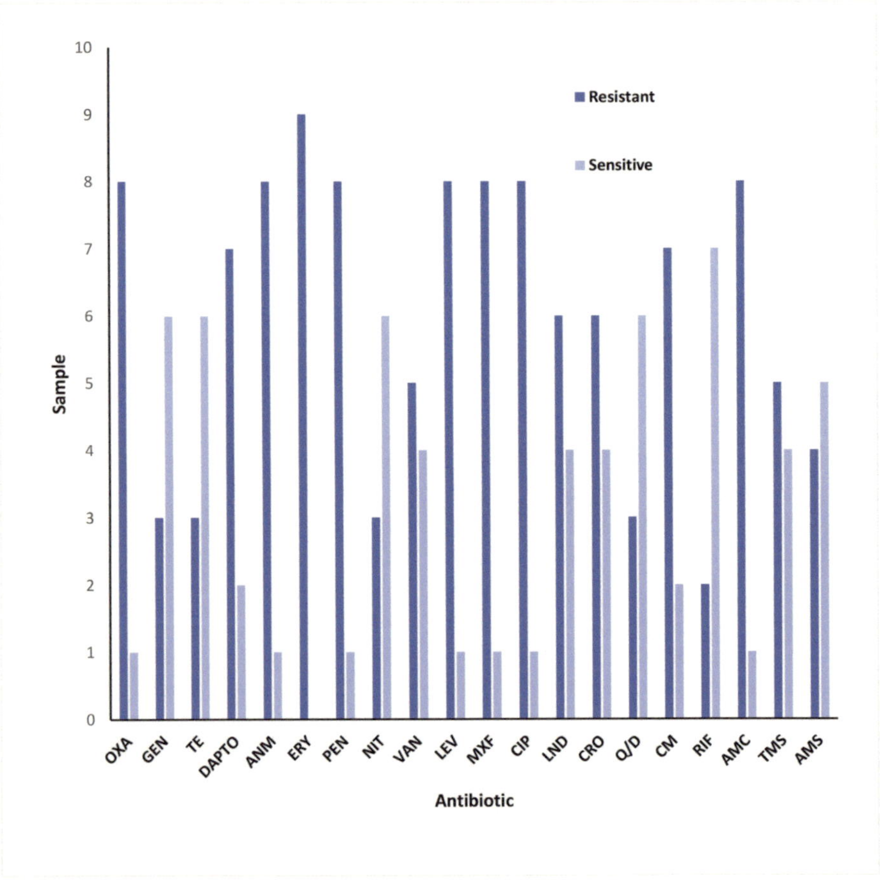

Figure 3. Antibiotic sensitivity and resistant toward *S. aureus*.

The most commonly used antibiotics for *S. aureus* treatments are vancomycin, linezolid, daptomycin, tigecycline, rifampin, clindamycin, cloxacillin, clindamycin, cotrimoxazol, and doxycycline [1]. Daptomycin has superior bactericidal action than other drugs against *S. aureus* [38]. Chirinos-Saldaña et al. [39] found that *S. aureus* isolated from conjunctivitis shows high sensitivity toward vancomycin, ciprofloxacin, and gentamicin. Antibiotic resistance is generated due to prolonged and inappropriate use of antibiotics [39]. Furthermore, if the bacterial population density in the infection is high, *S. aureus* can become resistant to most antibiotics used in monotherapy [40].

3.5. *S. aureus* sensitive chitosan membranes

The "*in vitro*" antimicrobial activity assays with chitosan membranes for *S. aureus* were carried out by the agar diffusion method. **Figure 4** presents the absence of microbial growth below the membranes. It was also observed that no inhibition halo or clear zones were formed around the membrane explained because chitosan is unable to diffuse through agar. However, chitosan membranes added with honey presented a small zone of inhibition, confirming that chitosan only has antimicrobial effect by direct contact and cannot migrate into the agar. Likewise, microbial growth occurred in both blank controls with acetic acid and sodium chloride, which means that the antimicrobial effect cannot be attributed to these chemicals.

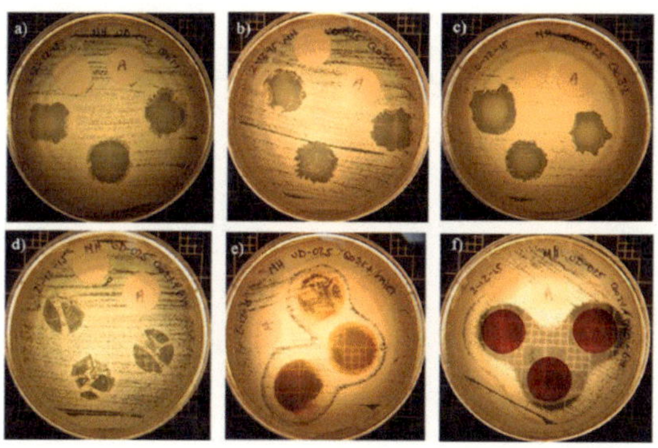

Figure 4. *S. aureus* susceptibility to chitosan membranes by agar diffusion method. Chitosan 1% (a), chitosan 2% (b), chitosan 3% (c), chitosan 2% + gly (d), chitosan 2% + honey (e), and chitosan 2% + honey + gly (f).

In a study by Hernández-Ochoa et al. [29], with *S. typhimurium*, *S. aureus*, and *Listeria monocytogenes*, results reported that chitosan membranes with essential oils (*Cuminum cyminum* and *Eugenia caryphyllata*) can present inhibition halos, while for pure chitosan membranes, the effect is shown only by direct contact.

The antimicrobial properties of chitosan mainly depend on the degree of deacetylation and molecular weight, as well as pH and ionic strength of the medium [41]. El-tahlawy et al. [42] and Hosseinnejad and Jafari [43] reported that low molecular weight chitosan can penetrate into the cell and inhibits mRNA and protein synthesis. Chitosan oligomers have higher antimicrobial effect due to their shorter chain and free amino groups from D-glucosamine [44].

Similarly, Champer et al. [45] reported that the amount of free amino groups influence the antibacterial properties of chitosan. Likewise, Wang et al. [46] state that all bacteria possess negative charges; therefore, they are easily captured by the protonated amine groups of chitosan and lose their reproductive functions and bioactivity. Acetic acid has an effect on the solubility of the polymer and on the protonation of the amino groups.

Kim et al. [47] evaluated the antimicrobial activity of chitosan membranes of different molecular weights with *L. monocytogenes, E. coli,* and *Salmonella typhimutium* and found that chitosan with low molecular weight has better effect. No et al. [48] reported that chitosan (1671, 746, 224, and 28 kDa) and chitosan oligomers (22, 10, 7, 3, 2, and 1 kDa) can inhibit the growth of *L. monocytogenes, Bacillus megaterium, Bacillus cereus, S. aureus,* and *Lactobacillus bulgaricus.*

Additionally, it was observed that the membranes tend to increase their diameter by staying in contact with the agar, thus increasing the antimicrobial effect by contact. **Table 2** presents the increase in diameter and area of the membranes at the end of agar diffusion assay. For pure chitosan membranes, it was found that an increase in size is directly proportional to its concentration. It was also observed that the addition of glycerin or honey increases the size of the chitosan membranes by 2%. The 2% chitosan membranes mixed with honey and glycerin showed the greatest increase, however, bacterial growth was observed.

Membranes	Increased radius (mm)[a]	Increase in contact area (%)[b]
Qo 1%	9.01 ± 4.97	20.03 ± 14.90
Qo 2%	9.39 ± 6.48	30.61 ± 17.33
Qo 3%	9.70 ± 9.58	39.80 ± 25.80
Qo 2% + gly	9.74 ± 6.34	40.34 ± 17.38
Qo 2% + miel	11.20 ± 4.65	65.38 ± 20.29
Qo 2% + miel + gly	11.20 ± 4.53	88.32 ± 21.73

[a]8.25 mm initial radius.
[b]213.82 mm^2 initial area.

Table 2. Comparison of the increase in radii and areas of chitosan membranes.

Vlacha et al. [49] reported that free hydroxyl groups from chitosan interact with the moist atmosphere increasing the diameter of the membrane. Also, Zamora-Mora et al. [50] mentioned that pure chitosan membranes show a higher water holding capacity due to the hydrophilicity of the chitosan. According to Estrada et al. [51], honey potentiates the antimicrobial activity of chitosan due to chemical action of its components; hydrogen peroxide, organic acids and flavonoids, nectar, pollen, and propolis. For Grade et al. [52], plasticizers provide flexibility to the membranes, but weaken the intermolecular forces and cause the penetration of water through the membrane increasing its size [23].

http://dx.doi.org/10.5772/65980

4. Conclusion

Different types of chitosan-based membranes mixed with glycerol and honey were developed and characterized. These membranes showed antimicrobial activity against *S. aureus* of clinical origin. Additionally, strains of *S. aureus* isolated from infected ulcers were found to have multidrug resistance to antibiotics. For future research where these materials will be applied in the treatment of chronic ulcers, it is important to recognize that the antimicrobial effect is given by direct contact in order to ensure that ulcers are completely covered with the membranes. These materials are an alternative for controlling intrahospital microorganisms without toxic hazards from antibiotics.

Acknowledgements

AA Escárcega-Galaz gratefully acknowledges the Consejo Nacional de Ciencia y Tecnología (CONACYT) by PhD scholarship: 417707. This research was funded by the Instituto Tecnológico de Sonora (Project PROFAPI-00471) and by the Consejo Nacional de Ciencia y Tecnología (PDCPN2014: 248160).

Author details

Ana A. Escárcega-Galaz[1], Jaime López-Cervantes[1], Dalia I. Sánchez-Machado[1*], Olga R. Brito-Zurita[2] and Olga N. Campas-Baypoli[1]

*Address all correspondence to: dalia.sanchez@itson.edu.mx

1 Department of Biotechnology and Food Sciences, Technological Institute of Sonora, Cd. Obregon, Sonora, Mexico

2 Medical Research Unit in Clinical Epidemiology, High Speciality Medical Unit, North-Western National Medical Center, Mexican Social Security Institute, Ciudad Obregón, Sonora, México

References

[1] Mensa J, Barberán J, Llinares P, Picazo JJ, Bouza E, Älvarez F, Borges M, Serrano R, León C, Guirao X, Arias J, Carreras E, Sanz MA, García JA. Guidelines for the treatment on infections caused by methicillin-resistant Staphylococcus aureus. Rev Esp Quimioter. 2008;21(4):234–258. ISSN-e: 0214–3429.

[2] Velazco E, Nieves B, Araque M, Calderas Z. Epidemiology of Staphylococcus aureus nosocomial infections in a high-risk neonatal unit. Enf Infecc Microbiol Clin. 2002;20(7): 321–325 doi:10.1016/S0213-005X(02)72808-5.

[3] Anisha BS, Sankar D, Mohandas A, Chennazhi KP, Nair SV, Jayakumar R. Chitosan-hyaluronan/nano chondroitin sulfate ternary composite sponges for medical use. Carbohyd Polym. 2013;92:1470–1476. doi:10.1016/j.carbpol.2012.10.058

[4] Dantas MDM, Cavalcante DRR, Araújo FEN, Barreto SR, Aciole GTS, Pinheiro ALB, Ribeiro MAG, Lima-Verde IB, Melo CM, Cardoso JC, Albuquereque RLC. Improvement of dermal burn healing by combining sodium alginate/chitosan-based films and low level laser therapy. J Photochem Photobiol B. 2011;105:51–59. doi:10.1016/j.jphotobiol.2011.06.009

[5] Mi F-L, Shyu S-S, Wu Y-B, Lee S-T, Shyong J-Y, Huang R-N. Fabrication and characterization of a sponge-like asymmetric chitosan membrane as a wound dressing. Biomaterials. 2001;22:165–173. doi:10.1016/S0142-9612(00)00167-8

[6] Sánchez-Saldaña L, Sáenz-Anduaga E. Bacterial cutaneous infections. Dermatol Peru. 2006;16(1):7–31.

[7] Abbaspour M, Makhmalzadeh BS, Rezaee B, Shoja S, Ahangari Z. Evaluation of the antimicrobial effect of chitosan/polyvinyl alcohol electrospun nanofibers containing mafenide acetate. Jundishapur J Microbiol. 2015;8(10):e24239. doi: 10.5812/jjm.24239

[8] Corrales L, Castillo A, Melo A. In vitro evaluation of antibacterial potential of Croton lechleri against bacterial isolates from patients with skin ulcers. NOVA. 2013;11(19):51–63. ISSN: 1794–2470.

[9] Flores-Reyes M, Camarillo-Romero MS, Flores-Estrada J, Flores-Merino MV. Polymeric skin substitutes for the treatment of diabetic foot ulcer. Medicina e Investigación. 2015;3(1):74–78. http://dx.doi.org/10.1016/j.mei.2015.02.006.

[10] Tavaria FK, Soares JC, Reis IL, Paulo MH, Malcata FX, Pintado ME. Chitosan: antimicrobial action upon *staphylococi* after impregnation onto corron fabric. J App Microbiol. 2012;112:1034–1041. ISSN: 1364-5072

[11] Didenko LV, Gerasimenko DV, Konstantinova ND, Silkina TA, Avdienko ID, Bannikova GE, Varlamov VP. Ultrastructural study of chitosan effect on *Klebsiella* and *Staphylpcocci*. Bull Exp Biol Med. 2005;140(3):356–360. DOI: 10.1007/s10517-005-0489-6

[12] Woo CH, Choi YC, Choi JS, Lee HY, Cho YW. A bilayer composite composed of TiO2-incorporated electrospun chitosan membrane and human extracellular matrix sheet as a wound dressing. J Biomater Sci Polym Ed. 2015;26(13):841–854. http://dx.doi.org/10.1080/09205063.2015.1061349.

[13] Sánchez-Duarte RG, Sánchez-Machado DI, López-Cervantes J, Correa-Murrieta M.A. Adsorption of allura red dye by cross-linked chitosan from shrimp waste. Wat Sci Technol. 2012;48:618–623. doi: 10.2166/wst.2012.900

[14] AOAC. Official methods of analysis.18th ed. In: Williams S, editor. Arlington, VA: Association of Official Analytical Chemists. 2005.

[15] Liu D, Wei Y, Yaob P, Jiang L. Determination of the degree of acetylation of chitosan by UV spectrophotometry using dual standards. Carbohyd Res. 2006;341:782–785. doi: 10.1016/j.carbpol.2005.11.007

[16] Solis Y, Peniche C, García N, Davidenko N. Un procedimeinto biomimético novedoso para obtener composites de quitosanahidroxipatita. VII Congreso de la Sociedad Cubana de Bioingenieria. 2007.

[17] Beil S, Schamberger A, Naumann W, Machill S, Van Pée K.H. Determination of the degree of N-acetylation (DA) of chitin and chitosan in the presence of water by first derivative ATR FTIR spectroscopy. Carbohyd Polym. 2012;87:117–122. doi:10.1016/j.carbpol.2011.07.025

[18] Pérez A, Rojas J, Rodriguez J, Arrieta I, Arrieta Y, Rodríguez A. Antibacterial activity of chitosan acid solutions obtained from shrimp exoskeleton. Rev Colomb Biotecnol. 2014;16(1):104–110. http://dx.doi.org/10.15446/rev.colomb.biote.v16n1.44251

[19] Mármol Z, Gutierrez E, FerrerJ, Rincin M. Desacetilación termoalcalina de quitina de conchas de camarón. Multiciencias. 2004;4(2):91–95. ISSN: 1317–2255

[20] Colina M, Ayala A, Roncón D, Molina J, Medina J, Ynciarte R, Vargas J, Montilla B. Enaluación de los procesos para la obtención química de quitina y quitosano a partir de desechos de cangrejos. Escala piloto e industrial. Rev Iberoam Polím. 2014;15(1):21–43. ISSN-e:01216651

[21] Gildberg A, Stenberg E. A new process for advanced utilisation of shrimp waste. Process Biochem. 2001;36. 809–812. 10.1016/s0032-9592(00)00278-8

[22] Sini T, Santhosh S, Mathew P. Study on the production of chitin and chitosan from shrimp shell by using Bacillus subtilis fermentation. Carbohyd Res. 2007;342:2423–2429. doi:10.1016/j.carres.2007.06.028

[23] Rodríguez-Núñez JR, Madera-Santa TJ, Sánchez-Machado DI, López-Cervantes J. Chitosan/hydrophilic plasticizer-based films: preparation, physicochemical and antimicrobial properties. J Polym Environ. 2014;22:41–51. DOI 10.1007/s10924-013-0621-z

[24] Fernández-Pan I, Maté JI, Gardrat C, Coma V. Effect of chitosan molecular weight on the antimicrobial activity and release rate of carvacrol-enriched films. Food Hydrocolloid. 2015; 51:60–68. http://dx.doi.org/10.1016/j.foodhyd.2015.04.033

[25] Bierhalz AC, Westin CB, Moraes AM. Comparison of the properties of membranes produced with alginate and chitosan from mushroom and from shrimp. Int J Biol Macromol. 2016; 91:496–504. http://dx.doi.org/10.1016/j.ijbiomac.2016.05.095

[26] Qun C, Li H, Xiao Q, Lu Y, Zhu J, Du Y. Water-solubility of chitosan and its antimicrobial activity. Carbohyd Polym. 2006;63:367–374. doi:10.1016/j.carbpol.2005.09.023

[27] Yen MT, Yang JH, Mau JL. Physicochemical characterization of chitin and chitosan from crab shells. Carbohyd Polym. 2009;75:15–21. doi:10.1016/j.carbpol.2008.06.006

[28] Davoodbasha M, Kim AC, Lee SY, Kim JW. The facile synthesis of chitosan-based silver nano-biocomposites via a solution plasma process and their potential antimicrobial efficacy. Arch of Biochem Biophys. 2016;605:49–58. http://dx.doi.org/10.1016/j.abb.2016.01.013

[29] Hernández-Ochoa L, Gonzales-Gonzales A, Gutiérrez-Mendez N, Muñoz-Castellanos LN, Quintero-Ramos A. Study of the antibacterial activity of chitosan–based films prepared with different molecular weights including spices essential oils and functional extracts as antimicrobial agents. Rev Mex Ing Quím. 2011;10(3):455–463. ISSN: 1665–2738

[30] Baskar D, Sampath Kumar TS. Effect of deacetylation time on the preparation, properties and swelling behavior of chitosan films. Carbohyd Polym. 2009; 78:767–772. doi: 10.1016/j.carbpol.2009.06.013

[31] Alvarenga ES, Olivera CP, Bellato CR. An approach to understanding the deacetylation degree of chitosan. Carbohyd Polym. 2010;80:1155–1160. doi:10.1016/j.carbpol.2010.01.037

[32] Correa LS, Zuluaga F, Valencia C, Godoy JE. Elaboración de andamios porosos osteoinductivos de poli(ácido L-láctico)/quitosano para la regeneración de tejido ósea. Revista Colombiana de Materiales. 2015;6:34–53. ISSN: 2256-1013

[33] Ayala G. Antimicrobial effect of chitosan: a review. Revista Scientia Agroalimentaria. 2015;2:32–38. ISSN: 2339–4684

[34] Barros I, Guzmán L, Tarón A. Extraction and quantitative comparison of chitin obtained from the shell of Callinectes sapidus and Penaeus vannamei. Rev UDCA Act Div. 2015;18(2):227–234. ISSN:0123–4226

[35] Shigemasa Y, Matsuura H, Sashiwa H, Saimoto H. Evaluation of different absorbance ratios from infrared spectroscopy for analyzing the degree of deacetylation in chitin. Int J Biol Macromol. 1996;18:237–242. doi:10.1016/0141-8130(95)01079-3

[36] Cárcamo CA. Preparación de films de complejo polieletrolito quitosano-alginato y comparación de sus propiedades mecánicas y biológicas con films de quitosano [Tesis]. Santiago, Chile: 2005.

[37] Sarratea MPF. Manejo diagnóstico y terapéutico de las úlceras cutáneas crónicas infectadas. Jano: Medicina y humanidades. 2011;1767:61–65.

[38] Barberán J, Fariñas MC. Daptomycin in complicated skin and soft tissue infections. Enferm Infecc Microbiol Clínica. 2012; 30(1):33–37. doi:10.1016/S0213-005X(12)70069-1

[39] Chirinos-Saldaña P, Graue-Hernández EO, Hernández-Camarena JC, Navas A,Ramírez-Miranda A, Romero-Díaz L, Vizuet-García L, Ortiz-Casas M, López-Espinosa NL, Gaona-Juárez C, Bautista-Hernández LA, Bautista-de Lucio VM. Microbiological profile and antibacterial sensitivity of conjunctival infections isolated microorganisms from the Fundación Conde de Valenciana Ophthalmological Institute. Report of the year 2012. Rev Mex Oftalmo. 2014;88(2):73–77. http://dx.doi.org/10.1016/j.mexoft.2014.01.001

[40] Espinosa LE, Vega ME, Rodríguez AA, Jiménez LV, Morales E. Caracterización de *Staphylococcus aureus* resistente a meticilina aislado de pacientes con piodermitis. Dermatol Rev Mex. 2013;57:165–170.

[41] Chung YC, Wang HL, Chen YM, Li SL. Effect of abiotic factors on the antibacterial activity of chitosan against waterborne pathogens. Bioresour Technol. 2003;88:179–184. doi:10.1016/S0960-8524(03)00002-6

[42] El-tahlawy KF, El-Bendary MA, Elhendawy AG, Hudson SM. The antimicrobial activity of cotton fabrics treated with different crosslinking agents and chitosan. Carbohyd Polym. 2005;60:421–430. doi:10.1016/j.carbpol.2005.02.019

[43] Hosseinnejad M, Jafari SM. Evaluation of different factors affecting antimicrobial properties of chitosan. Int J Biol Macromol. 2016;85:467–475. http://dx.doi.org/10.1016/j.ijbiomac.2016.01.022

[44] Xia W, Liu P, Zhang J, Chen J. Biological activities of chitosan and chitooligosacharides. Food Hydrocolloid. 2011;25:170–179. doi:10.1016/j.foodhyd.2010.03.003

[45] Champer J, Patel J, Fernando N, Salehi E, Wong V, Kim J. Chitosan against cutaneous pathogens. AMB Express. 2013;3(37):1–8. doi:10.1186/2191-0855-3-37

[46] Wang T, Zhu XK, Xue XT, Wu DY. Hydrogel sheets of chitosan, honey and gelatin as burn wound dressings. Carbohyd Polym. 2012;88:75–83. doi:10.1016/j.carbpol.2011.11.069

[47] Kim KW, Min BJ, Kim YT, Kimmel RM, Cooksey K, Park SI. Antimicrobial activity against foodborne pathogens of chitosan biopolymer films of different molecular weights. Food Sci Technol. 2011;44:565–569. doi:10.1016/j.lwt.2010.08.001

[48] No HK, Park NY, Lee SH, Meyers SP. Antibacterial activity of chitosans and chitosan oligomers with different molecular weights. Int J Food Microbiol. 2002;74:65–72. doi:10.1016/S0168-1605(01)00717-6

[49] Vlacha M, Giannakas A, Katapodis P, Stamatis H, Ladavos A, Barkoula NM. On the efficiency of oleic acid as plasticizer of chitosan/clay nanocomposites and its role on

thermo-mechanical, barrier and antimicrobial properties – comparison with glicerol. Food Hydrocolloid. 016;57:10–19. http://dx.doi.org/10.1016/j.foodhyd.2016.01.003

[50] Zamora-Mora V, Sibaja M, Vega-Baudrit J. Diseño de un biofilm a partir de colágeno de pieles de tilapia y de quitosano de camarón como soporte para aplicaciónes en ingeniería de tejidos. Revista iberoamericana de polímeros. 2010;11(7):607–619.

[51] Estrada H, Gamboa MM, Chaves C, Arias ML. Evaluation of the antimicrobial action of honey against Staphylococcus aureus, Staphylococcus epidermidis, Pseudomonas aeruginosa, Escherichia coli, Salmonella enteritidis, Listeria monocytogenes and Aspergillus niger. Evaluation of its microbiological charge. Arch Latinoam Nutr. 2005;55(2):161–171. ISSN: 0004–0622

[52] Grade R, Pessan LA, Carvalho A. Ternary melt blends of poly(lactic acid)/poly(vinyl-alcohol)-chitosan. Ind Crrrop Prod. 2015;72:159–165. http://dx.doi.org/10.1016/j.indcrop.2014.12.041

Section 2

Staphylococcus aureus Virulence Factors

Chapter 8

Exfoliative Toxins of *Staphylococcus aureus*

Ricardo B. Mariutti, Natayme R. Tartaglia,
Núbia Seyffert, Thiago Luiz de Paula Castro,
Raghuvir K. Arni, Vasco A. Azevedo, Yves Le Loir and
Koji Nishifuji

Additional information is available at the end of the chapter

http://dx.doi.org/10.5772/66528

Abstract

Virulent strains of *Staphylococcus aureus* secrete exfoliative toxins (ETs) that cause the loss of cell-cell adhesion in the superficial epidermis. *S. aureus* ETs are serine proteases, which exhibit exquisite substrate specificity, and their mechanisms of action are extremely complex. To date, four different serotypes of ETs have been identified and three of them (ETA, ETB and ETD) are associated with toxin-mediated staphylococcal syndromes related to human infections leading to diseases of medical and veterinary importance.

Keywords: epidermolytic diseases, *Staphylococcus aureus*, exfoliative toxins, Desmoglein 1, keratinocytes

1. Introduction

Staphylococcus aureus, a commensal and opportunistic microorganism, is capable of colonizing the skin and mucous of individuals and represents a global public health problem [1–3]. It has been described as the etiological agent of various diseases both in humans and animals and is the main representative bacteria of the genus Staphylococcus [4]. *S. aureus* is a versatile microorganism and is capable of quickly adapting to different environmental conditions [5, 6]. This microorganism secretes several virulence factors that are associated with its pathogenesis [2] and in facilitating access to sites in the host that are normally sterile [7]. Diseases caused by *S. aureus* do not necessarily originate only by direct tissue invasion, but may be due to the action of more than 30 exoproteins codified by the pathogen [8, 9].

The exfoliative toxins (ETs) also known as epidermolytic toxins, are serine proteases secreted by *S. aureus* that recognize and hydrolyze desmosome proteins in the skin. ETs have been described as exotoxins produced by certain *S. aureus* strains, in the epidermis of the host, that have been associated with the loss of keratinocytes and with the cell-cell adhesion, inducing peeling of the skin and blister formation [10–13].

In 1878, Baron Gottfried Rotter Von Rittershain described the clinical features of epidermal exfoliation in newborns [14]. The relationship between skin exfoliation and *S. aureus* was established in 1967 by Lyell [14–16] and in 1972 [17] epidermal detachment at the stratum granulosum was established by electron microscopy. The pathogenic role of those toxins was demonstrated in 1970 by Melish and Glasgow by using newborn mice as experimental models [18]. However, the protein capable of causing generalized exfoliation in mice, denominated as exfoliatin, was not isolated and purified until 1971 [19] and subsequently serotypes have been identified [20, 21].

The principal isoforms of exotoxins implicated in human skin damage are exfoliative toxin A (ETA) and exfoliative toxin B (ETB) [22]. Exfoliative toxin C (ETC) isolated from a horse infection has not been associated with human disease. In 2002, a new exfoliative toxin (ETD) was identified in a clinical sample of *S. aureus* [13]. Recent crystallographic studies indicated that the ETD-like protein isolated from ewe mastitis [23] is structurally homologous to ETA and ETB [24]. ETA is codified by the *eta* gene on chromosomal DNA, carried on the genome on a temperate phage, and ETB by the *etb* gene on a large plasmid DNA [22, 25, 26]. ETD is codified by the *etd* gene which is located chromosomally on a pathogenicity island [13].

The ETA and ETB serotypes are homologous, have molecular masses of approximately 27 kDa, and contain 242 and 246 amino acids, respectively [22] and present identical dermatologic symptoms [26, 27].The ETA serotype was described as being heat stable whereas the ETB serotype has been demonstrated to be heat labile. The ETC serotype with a molecular mass of 27 kDa is also heat labile and causes exfoliation in mice and chickens [28].

2. Exfoliative toxins and associated diseases

ET-producing strains of *S. aureus* are related to localized epidermal infections such as bullous impetigo and generalized diseases like Staphylococal scalded skin syndrome (SSSS). Approximately 5% of all *S. aureus* strains produce exfoliative toxins, with ETA being most prevalent in Europe, Africa, and America and ETB being more common in Japan [26]. Most strains of *S. aureus* associated with SSSS in Europe and the United States belong to the type II phage group, such as 71 and 55/71, however, in Japan; most of the strains belong to other groups [15, 29]. In France, based on a retrospective study conducted between 1997 and 2007 [30], the mean incidence of SSSS cases was estimated to be 0.56 cases/year/million inhabitants.

Both ETA and ETB are distinguished by the extent of the damage caused in the epidermis [29, 30]. SSSS clinical manifestations involve fever, skin hypersensitivity, and erythema followed by superficial blister formation and skin separation, leaving long areas of denuded skin [10, 31]. In the localized form, toxin production and formation of flaccid blisters with purulent fluid occur [12, 30]. SSSS occurs mainly in newborns and children with occurrences in adults being rare [11, 32]. The mortality rate in children submitted to immediate treatment is low [33].

The greater susceptibility of children has been attributed to the immature immune system, weak renal clearance of the toxin, and the fact that children are common carriers of microorganisms [30]. In the most severe cases, exfoliation may affect the entire corporal surface [33]. The quick and sensitive diagnosis of those infections may be performed using radioimmunoassays, enzyme-linked immunosorbent assays, the reverse passive latex agglutination assay [26] as well as the polymerase chain reaction (PCR) to amplify the genes that codify ETs.

When the ET serotypes and the clinical forms of the disease were correlated, the ETA toxin was found to be associated with bullous impetigo formation, whereas ETB was found to be associated with SSSS, a generalized manifestation [34]. The ETB plasmid has multiple genes that confer antibiotic resistance, which contributes to the increased resistance of *etb*-positive *S. aureus* strains [35]. The *etd*-positive strains have been isolated mainly from patients with deep pyoderma [12].

In addition to *S. aureus*, *Staphylococcus hyicus* and *Staphylococcus chromogenes* are also associated with skin infections and produce exfoliative toxins [36]. In *S. hyicus*, ET production has been associated with exudative epidermitis (EE) in pigs [37]. The toxin also has the capacity to cleave swine desmoglein [38, 39]. Clinical manifestations are characterized by exfoliation accompanied by epidermal cell separation, erythema, and serous exudation [40]. The isolated toxins of these clinical manifestations have been denominated as SHETA and SHETB [41] and ExhA, ExhB, ExhC [41], and ExhD [38, 42]. In 2007, a *Staphylococcus sciuri* strain, highly pathogenic and *ExhC*-positive, was described as the etiological agent of EE in pigs in China [43]. The ExhC recombinant protein (rExhC) has induced necrosis *in vitro* and has caused skin lesions in newborn mice [44].

Currently many phylogenetically distant hosts are described as being susceptible to exfoliation caused by the same isoforms of ET, revealing a certain specificity for various host organisms [29]. Among six different ETs (SHETA, SHETB, ExhA, ExhB, ExhC, and ExhD) codified by *S. hyicus*, SHET toxins caused exfoliation in piglets and chicks, but not in mouse, rat, guinea pig, hamster, dog, or cat [30]. All four Exh toxins cause exfoliation in pigs, but only ExhA and ExhC cause it in neonatal mice [40, 42]. SCET exfoliative toxin of *Staphylococcus chromogenes* also induces exfoliation in two different hosts; pigs and chicks. Different hosts are also susceptible to EXI exfoliative toxin of *Staphylococcus pseudintermedius* that induces exfoliation in dogs and mice.

Infections by *et*-positive *Staphylococcus intermedius* in dogs can also cause a pathology that resembles SSSS and EE [45]. A previous study described the distribution of toxin genes among phage types of animal isolates of *S. aureus* and the canine isolates of phage group II that harbored the *eta* gene [46].

In Japan, hospital-acquired methicillin-resistant *S. aureus* (HA-MRSA) strains frequently carry the *etb* gene [47] and, isolated samples of *etb*-positive *S. aureus* have been encountered in strains with mecA, contrary to the isolated samples of *eta*-positive *S. aureus* [48].

ET-producing *S. aureus* strains (*eta* and *etb*) are related to the clonal complex CC121 [49]. Infections with Staphylococci of this complex are associated with clinical features like impetigo, staphylococcal scalded skin syndrome, conjunctivitis, and exfoliative dermatitis [50].

3. Structural biology and mechanism of exfoliative toxins

The crystal structure of ETA was the first to be determined in atomic detail [51], followed by ETB [52] and by ETD [24] and currently, the atomic coordinates of six ET structures have been deposited with the Protein Data Bank (www.rcsb.org). The crystallographic structures of ETs have revealed much about their mechanisms of action, lack of hydrolytic activity against substrates in the native state, and the susceptibility of certain constituent layers of the epidermis to disruption by ETs.

4. Similarities and differences among ETs and other serino proteinases

Exfoliative toxins are glutamic-acid specific trypsin-like serine proteinases that share 50% sequence identity but display very low sequence identity with other serine proteases. The significant sequence identity of ETs is also reflected in the high structural similarity as evidenced by the low RMSD values of the superposed structures (ETA-ETB: 0.9, ETA-ETD: 1.3, and ETB-ETD: 0.6). Similar to other trypsin-like serine-proteinases, the three-dimensional structures of ETs are characterized by two six-stranded β-barrels domains, S1 and S2, whose axes lie roughly perpendicular to each other, a Greek key motif consisting of four antiparallel strands and N- and C-terminal extensions. The amino acids constituting the catalytic triad (His-Ser-Asp) and Thr190 and His213 which are characteristic of glutamate-specific serine proteinases are located at the junction of the S1 and S2 domains [51, 53].

ETs specifically cleave both mouse and human desmoglein 1 following glutamic acid 381, however only the presence of the Glu^{381}–Gly^{382} bond, highly conserved in desmogleins, does not guarantee hydrolysis. The prerequisites for the exquisite specificity exhibited by ETs involves not only the presence of this cleavage site, but, also (1) the presence of the highly charged N-terminal alpha-helix, (2) the calcium dependent conformation of its substrate Dsg-1, and (3) existence of a specific sequence 110 residues upstream of the cleavage site of the substrate Dsg-1, characteristics that differentiate them from other typical glutamic-acid-specific serine proteinases of the chymotrypsin family.

(1) The highly charged N-terminal alpha-helix of ETs: The charge profile of N-terminal alpha-helix is significantly different, principally between ETD/ETA and ETB (**Figure 1D**) and its size also varies, containing 15, 11 and 12 residues in ETA, ETB and ETD, respectively.

This N-terminal extension which is unique to ETs and its deletion results in an inactive protein [53, 54] that interacts with residues in loop 2 thereby coordinating and determining the architecture of the S1 pocket and hence contributing to substrate specificity [51–53] by modifying the pocket entrance. The amino acid sequences (**Figure 1D**) and the conformations in loop2 (**Figure 1E**) are different in the ETs. In ETA (**Figure 1E**), this loop is longer than in ETB and ETD, additionally its Trp14 and Tyr18 present in the N-terminal

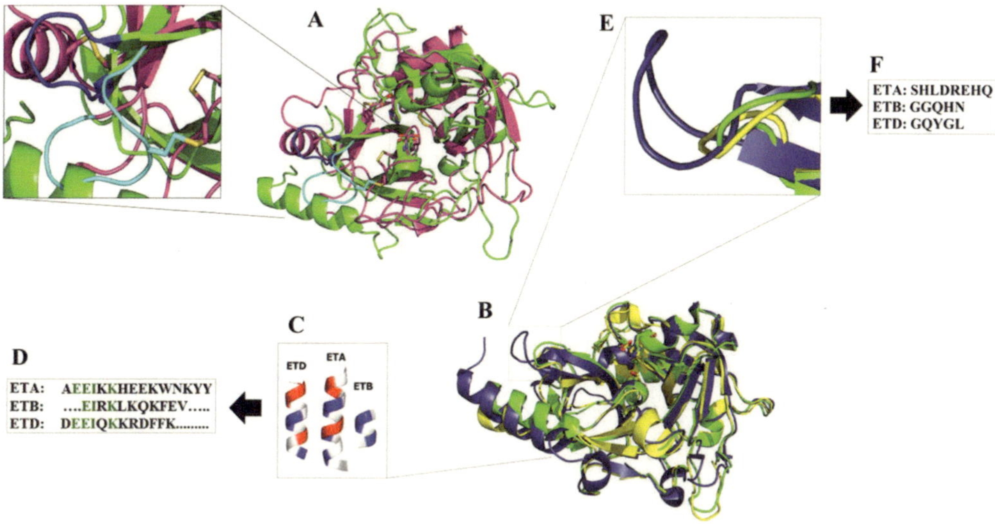

Figure 1. Results of superpositioning of the three-dimensional structures: (A) ETD in green and a serine proteinase [PDB:2AIP] of the trypsin subfamily in pink. The loop 2 is dark blue in ETD, and the equivalent loop of serine proteinase is light blue. (B) ETA (blue), ETB (yellow) and ETD (green); amino acid sequences (C) and charge profile of the N-terminal helices (D) and its variation in the amino acid sequences. (E) The lengths of loop 2 in ETA (blue), ETB (yellow) and ETD (green) and its variation in the amino acid sequences (F).

helix are buried deeper in the S1 pocket than in ETB which contains Lys and Glu and in ETD with Arg and Lys at these equivalent positions. In the other trypsin-like serine proteinases, the presence of a disulfide bridge determines the conformation of the pocket (**Figure 1A**).

(2) **Calcium dependent conformation of Dsg-1:** Dsg1 is a member of the cadherin super-gene family [55] and most of these proteins require calcium to promote cell–cell adhesion and to ensure the proper conformation [56, 57]. Unlike trypsin, ETs are not capable of cleaving heat-denatured Dsg1 or Ca^{2+} depleted Dsg1 [58] and circular dichroism demonstrates that ET specificity is dependent on calcium-stabilized conformation of Dsg1.

(3) **Residues upstream of the Dsg-1 cleavage site are critical for its hydrolysis by ETA**: ETA is able to bind but is unable to cleave canine Dsg1 and a sequence of 5 amino acids 110 residues upstream of the cleavage site are essential for the hydrolysis of Dsg1 by ETA [59]. Four of five of these critical residues are identical in human and mouse Dsg-1(**Figure 2**) and when replaced in canine Dsg-1 at its same position, the cleavage by ETA becomes susceptible. The recognition of this peculiar sequence (Q271-x-x-Y274-T275-I276-E277) is one of the factors that make ETs highly specific in Dsg cleavage, even among homologous Dsg-1s. This also demonstrated that E5 and EC4 do not exert any influence on the cleavage of the substrate and the chimeric human Dsg-3 containing swapped amino acids 214-398 of Dsg-1was cleaved by ETA.

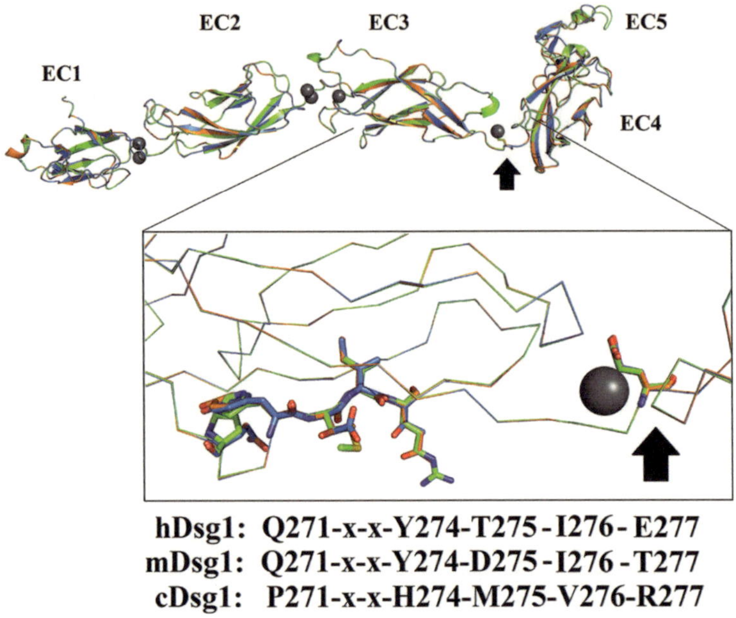

Figure 2. Results of superpositioning of the structural model of human Dsg1(orange), canine Dsg1 (green) and mouse Dsg1 (blue), purple spheres represent bound Ca2+, the susceptible glutamic acid is indicated by an arrow; amino acids sequence of the human, mouse, and canine Dsg1s upstream of the cleavage site; upstream location of the recognition sequence and the susceptible glutamic acid.

5. Tyrosines 157 and 159 are essential for ETB activity

Based on the results of site-directed mutagenesis, Sakurai et al. [60] concluded that the substitution of either Tyr 157 or 159 in ETB decreased exfoliative activity and the double mutation resulted in the complete loss of exfoliative activity and antigenicity. Interestingly, ETA does not possess either one of these tyrosines but contains Phe and His at these positions and in ETD these positions are occupied by Tyr and Thr.

6. Why are the exfoliative toxins inactive in the native states?

Gly193 is highly conserved in serine proteinases, however, in structures of ETs the peptide bond between residues 192 and 193 (chymotrypsin numbering) is flipped 180° relative to the other serine proteases. Pro192 in ETA and ETD and Val192 (ETB) form hydrogen bonds with both the amide nitrogen atoms and the hydroxyl oxygen atoms of the catalytic serine residues interrupting the charge-relay-network. These enzymes can only be functional if this bond is ruptured and the conformation is restored as in other serine proteinases.

http://dx.doi.org/10.5772/66528

7. Molecular mechanisms of the *S. aureus* exfoliative toxin

7.1. *S. aureus* exfoliative toxins selectively and directly solubilize mouse and human desmoglein 1

In 1970, Melish and Glasgow first investigated mechanisms of action of the exfoliative toxin (ET)-producing *S. aureus* in SSSS [11]. When the organisms isolated from SSSS patients were injected into neonatal mice, they cause epidermal blisters resembling those in the naturally occurred human disease. Several years later, two serotypes of ETs, ETA and ETB, which are capable of inducing epidermal blisters, were identified [21]. However, the exact molecular mechanisms of ET-causing epidermal blisters had long been unknown over the three decades.

In 2000, Amagai and colleagues established desmoglein 1 (Dsg1), a desmosomal cadherin-type adhesion molecule and also known as pemphigus foliaceus autoantigen, as the target of *S. aureus* ETs [61]. They advocate this hypothesis based on the fact that histopathology of superficial epidermal blisters created by ET injection in mice resembles to those created by pemphigus foliaceus IgG. They revealed that immunostaining for the extracellular domain of Dsg1, but not that for Dsg3, is abolished in ETA-injected mouse skin. Moreover, an *in vitro* analysis revealed that ETA selectively solubilize the recombinant extracellular segments of human and mouse Dsg1 (α) produced by baculovirus. The same group also identified that *S. aureus* ETB and a newly identified ETD have similar enzymatic activity to solubilize Dsg1 [10, 12].

The site of blister formation by ETs could be explained in the context of tissue distribution of desmosomal cadherins (**Figure 3**) [13, 62].

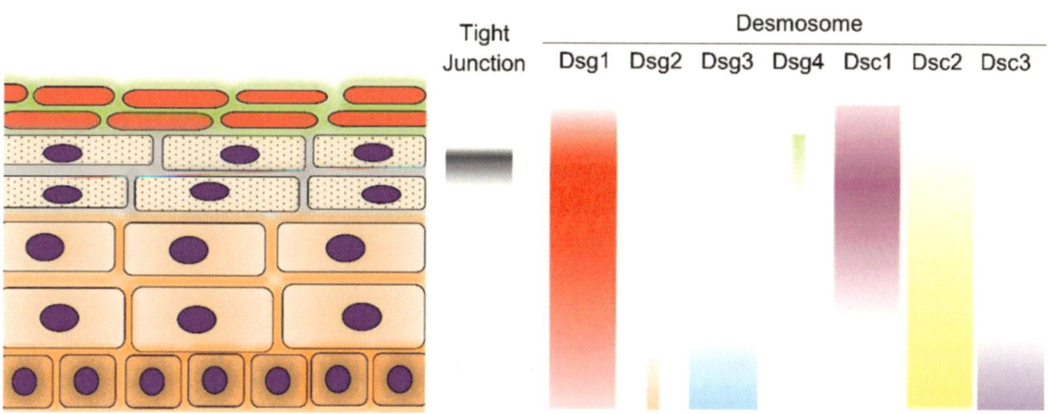

Figure 3. Distribution of functional tight junction and desmosomalcadherins in the epidermis. Dsg, desmoglein; Dsc, desmocollin. Functional tight junctions are located in the upper granular layer. Expression pattern of four isoforms of desmogleins (Dsg) and three isoforms of desmocollins (Dsc) is associated with differentiation level of keratinocytes.

In humans, there are four subclasses of Dsg with different tissue distributions. Among them, Dsg2 is expressed in all desmosome-bearing tissues, whereas Dsg1 and Dsg3 are expressed preferentially in stratified squamous epithelia [63]. Dsg1 and Dsg3 are hypothesized to have compensatory effects [64]. For example, if both Dsg1 and Dsg3 express in the same epithelial cells, and adhesive function by Dsg1 is abolished, the loss of adhesive function can be compensated by intact Dsg3. In the epidermis, Dsg1 is expressed in the whole layers, whereas Dsg3 is expressed in basal and immediate suprabasal layers [65]. In contrast, in oral mucous membrane, both Dsg1 and Dsg3 are expressed in the whole layer, but the expression level of Dsg1 is relatively low compared with that of Dsg3 [63]. As Dsg2 and Dsg4 are expressed weakly in basal and upper granular layers, respectively [65], these molecules may have less ability to compensate the loss of Dsg1 function.

Desmocollin (Dsc) 1, another desmosomal cadherin is also expressed in superficial epidermis. It is hypothesized that Dsg1 and Dsc1 may have combinational effect on integrity of keratinocyte cell adhesion [66]: Abolishment of either Dsg1 by ETs or genetic ablation of Dsc1 causes dissociation of keratinocytes in the superficial layer of mouse epidermis [10, 13, 59, 67]. If adhesive function of Dsg1 is abolished by ETs, it may cause keratinocyte separation only in spinous-to-granular layers of epidermis, in which loss of adhesive function by Dsg1 could not be compensated by other Dsgs. This could be a reasonable explanation why ETs cause only superficial epidermal blisters in SSSS patients, although ETs produced in upper respiratory organs (e.g., tonsils), enter the circulatory system and induce toxemia [27].

7.2. *S. aureus* ETs are unique glutamate-specific serine proteases that hydrolyze a single peptide bond within the extracellular segment of Dsg1

Hanakawa et al. demonstrated that substitution of catalytic serine in ETA, ETB and ETD to alanine causes loss of their functions to solubilize Dsg1 [59]. Kinetic analysis of three ETs revealed kcat/Km values in the range of 2–6 × 104 M^{-1} s^{-1}, suggesting their efficient enzymatic activity to digest relatively large molecules. These findings indicate that three known *S. aureus* ETs are serine proteases that efficiently solubilize the extracellular segment of Dsg1.

The same group also investigated substrate-specificity of *S. aureus* ETs [58]. All three ETs cleave human and mouse Dsg1 (α) into two segments. Moreover, mouse has three isoforms of Dsg1 (Dsg1-α, -β and -γ) [65, 68], and ETA solubilize the extracellular segments of mouse Dsg1-α and -β, but not that of Dsg1-γ in which glutamic acid residue 381 is substituted by lysine [66, 68]. These findings indicate the specificity of the glutamic acid residue as the cleavage site of Dsg1 by ET.

S. aureus ETs are unique serine proteases that specifically and efficiently cleave only one peptide bond in the extracellular segment of Dsg1. The enzymatic properties of *S. aureus* ETs cause efficient and specific abolishment of a major epidermal adhesion molecule in selected mammalian species.

7.3. Possible mechanisms of ET-associated keratinocyte dissociation

Desmosomes composed of two major transmembrane cadherin-type adhesion molecules (Dsg and Dsc) and cytoplasmic plaque proteins that link between desmosomal cadherins and intracellular cytoskeletons. It has been long debated questions whether disruption of Dsgs alone by pemphigus autoantibodies is sufficient to cause keratinocyte dissociation, or subsequent disorganization of other desmosomal consituents in plasma membrane of keratinocytes is necessary [69].

To determine whether cleavage of the extracellular segment of Dsg1 by *S. aureus* ETs is sufficient to cause keratinocyte dissociation, our group has investigated the fate of desmosomal constituents in ETA-injected mouse skin [66]. We found that the amino-termini of Dsg1 is abolished in plasma membrane of murine epidermal keratinocytes, whereas cleaved carboxyl-termini of Dsg1 and the extracellular segment of Dsc1 remained on the surface of keratinocytes faced to blister cavity in the early phase of keratinocyte dissociation. Based on these findings, we proposed a theory that removal of the amino-termini of Dsg1 by ETs is sufficient to initiate *in vivo* keratinocyte dissociation.

Meanwhile, Simpson et al. proposed another theory for ET-induced keratinocyte dissociation through sequestration of plakoglobin (PG), a member of catenin family cytoplasmic protein, by ectodomain-deleted Dsg1 [70]. When truncated Dsg1, in which amino acids 1–381 were spliced to mimic ET-cleaved carboxy-termini of Dsg1, was expressed in primary human keratinocytes, it reduced mechanical strength of keratinocyte sheets in a dose-dependent manner, implicating a dominant-negative effect by truncated Dsg1. Truncated Dsg1 localized in close to intercellular borders and reduce endogenous desmosomal cadherin Dsc3 and desmosomal plaque protein desmoplakin in intercellular borders. In the same cells, PG localized in intercellular borders and seem to be associated with truncated Dsg1. Remarkably, triple-point mutation of the PG-binding region in the truncated Dsg1 restored mechanical integrity of keratinocyte sheets, implicating that PG binding to truncated Dsg1 is essential in disruption of desmosomes and subsequent keratinocyte dissociation.

Putting all these findings together, the authors advocate a theory that cleavage of Dsg1 by ETs initiate keratinocyte dissociation, while subsequent PG sequestration may contribute to the expansion of intercellular spaces between keratinocytes (**Figure 4**). Further accumulation of *in vivo* evidences to elucidate the role of PG in ET-inducing keratinocyte dissociation will be expected.

7.4. How ET-producing *S. aureus* penetrate the epidermis through firm keratinocyte adhesion in the upper stratum granulosum?

The aforementioned theory can satisfactorily explain how ETs cause blistering in SSSS, in which ETs access to the skin from dermal side. However, this theory cannot explain the mechanisms of blistering in bullous impetigo, in which ET-producing *S. aureus* enter the epidermis from the skin surface. It has been reported that ETs do not penetrate tight junction, an occlusive adhesive structure located at the upper granular layer (**Figure 5**) [71]. Then the question arises how ET-producing *S. aureus* invade the epidermis apart from a route of microwounds on the skin.

To address this issue, we recently established a mouse model of bullous impetigo [72]. *S. aureus* harboring *etb* gene was inoculated epicutaneously to murine inner pinnae after the stratum corneum was partially removed by tape stripping. Intraepidermal neutrophilic pustules containing intercellular staphylococci were successfully created in the mouse skin by 6

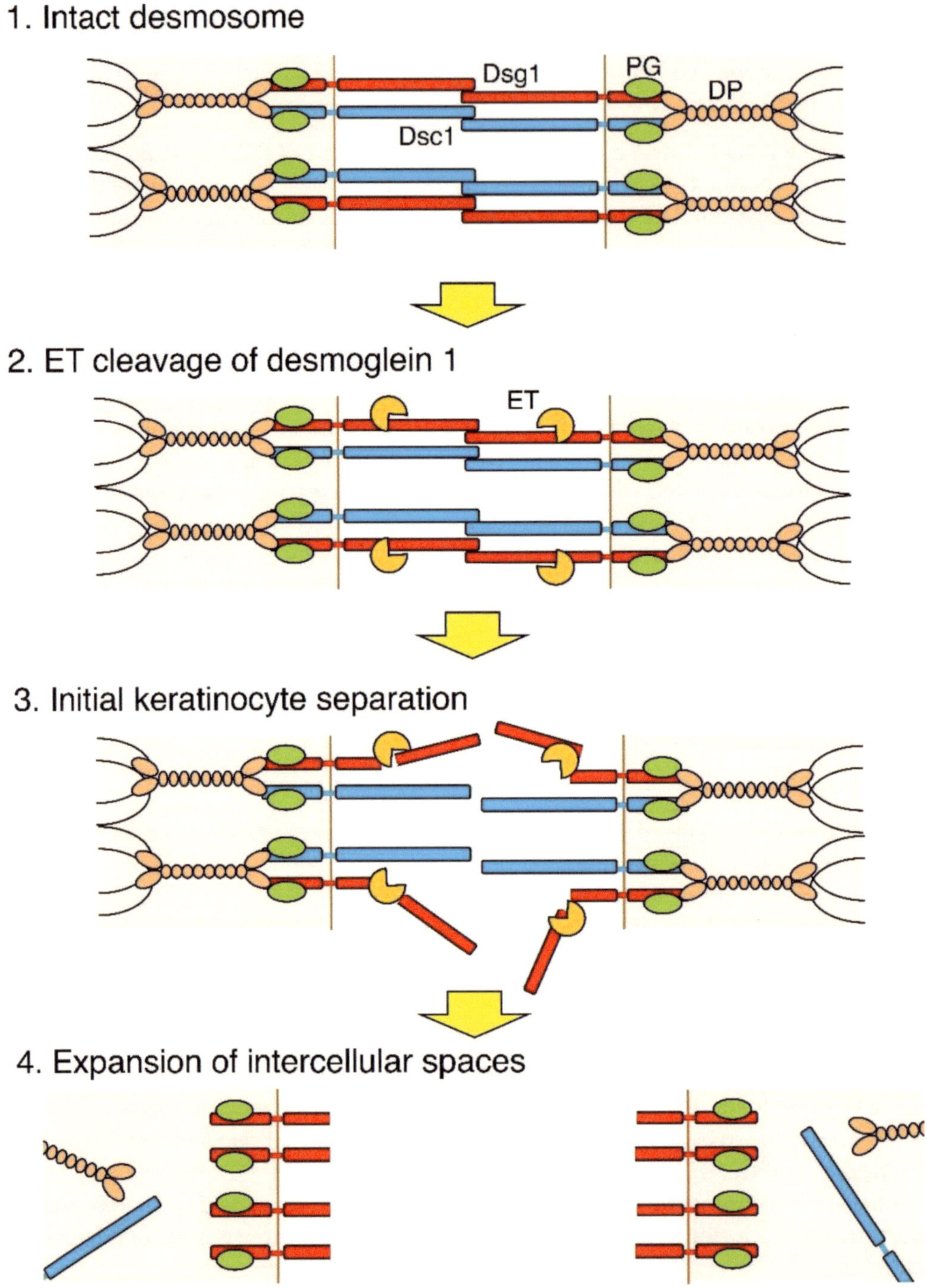

Figure 4. Possible mechanisms of ET-induced keratinocyte dissociation. PG, plakoglobin. Cleavage of the extracellular segment of Dsg1 initiates keratinocyte separation. Sequestration of PG by truncated Dsg1 and disintegrity of other desmosomal components are associated with expansion of the intercellular spaces between keratinocytes.

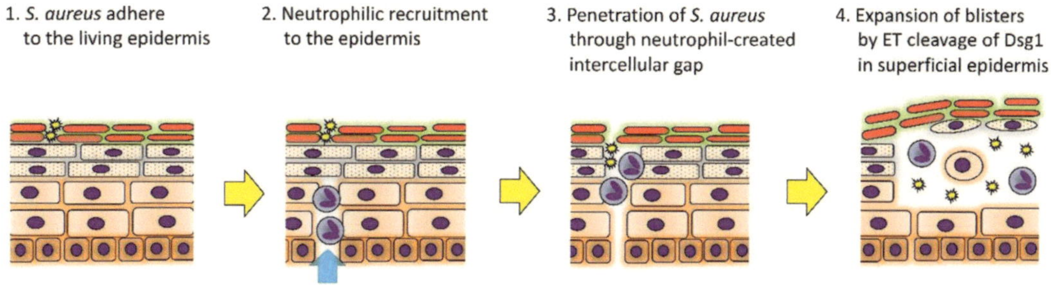

Figure 5. Proposed theory for bacterial cutaneous invasion and blistering in bullous impetigo. *S. aureus* harboring at gene adhere to the living epidermis recruits neutrophils. When neutrophils create intercellular gap between superficial keratinocytes, *S. aureus* produce ET to expand the blisters by cleavage of Dsg1.

hours after the inoculation. The size of intraepidermal pustules created by *etb* gene-harboring strains was significantly larger than those created by et gene-negative strains. Chronological study revealed that staphylococci invaded the epidermis after neutrophils infiltrated the skin. Moreover, if the neutrophilic infiltration was blocked by injection of cyclophosphamide, staphylococci in the epidermis were not recognized at all.

Based on these findings, we propose a novel hypothesis for percutaneous entry of ET-producing *S. aureus* in bullous impetigo. These strains may invade the epidermis through intercellular spaces created by skin-infiltrated neutrophils. In addition, once *S. aureus* invade the epidermis, ETs expand the interkeratinocyte spaces, which allows bacteria to skew neutrophils attack in blister cavity. Future studies to elucidate the molecular interactions that underlie neutrophilic epidermal infiltration in response to *S. aureus* adhere to living keratinocytes. In addition, the mechanisms how ET-producing penetrate the stratum corneum remains to be elucidated.

Author details

Ricardo B. Mariutti[1], Natayme R. Tartaglia[2, 3], Núbia Seyffert[4], Thiago Luiz de Paula Castro[2], Raghuvir K. Arni[1], Vasco A. Azevedo[2], Yves Le Loir[3] and Koji Nishifuji[5]*

*Address all correspondence to: kojimail@cc.tuat.ac.jp

1 Multiuser Center for Biomolecular Innovation, IBILCE/UNESP, São José do Rio Preto, SP, Brazil

2 Federal University of Minas Gerais, Belo Horizonte, MG, Brazil

3 Institut National de la Recherche Agronomique, Rennes, France

4 Federal University of Pará, Belém, Brazil

5 Tokyo University of Agriculture and Technology, Tokyo, Japan

References

[1] Gordon, R.J., Lowy, F.D. Pathogenesis of methicillin resistant *Staphylococcus aureus* infection. Clin. Infect. Dis. 2008,**46**:S350–S359. DOI:10.1086/533591

[2] Ortega, E., Abriouel, H., Lucas, R., Gálvez, A. Multiple roles of *Staphylococcus aureus* enterotoxins: pathogenicity, superantigenic activity, correlation to antibiotic resistance. Toxins. 2010,**2**:2117–2131. DOI:10.3390/toxins2082117

[3] Popov, L., Kovalski, J., Grandi, G., Bagnoli, F., Amieva, M.R. Three-dimensional human skin models to understand *Staphylococcus aureus* skin colonization and infection. Front. Immunol. 2014,**5**:41. DOI:10.3389/fimmu.2014.00041

[4] Ishii, Y. Identification of biochemically atypical *Staphylococcus aureus* clinical isolates with three automated identification systems. J. Med. Microbiol. 2006,**55**:387–392. DOI:10.1099/jmm.0.46231-0

[5] Cepeda, J.A., Whitehouse, T., Cooper, B., Hails, J., Jones, K., Kwaku, F., Kibbler, C. Isolation of patients in single rooms or cohorts to reduce spread of MRSA in intensive-care units: prospective two centre study. Lancet. 2005,**365**:295–304. DOI:10.1016/S0140-6736(05)17783-6; 10.1016/S0140-6736%2805%2917783-6

[6] Kniehl, E., Becker, A., Forster, D.H. Bed, bath and beyond: pitfalls in prompt eradication of methicillin-resistant *Staphylococcus aureus* carrier status in healthcare workers. J. Hosp. Infect. 2005,**59**:180–187. DOI:10.1016/j.jhin.2004.06.016

[7] Feil, E.J., Cooper, J.E., Grundmann, H., Robinson, D.A., Enright, M.C., Berendt, T., Peacock, S.J., Smith, J.M., Murphy, M., Spratt, B.G. How clonal is *Staphylococcus aureus*? J. Bacteriol. 2003,**185**:3307–3316. DOI:10.1128/JB.185.11.3307-3316

[8] Iandolo, J.J. Genetic analysis of extracellular toxins of *Staphylococcus aureus*. Ann. Rev. Microbiol. 1989,**43**(1):375–402. DOI:10.1128/MMBR.00055-13

[9] Marrack, P., Blackman, M., Kushnir, E., Kappler, J. The toxicity of staphylococcal enterotoxin B in mice is mediated by T cells. J. Exp. Med. 1990,**1712**:455–464. PMCID: PMC2187711

[10] Amagai, M., Yamaguchi, T., Hanakawa, Y., Nishifuji, K., Sugai, M., Stanley, J.R. Staphylococcal exfoliative toxin B specifically cleaves desmoglein 1. J. Invest. Dermatol. 2002,**118**:845–850. DOI:10.1046/j.1523-1747·2002.01751.x

[11] Melish, M.E., Glasgow, L.A. Staphylococcal scalded skin syndrome: the expanded clinical syndrome. J. Pediatr. 1971,**78**:958–967. DOI:10.1016/S0022-3476(71)80425-0; 10.1016/S0022-3476%2871%2980425-0

[12] Yamaguchi, T., Nishifuji, K., Sasaki, M., Fudaba, Y., Aepfelbacher, M., Takata, T., Ohara, M., Komatsuzawa, H., Amagai, M., Sugai, M. Identification of the *Staphylococcus aureus* etd pathogenicity island which encodes a novel exfoliative toxin, ETD, and EDIN-B. Infect. Immun. 2002,**70**:5835–5845. DOI:10.1128/IAI.70.10.5835-5845.2002

[13] Nishifuji, K., Sugai, M., Amagai, M. Staphylococcal exfoliative toxins: molecular scissors of bacteria that attack the cutaneous defense barrier in mammals. J. Dermatol. Sci. 2008,**49**:21–31. DOI:10.1016/j.jdermsci.2007.05.007

[14] Lyell, A. The staphylococcal scalded skin syndrome in historical perspective: emergence of dermopathic strains of *Staphylococcus aureus* and discovery of the epidermolytic toxin. A review of events up to 1970. J. Am. Acad. Dermatol. 1983,**9**:285–294. PMID: 6350386

[15] Lyell, A. A review of toxic epidermal necrolysis in Britain. Br. J. Dermatol. 1967,**79**:662–671. DOI:10.1111/j.1365-2133.1967.tb11434.x

[16] Lyell, A. Toxic epidermal necrolysis the scalded skin syndrome: a reappraisal. Br. J. Dermatol. 1979,**100**:69–86.DOI:10.1111/j.1365-2133.1979.tb03571.x

[17] Lillibridge, C.B., Melish, M.E., Glasgow, L.A. Site of action of exfoliative toxin in the staphylococcal scaled-skin syndrome. Pediatrics. 1972,**50**:728–738. PMID: 4263751

[18] Melish, M.E., Glasgow, L.A. The staphylococcal scalded-skin syndrome: development of an experimental model. N. Engl. J. Med. 1970,**282**:1114–1119. DOI:10.1084/jem.20111718

[19] Kapral, F.A., Miller, M.M. Product of *Staphylococcus aureus* responsible for the scalded-skin syndrome. Infect. Immun. 1971,**4**:541–545. PMCID: PMC416349

[20] Kondo, I., Sakurai, S., Sarai, Y. Purification of exfoliatin produced by *Staphylococcus aureus* of bacteriophage group 2 and its physicochemical properties. Infect. Immun. 1973,**8**:156–164.

[21] Kondo, I., Sakurai, S., Sarai, Y. New type of exfoliatin obtained from staphylococcal strains, belonging to phage groups other than group II, isolated from patients with impetigo and Ritter's disease. Infect. Immun. 1974,**10**:851–861. PMCID: PMC423032

[22] Lee, C.Y., Schmidt, J.J., Johnson-Winegar, A.D., Spero, L., Iandolo, J.J. Sequence determination and comparison of the exfoliative toxin A and toxin B genes from *Staphylococcus aureus*. J. Bacteriol. 1987,**1699**:3904–3909. PMCID: PMC213685

[23] Le Maréchal, C., Jardin, J., Jan, G., Even, S., Pulido, C., Guibert, J.M., Hernandez, D., François, P., Schrenzel, J., Demon, D., Meyer, E., Berkova, N., Thiéry, R., Vautor, E., Le Loir, Y. *Staphylococcus aureus* seroproteomes discriminate ruminant isolates causing mild or severe mastitis. Vet. Research. 2011,**421**:35–55. DOI:10.1186/1297-9716-42-35

[24] Mariutti, R.B., Souza, T.A.C.B., Ullah, A., Caruso, I.P., de Moraes, F.R., Zanphorlin, L.M., Tartaglia, N.R., Seyffert, N., Azevedo, V.A., Le Loir, Y., Murakami, M.T., Arni, R.K. Crystal structure of *Staphylococcus aureus* exfoliative toxin D-like protein: structural basis for the high specificity of exfoliative toxins. Biochem. Biophys. Res. Commun. 2015,**467**:171–177. DOI:10.1016/j.bbrc.2015.08.083.

[25] O'Toole, P.W., Foster, T.J. Molecular cloning and expression of the epidermolytic toxin a gene of *Staphylococcus aureus*. Microbial. Pathogenesis. 1986,**1**(6):583–594. PMID:3508500

[26] Ladhani, S. Recent developments in staphylococcal scalded skin syndrome. Clin. Microbiol. Infect. Off. Publ. Eur. Soc. Clin. Microbiol. Infect. Dis. 2001,**7**:301–307. PMID: 11442563

[27] Bailey, C.J., de Azavedo, J., Arbuthnott, J.P. A comparative study of two serotypes of epidermolytic toxin from *Staphylococcus aureus*. Biochim. Biophys. Acta. 1980;**624**:111–120. PMID: 6773585

[28] Sato, H., Matsumori, Y., Tanabe, T., Saito, H., Shimizu, A., Kawano, J. A new type of staphylococcal exfoliative toxin from a *Staphylococcus aureus* strain isolated from a horse with phlegmon. Infect. Immun. 1994,**62**:3780–3785. PMCID: PMC303031

[29] Bukowski, M., Wladyka, B., Dubin, G. Exfoliative toxins of *Staphylococcus aureus*. Toxins. 2010,**2**:1148–1165. DOI:10.3390/toxins2051148

[30] Ladhani, S. Understanding the mechanism of action of the exfoliative toxins of *Staphylococcus aureus*. FEMS Immunol. Med. Microbiol. 2003,**39**:181–189. DOI:10.1016/S0928-8244(03)00225-6

[31] Mueller, E., Haim, M., Petnehazy, T., Acham-Roschitz, B., Trop, M. An innovative local treatment for staphylococcal scalded skin syndrome. Eur. J. Clin. Microbiol. Infect. Dis. Off. Publ. Eur. Soc. Clin. Microbiol. 2010,**29**:893–897. DOI:10.1007/s10096-010-0927-x.

[32] Cribier, B., Piemont, Y., Grosshans, E. Staphylococcal scalded skin syndrome in adults. A clinical review illustrated with a new case. J. Am. Acad. Dermatol. 1994,**30**:319–324. PMID:8294590

[33] Jeyakumari, D., Gopal, R., Eswaran, M., Maheshkumar, C. Staphylococcal scalded skin syndrome in a newborn. J. Glob. Infect. Dis. 2009,**1**:45–47. DOI:10.1155/2015/901968

[34] Yamasaki, O., Yamaguchi, T., Sugai, M., Chapuis-Cellier, C., Arnaud, F., Vandenesch, F., Etienne, J., Lina, G. Clinical manifestations of staphylococcal scalded-skin syndrome depend on serotypes of exfoliative toxins. J. Clin. Microbiol. 2005,**43**:1890–1893. DOI:10.1128/JCM.43.4.1890–1893.2005

[35] Hisatsune, J., Hirakawa, H., Yamaguchi, T., Fudaba, Y., Oshima, K., Hattori, M., Kato, F., Kayama, S., Sugai, M. Emergence of *Staphylococcus aureus* carrying multiple drug resistance genes on a plasmid encoding exfoliative toxin B. Antimicrob. Agents Chemother. 2013,**57**:6131–6140. DOI:10.1128/AAC.01062-13

[36] Futagawa-Saito, K., Makino, S., Sunaga, F., Kato, Y., Sakurai-Komada, N., Ba-Thein, W., Fukuyasu, T. Identification of first exfoliative toxin in *Staphylococcus pseudintermedius*. FEMS Microbiol. Lett. 2009,**301**:176–180. DOI:10.1111/j.1574-6968.2009.01823.x

[37] Wegener, H.C., Andresen, L.O., Bille-Hansen, V. *Staphylococcus hyicus* virulence in relation to exudative epidermitis in pigs. Can. J. Vet. Res. Rev. Can. Rech. Vét. 1993,**57**:119–125. PMCID:PMC1263605

[38] Fudaba, Y., Nishifuji, K., Andresen, L.O., Yamaguchi, T., Komatsuzawa, H., Amagai, M., Sugai, M. *Staphylococcus hyicus* exfoliative toxins selectively digest porcine desmoglein 1. Microb. Pathog. 2005,**39**:171–176. DOI:10.1016/j.micpath.2005.08.003

[39] Nishifuji, K., Fudaba, Y., Yamaguchi, T., Iwasaki, T., Sugai, M., Amagai, M. Cloning of swine desmoglein 1 and its direct proteolysis by *Staphylococcus hyicus* exfoliative toxins isolated from pigs with exudative epidermitis. Vet. Dermatol. 2005,**16**:315–323. DOI:10.1111/j.1365-3164.2005.00474.x

[40] Ahrens, P., Andresen, L.O. Cloning and sequence analysis of genes encoding *Staphylococcus hyicus* exfoliative toxin types A, B, C, and D. J. Bacteriol. 2004,**186**:1833–1837. PMCID:PMC355961

[41] Sato, H., Watanabe, T., Higuchi, K., Teruya, K., Ohtake, A., Murata, Y., Saito, H., Aizawa, C., Danbara, H., Maehara, N. Chromosomal and extrachromosomal synthesis of exfoliative toxin from *Staphylococcus hyicus*. J. Bacteriol. 2000,**182**:4096–4100. DOI:10.1128/JB.182.14.4096-4100.2000

[42] Andresen, L.O. Differentiation and distribution of three types of exfoliative toxin produced by *Staphylococcus hyicus* from pigs with exudative epidermitis. FEMS Immunol. Med. Microbiol. 1998,**20**:301–310. DOI:10.1111/j.1574-695X.1998.tb01140.x

[43] Chen, S., Wang, Y., Chen, F., Yang, H., Gan, M., Zheng, S.J. A highly pathogenic strain of *Staphylococcus sciuri* caused fatal exudative epidermitis in piglets. PLoS One 2007,**2**:147. DOI:10.1371/journal.pone.0000147

[44] Li, H., Wang, Y., Ding, L., Zheng, S.J. *Staphylococcus sciuri* exfoliative toxin C ExhC is a necrosis-inducer for mammalian cells. PLoS One. 2011,**6**:23145. DOI:10.1371/journal.pone.0023145.

[45] Terauchi, R., Sato, H., Endo, Y., Aizawa, C., Maehara, N. Cloning of the gene coding for *Staphylococcus intermedius* exfoliative toxin and its expression in *Escherichia coli*. Vet. Microbiol. 2003,**94**:31–38. DOI:10.1016/S0378-1135(03)00047-6

[46] Garbacz, K., Piechowicz, L., Mroczkowska, A. Distribution of toxin genes among different spa types and phage types of animal *Staphylococcus aureus*. Arch. Microbiol. 2015,**197**:935–940. DOI:10.1007/s00203-015-1127-y

[47] Motoshima, M., Yanagihara, K., Morinaga, Y., Matsuda, J., Sugahara, K., Yamada, Y., Kohno, S., Kamihira, S. Genetic diagnosis of community-acquired MRSA: a multiplex real-time PCR method for Staphylococcal cassette chromosome mec typing and detecting toxin genes. Tohoku J. Exp. Med. 2010,**220**:165–170. DOI:10.1620/tjem.220.165

[48] Nakaminami, H., Noguchi, N., Ikeda, M., Hasui, M., Sato, M., Yamamoto, S., Yoshida, T., Asano, T., Senoue, M., Sasatsu, M. Molecular epidemiology and antimicrobial susceptibilities of 273 exfoliative toxin-encoding-gene-positive *Staphylococcus aureus* isolates from patients with impetigo in Japan. J. Med. Microbiol. 2008,**57**:1251–1258. DOI:10.1099/jmm.0.2008/002824-0.

[49] Larsen, A.R., Skov, R.L., Jarlier, V., Henriksen, A.S. Epidemiological differences between the UK and Ireland versus France in *Staphylococcus aureus* isolates resistant to fusidic acid from community-acquired skin and soft tissue infections. J. Antimicro. Chemother. 2008,**613**:589–594. DOI:10.1093/jac/dkm532

[50] Kurt, K., Rasigade, J.P., Laurent, F., Goering, R.V., Žemličková, H., Machova, I., Ritchie, S. Subpopulations of *Staphylococcus aureus* clonal complex 121 are associated with distinct clinical entities. PLoS One. 2013,**83**:58155. DOI:10.1371/journal.pone.0058155

[51] Vath, G.M., Earhart, C.A., Rago, J.V., Kim, M.H., Bohach, G.A., Schlievert, P.M., Ohlendorf, D.H. The structure of the superantigen exfoliative toxin A suggests a novel regulation as a serine protease. Biochemistry. 1997,**36**:1559–1566. DOI:10.1021/bi962614f

[52] Vath, G.M., Earhart, C.A., Monie, D.D., Iandolo, J.J., Schlievert, P.M., Ohlendorf, D.H. The crystal structure of exfoliative toxin B: a superantigen with enzymatic activity. Biochemistry. 1999,**38**:10239–10246. DOI:10.1021/bi990721e

[53] Cavarelli, J., Prévost, G., Bourguet, W., Moulinier, L., Chevrier, B., Delagoutte, B., Moras, D. The structure of *Staphylococcus aureus* epidermolytic toxin A, an atypic serine protease, at 1.7 Å resolution. Structure. 1997,**56**:813–824. PMID:9261066

[54] Prévost, G., Couppié, P., Monteil, H. Staphylococcal epidermolysins. Curr. Opin. Infect. Dis. 2003,**16**(2):71–76. DOI:10.1097/01.aco.0000065073.06965.58

[55] Angst, B.D., Marcozzi, C., Magee, A.I. The cadherin superfamily: diversity in form and function. J. Cell Sci. 2001,**114**(4):629–641. PMID:11171368

[56] Kemler, R. From cadherins to catenins: cytoplasmic protein interactions and regulation of cell adhesion. Trends Genet. 1993,**9**(9):317–321. PMID:8236461

[57] Steinberg, M.S., McNutt, P.M. Cadherins and their connections: adhesion junctions have broader functions. Curr. Opin. Cell Biol. 1999,**11**(5):554–560. DOI:10.1016/S0955-0674(99)00027-7

[58] Hanakawa, Y., Selwood, T., Woo, D., Lin, C., Schechter, N.M., Stanley, J.R. Calcium-dependent conformation of desmoglein 1 is required for its cleavage by exfoliative toxin. J. Invest. Dermatol. 2003,**121**:383–389. DOI:10.1046/j.1523-1747.2003.12362.x

[59] Hanakawa, Y., Schechter, N.M., Lin, C., Nishifuji, K., Amagai, M., Stanley, J.R. Enzymatic and molecular characteristics of the efficiency and specificity of exfoliative toxin cleavage of desmoglein 1. J. Biol. Chem. 2004,**279**:5268–5277. DOI:10.1074/jbc.M311087200

[60] Sakurai, S., Suzuki, H., Saito, S., Konishi, Y., Machida, K., Kohno, M. New evidence that the Tyr-157 and Tyr-159 residues of Staphylococcal exfoliative toxin B are essential for its toxicity. Microbiol. Immunol. 1998,**42**:829–836. DOI:10.1111/j.1348-0421.1998.tb02358.x

[61] Amagai, M., Matsuyoshi, N., Wang, Z.H., Andl, C., Stanley, J.R. Toxin in bullous impetigo and staphylococcal scalded-skin syndrome targets desmoglein 1. Nat. Med. 2000,**6**:1275–1277. DOI:10.1038/81385

[62] Getsios, S., Huen, A.C., Green, K.J. Working out the strength and flexibility of desmosomes. Nat. Rev. Mol. Cell Biol. 2004,**5**:271–281. DOI:10.1038/nrm1356

[63] Shirakata, Y., Amagai, M., Hanakawa, Y., Nishikawa, T., Hashimoto, K. Lack of mucosal involvement in pemphigus foliaceus may be due to low expression of desmoglein 1. J. Invest. Dermatol. 1998,**10**:76–78. DOI:10.1046/j.1523-1747.1998.00085.x

[64] Amagai, M. Autoimmunity against desmosomalcadherins in pemphigus. J. Dermatol. Sci. 1999,**20**:92–102. PMID: 10379702

[65] Mahoney, M.G., Hu, Y., Brennan, D., Bazzi, H., Christiano, A.M., Wahl, J.K. 3rd. Delineation of diversified desmoglein distribution in stratified squamous epithelia: implications in diseases. Exp. Dermatol. 2006,**15**:101–109. DOI:10.1111/j.1600-0625.2006.00391.x

[66] Nishifuji, K., Shimizu, A., Ishiko, A., Iwasaki, T., Amagai, M. Removal of amino-terminal extracellular domains of desmoglein 1 by staphylococcal exfoliative toxin is sufficient to initiate epidermal blister formation. J. Dermatol. Sci. 2010,**59**:184–191. DOI:10.1016/j.jdermsci.2010.07.010

[67] Chidgey, M., Brakebusch, C., Gustafsson, E., Cruchley, A., Hail, C., Kirk, S., Merritt, A., North, A., Tselepis, C., Hewitt, J., Byrne, C., Fassler, R., Garrod, D. Mice lacking desmocollin 1 show epidermal fragility accompanied by barrier defects and abnormal differentiation. J. Cell Biol. 2001,**155**:821–832. DOI:10.1083/jcb.200105009

[68] Brennan, D., Hu, Y., Kljuic, A., Choi, Y., Joubeh, S., Bashkin, M., Wahl, J., Fertala, A., Pulkkinen, L., Uitto, J., Christiano, A.M., Panteleyev, A., Mahoney, M.G. Differential structural properties and expression patterns suggest functional significance for multiple mouse desmoglein 1 isoforms. Differentiation. 2004,**72**:434–449. DOI:10.1111/j.1432-0436.2004.07208009.x

[69] Amagai, M., Stanley, J.R. Desmoglein as a target in skin disease and beyond. J. Invest. Dermatol. 2012,**132**:776–784. DOI:10.1038/jid.2011.390

[70] Simpson, C.L., Kojima, S., Cooper-Whitehair, V., Getsios, S., Green, K.J. Plakoglobin rescues adhesive defects induced by ectodomain truncation of the desmosomal cadherin desmoglein 1: implications for exfoliative toxin-mediated skin blistering. Am. J. Pathol. 2010,**177**:2921–2937. DOI:10.2353/ajpath.2010.100397

[71] Ouchi, T., Kubo, A., Yokouchi, M., Adachi, T., Kobayashi, T., Kitashima, D.Y., Fujii, H., Clausen, B.E., Koyasu, S., Amagai, M., Nagao, K. Langerhans cell antigen capture through tight junctions confers preemptive immunity in experimental staphylococcal scalded skin syndrome. J. Exp. Med. 2011,**208**:2607–2613. DOI:10.1084/jem.20111718

[72] Imanishi, I., Hattori, S., Hisatsune, J., Ide, K., Sugai, M., Nishifuji, K. Staphylococcus aureus penetrate the inter-keratinocyte spaces created by skin-infiltrating neutrophils in the mouse model of impetigo. Vet Dermatol. 2016 Nov 13. doi: 10.1111/vde.12398. [Epub ahead of print]

Chapter 9

Staphylococcus aureus Enterotoxin Production in Relation to Environmental Factors

Alžbeta Medved'ová, Adriana Havlíková and Ľubomír Valík

Additional information is available at the end of the chapter

http://dx.doi.org/10.5772/66736

Abstract

Staphylococcal enterotoxins (SEs) and SE-like toxins (SEls) are the most notable virulence factors associated with *Staphylococcus aureus*. They are involved in food poisoning, toxic shock syndrome and staphylococcal infectious diseases in human. In dairy practise, the initial numbers of *S. aureus* play an important role especially at the beginning of the milk fermentation within the first 6 h or in 24-h-old cheese. As we presented in our previous works, one of the most effective tools to inhibit *S. aureus* growth is by adding a sufficient amount of active dairy starters, which are able to produce lactic acid very rapidly. Thus, by inhibiting the growth of *S. aureus* the production of SEs may be reached. Based on this study focusing on the effect of temperature, pH, water activity and initial numbers of lactic acid bacteria on the growth and the ability of *S. aureus* 14733 to produce SED, we consider it as a strong SED producer. The SED production was not limited with the incubation temperatures and the NaCl addition related to traditional cheese manufacture. As this isolate comes originally from such an artisanal cheese production, we can expect that other strong SE producer could be present in milk or environment. Besides strict prerequisites approach in production hygiene, it is necessary to add the starters ensuring the initial dominance of lactic acid bacteria (LAB) and supporting the growth of the natural LAB present in raw milk.

Keywords: staphylococcal enterotoxins, growth inhibition, water activity, lactic acid bacteria, predictive microbiology

1. Introduction

In Slovakia, the manufacture of "Bryndza" cheese from ewes' lump cheese is of great importance to preserve the national gastronomic heritage. In the traditional way of production, it is produced immediately after milking from raw milk in upland cottages. The cheese is curdled with rennet, fermented by native lactic acid bacteria (LAB) and ripened for 7–10 days. Then, it is usually sent to a cheese factory, where the next technology processes (including salting) take part resulting in the production of the final soft "Bryndza" cheese [1, 2].

As coagulase-positive staphylococci are ubiquitous in milk, the control of *Staphylococcus aureus* growth during the fermentation of young raw milk cheese means prevention against staphylococcal enterotoxins (SEs) production. During milk fermentation and cheese production, *S. aureus* is exposed to growth competition with LAB and the effect of their metabolites during artisanal raw milk cheese manufacture. However, *S. aureus* is competitive in milk and dairy products; it is quite sensitive to higher lactic acid concentration.

The growth of *S. aureus* and potential production of heat-stable staphylococcal enterotoxins (SEs) with respect to the food matrices and conditions of food preparation represent a potential, even actual threat of a public health menace residing in food-poisoning outbreaks. From the food point of view, the production of one or more SEs is the most crucial, because they are causative agents of staphylococcal food-poisoning outbreaks.

As a pathogen, *S. aureus* disposes of remarkable wide range of virulent factors causing different infectious and food-borne outbreaks. Due to the production of surface-associated factors, *S. aureus* can avoid opsonophagocytosis, form biofilm and adhere to the host cell matrix [3, 4]. Following colonization, *S. aureus* secretes various toxins and enzymes that are responsible for the lesions. Once *S. aureus* penetrates the subcutaneous tissues and reaches the blood stream, it can infect almost any organ, most notably bone tissue and cardiac valves [4]. The role of enzymes is to disrupt cell structure, degrade cell lipids and hyaluronic acid, and to convert fibrinogen to fibrin. All those activities promote *S. aureus* to affect leukocytes, sebaceous glands, subcutaneous tissues and to increase propagation of infection [3, 5]. On the other hand, toxins (leukocidins, haemolysins and epidermolytic toxin) are able to paralyse smooth and skeletal muscles, damage blood vessels, cause extensive lesions on the skin and reveal a moist glistering surface and finally have a toxic effect on the central nervous system [3, 6, 7].

In addition, some strains of *S. aureus* are also equipped with superantigenic toxins, including shock syndrome toxin-1 (TSST-1) and SEs. They not only modulate host immune response but are also able to cause food poisoning in human [3]. The release of TSST-1 into a bloodstream may give rise to a variety of severe clinical difficulties, such as toxic shock syndrome and sudden infant death syndrome [8]. Besides *S. aureus*, also some other staphylococcal species, including *S. intermedius*, *S. hyicus*, *S. xylosus* and *S. epidermidis*, are able to produce SEs [9].

1.1. Biological characteristics of staphylococcal enterotoxins

To date, 23 SEs and enterotoxin-like (SEls) types have been described based on their antigenicity. They have sequentially been assigned a letter of the alphabet in order of their discovery (SEA, SEB, ….., SElX) [10–12]. SEA and SEB were the first one SEs characterized by Casman and Bergdoll in 1959 and 1960. From the late 1990s, new toxins were discovered one after another by sequencing the entire genome of *S. aureus*, genomic DNA library screening and genetic analysis of plasmids and pathogenicity islands [10]. Besides classical enterotoxins

http://dx.doi.org/10.5772/66736

with emetic activity (SEA to SEE, SEG to SEI and SER to SET), there are also staphylococcal-like (SEl) proteins that exhibits vomiting activity in oral primate model (SElL and SElQ) or SElJ, SElK, SElM-SElP, SElU-SElX that have not been tested yet [10, 12–15].

SEs and SEls proteins are globular, single peptides with molecular weights ranging from 19 to 29 kDa [16, 19]. Their molecular composition is characterized by containing only two residues of half cystine and one or two residues of tryptophane [20]. They are rich in lysine, aspartic and glutamic acids and tyrosine. Most of them possess a cysteine loop required for proper conformation and which is probably involved in the emetic activity [21]. Overall, 15% of amino acid residues are entirely conserved in SEs and occurred in four stretches of primary sequence located either centrally or at the C-terminus [9].

As it is seen in **Table 1**, all genes for SEs and SEls are located on mobile genetic elements, including plasmids, transposons, prophages, *S. aureus* pathogenicity islands (SaPI), variable genomic region vSaβ, or next to the staphylococcal cassette chromosome (SCC) elements. Only the staphylococcal gene cluster *egc* is organized as an operon. Most of these are mobile elements, thus horizontal transfer between strains is not rare [15, 16, 18, 22].

Distribution of superantigens (SAg) gene is strain dependent. As reported by Jin and Yamada [17], 80% of human isolates contain at least one of these genes, including 50% which contain the *egc* cluster. In animal isolates, 57% contain at least one of the SAg genes and the *egc* cluster was detected in 30% of isolates [21]. No single SAg is encoded by more than 50% of strains and that some strains may not have superantigenic capacity at all [15]. Moreover, the production of specific SEs may depend on the host environment [17].

Staphylococcal enterotoxins (SEs) and SE-like toxins (SEls) are the most notable virulence factors associated with *S. aureus* and they are involved in food poisoning, toxic shock syndrome and staphylococcal infectious diseases in human. They belong to the broad family of pyrogenic toxin superantigens that stimulate non-specific T-cell proliferation. As superantigens, SEs bind directly to the outside of the major histocompatibility complex (MHC) class II molecules on antigen-presenting cells and cross-link it to T-cell antigen receptor variable β (Vβ)-chain, which initiates non-specific activation of the T-cell without proteolytic processing in antigen-presenting cells. Thanks to it, the massive release of chemokines and pro-inflammatory cytokine is followed after T-cell proliferation, resulting in systemic shock [12, 15, 19, 23, 24]. The interaction activates as many as one in five T-cells, whereas the conventional antigen presentation activates on in 10,000 T-cells [21].

Besides superantigen activity, SEs (but not SEls) act also as a potent gastrointestinal toxins causing emesis. SEs can penetrate the epithelium, accumulate in the submucosa, enter the blood stream and circulate through the body allowing activation of local and systemic immune response by their interaction with antigen-presenting- and T-cells [16, 25]. SEA binds in submucosa to the submucosal mast cells or directly to neuron cells [10, 26]. The binding of SEA to an unidentified receptor expressed on the surface of these cells induces the degranulation, resulting in the release of 5-hydroxytryptamine (5-HT). This stimulates 5-HT receptor on adjacent vagal afferent nerves in the intestine resulting in depolarization of the vagal nerves and stimulation of the vomiting centre in the brain [10, 16]. The release

Toxin	Molecular weight (kDa)	Emetic activity	Super-antigenic activity	gene	Genetic element	Accessory genetic element
SEA	27.1	+	+	*sea*	prophage	ΦSa3ms; ΦSa3mw; Φ252B; ΦNM3; ΦMu50a
SEB	28.4	+	+	*seb*	chromosome, SaPI, plasmid	pZA10; SaPI3
SEC1-SEC3	27.5-27.6	+	+	*sec*	SaPI	SaPIn1; SaPIm1; SaPImw2; SaPIbov1
SED	26.9	+	+	*sed*	plasmid (pIB485)	pIB485-like
SEE	26.4	+	+	*see*	prophage	ΦSa
SEG	27.0	+	+	*seg*	*egc*, chromosome	*egc*1(*v*Saβ I); *egc*2(*v*Saβ III); *egc*3; *egc*4
SEH	25.1	+	+	*seh*	transposon	MGEmw2/mssa476 *seh*/*Δseo*
SEI	24.9	+	+	*sei*	*egc*, chromosome	*egc*1(*v*Saβ I); *egc*2(*v*Saβ III); *egc*3
SElJ	28.6	n_d	+	*selj*	plasmid (pIB485, pF5)	pIB485-like; pF5
SElK	25.3	n_d	+	*selk*	SaPI	ΦSa3ms; ΦSa3mw; SaPI1; SaPI3; SaPIbov1; SaPI5
SElL	24.7	-	+	*sell*	SaPI	SaPIn1; SaPIm1; SaPImw2; SaPIbov1
SElM	24.8	n_d	+	*selm*	*egc*, chromosome	*egc*1(*v*Saβ I); *egc*2(*v*Saβ III)
SElN	26.1	n_d	+	*seln*	*egc*, chromosome	*egc*1(*v*Saβ I); *egc*2(*v*Saβ III); *egc*3; *egc*4
SElO	26.8	n_d	+	*selo*	*egc*, chromosome	*egc*1(*v*Saβ I); *egc*2(*v*Saβ III); *egc*3; *egc*4; MGEmw2/ mssa476 *seh*/*Δseo*
SElP	26.7	n_d	+	*selp*	prophage (Sa3n)	ΦN315; ΦMu3A
SElQ	25.2	-	+	*selq*	SaPI	ΦSa3ms; ΦSa3mw; SaPI1; SaPI3; SaPI5
SER	27.0	+	+	*ser*	plasmid (pIB485, pF5)	pIB485-like; pF5
SES	26.2	+	+	*ses*	plasmid (pF5)	pF5
SET	22.6	+	+	*set*	plasmid (pF5)	pF5
SElU	27.2	n_d	+	*selu*	*egc*, chromosome	*egc*2(*v*Saβ III); *egc*3
SElV	27.6	n_d	+	*selv*	*egc*, chromosome	*egc*4
SElW	23.2	n_d	n_d		chromosome	
SElX	19.3	n_d	+	*selx*	chromosome	*oriC*

Source: Argudín et al. [15], Hu et al. [10], Omoe et al. [16], Jin and Yamada [17].

Table 1. General properties of SEs and SEls and genomic location of the encoding genes.

of 5-HT can be direct after interaction of SEA with enterochromaffin cells or neurons or indirect through the release of pro-inflammatory molecules or free-radical formation [13, 26]. It appears that besides 5-HT, also the serotonin pathway is involved in emesis, since serotonin is an important signalling mediator in the gastrointestinal tract and can activate enteric neurons, stimulate muscle responses and enhance secretion [23]. Release of inflammatory mediators (histamine, leukotrienes and neuroenteric peptide substance P) is responsible for local damage of gastrointestinal tract. The most severe lesions appear in the stomach and the upper part of the small intestine. Due to the inhibition of water and electrolyte reabsorption in small intestine, diarrhoea may occur [16, 25]. The dose of SEs inducing emetic activity in monkeys after oral administration ranged from 5 to 600 μg/animal [10]. The minimal dose required for intoxication in human is 144 ± 50 ng/humans for SEA and 0.4 μg/humans for SEB. All the SEls that were tested induced emetic reaction in monkeys at a dose of 100 μg/kg [11].

Although emetic and superantigenic activities are two separate functions localized on separate domains of the proteins, there is a high correlation between these activities and in most cases a loss of superantigen activity results in loss of emetic activity as [11, 18]. However, the role of SEls in human food-poisoning outbreaks currently remains unclear [12].

1.2. Prevalence of staphylococcal enterotoxins in humans and animals

Approximately 20–60% of humans are permanent or intermittent carriers of *S. aureus*, which harbours SE genes in one- to two-thirds of cases [17]. Among SEs, SEA and SED are the most frequent agents in food-borne intoxications [27, 28]. The regulation of production of SE is SE-dependent, as well as strain- and environment-dependent. Under the same conditions, different strains may produce different amounts of SE and in different growth phases. This reflects also in considerable variability in amounts and types of SEs produced by *S. aureus* growing under optimal conditions.

For SEB and SEC, the amounts may exceed 100 μg/ml, compared with 1–10 μg/ml for SEA and SED. Some indications exists that low amounts of SEB are produced already in early exponential growth phase and it can appear in cultures as early as 4–6 h. However, SEA and SED are produced in foods under a wider range of pH, redox potential (E_h) and water activity (a_w) than are the other SEs, which explain why SEA and SED are principal toxins involved in staphylococcal food poisoning [11]. SEA is expressed from the mid-exponential growth phase, but is not regulated by the accessory gene regulator *agr*, unlike *seb*, *sec* and *sed*, which require a functional *agr* for maximal expression [18].

The ***sea*** gene was the most predominant (41%) among isolates from raw and pasteurized milk studied by Rall et al. [29]. In food samples analysed by Aydin et al. [30], the SEA was found in 38%. Also, SEA and also **SEB** were presented in bovine isolates in 5–19%, in ewes' and goats' isolates in about 2–11% [21]. SEA is predominantly produced by human strains, so the connection with food contamination during the manufacture is possible [31]. On the other hand, **SEC** is considered the most important cause of staphylococcal food poisoning associated with the consumption of dairy products [27]. In dairy goat herds, the most prevalent was SEC (71%), with overall 72% prevalence of enterotoxinogenic isolates [32]. Also in 152 *S. aureus* strains isolated from cheese samples, the SEC was detected in 44% [28]. In food samples, the SEC was the most prevalent (52%) [30]. In bovine isolates, the SEC occurred in 1–27%, 22–42% in ewes' isolates and 23% in caprine isolates. SED was produced by 6–35% of bovine isolates, by 2–35% of ewes' milk isolates and by 2% of caprine isolates [20].

1.3. Resistance of staphylococcal enterotoxins to environmental factors

SEs are highly stable, resist most proteolytic enzymes (pepsin or trypsin) thus keeping their activity in the digestive tract after ingestion. They are also resisting chymotrypsin, rennin and papain. Based on the poor ability of proteolytic enzymes to affect the biological activity of SEs, it is not surprising that SE levels are unaffected by proteolytic or enteric bacteria. Lactic acid bacteria (LAB), however, do decrease SE concentrations. It could not be accounted for the addition of lactic acid alone, suggesting the involvement of specific enzymes of other metabolites. Alternatively, selective physical adsorption of toxin to LAB may have occurred during removal of cells to obtain supernatants from toxin assays [9].

1.3.1. Heat resistance

SEs are in general produced in a temperature range of 10–46°C, with the optimum at 40–45°C. Their production is substantially reduced at 20–25°C and it is unlikely that they are produced at temperatures below 10°C [19, 33, 34]. They can resist both the process of milk pasteurization and sterilization of canned foods [20, 36]. The heat stability of SEs is not the same for all of them and depends on the food matrix and toxin concentration. It decreases in the order SEC>SEB>SEA and significantly reduces in acidic conditions [3].

The thermal inactivation can generally be described by *D*- and *z*-values representing the time (at certain temperature) and the increase of temperature responsible for decimal reduction of their activity, respectively. They are for SEs as follows: $D_{121°C}$ ranges from 8.3 to 34 min or $D_{100°C}$ is about 70 min and *z*-value is 25–33°C, with some differences among specific SEs [9, 36, 37]. The biological activity of SEB retains after heating at 60°C for 16 h and pH 7.3. Heating of SEC for 30 min at 60°C did not result in any change in serological reactions. However, the loss of serological reaction of SEA was noticed after its heating for 3 min at 80°C or for 1 min at 100°C. It should also be mentioned that even after SEs lose serological activity in detection of immunological assay, they can remain biologically active [11]. Heat stability seems to be dependent on the media the toxin is in, the pH, salt concentration and other environmental factors related to the level of toxin denaturation [18].

1.3.2. Acid tolerance

The pH range allowing the production of SEs is limited in higher degree as the growth of a producing strain. Optimum enterotoxin production occurs at pH 6–7 and it is influenced by environmental conditions, carbon and nitrogen source and salt level [33]. Already pH 5.0 is generally considered as a lower limit pH value. The SEA is produced under a wider range of pH than SEB or SEC [19, 38]. SEB can be destroyed by pepsin digestion at pH 2 but it is resistant at higher pHs, which are normal conditions in the stomach after food ingestion [9].

1.3.3. Salt resistance

A characteristic feature that distinguishes *S. aureus* from other pathogenic bacteria is its high tolerance to NaCl concentrations up to 20% which means high osmotic pressure and low water activity values. Generally, it is reported that the minimal water activity for the *S. aureus* growth is in the range of a_w from 0.83 to 0.86 [33–36].

With respect to enterotoxins production requirements, values of water activity for their production are mostly in the same range as for the growth of the producer. In food with decreased water activity and at aerobic conditions, the enterotoxins can be produced even if the a_w value is from 0.86 to 0.89 (at 22–17% NaCl). The production of SEB appears to be more sensitive to reduced water activity than SEA production. Whereas SEA is produced up to a_w 0.87–0.89 (20–17% NaCl), SEB is produced only in the narrow range of 2–5% NaCl (a_w 0.99-0.97) [34, 39].

2. Effect of intrinsic and extrinsic factors on the growth dynamics of *S. aureus* and enterotoxin D production

Many intrinsic and extrinsic factors affect not only the growth of food-borne microbial pathogens but also metabolism and production of toxins. As SEs are extremely heat-stable and cannot be inactivated by measures such as heating of food, it is crucial to prevent their formation by preventing *S. aureus* growth in food matrix. In this term, NaCl addition (expressed as water activity) and LAB are suggested as the most frequent, not only during the production of cheese. The inhibition of staphylococci by LAB is related to the poor competition of *S. aureus* with antagonistic activities of indigenous bacteria in raw milk.

2.1. Effect of temperature and water activity on the growth dynamics of *S. aureus* and enterotoxin D production

The growth of *S. aureus* 14733 isolate in nutrient broth in dependence on mutual effect of temperature and water activity in the range from 1.0 to 0.84 (adjusted by NaCl addition) is demonstrated in **Figure 1**. Corresponding growth parameters were calculated using DMFit tool [40] and further analysed by secondary models (**Figure 2**, **Table 2**). Characterization of *S. aureus* ability to grow and to produce SEs at such low water activity values is important in respect to cases when the competitive microbiota is inhibited by a_w down to 0.92 and the monoculture *S. aureus* growth may still occur following SEs production.

In general, a decrease of water activity prolonged the lag-phase duration and slowed down growth rate, until the minimal water activity was reached. At 18°C and a_w = 0.869 (18.17% NaCl), there was no upgrowth observed and even more, the slow reduction ($\mu = -0.007$ h^{-1}) of *S. aureus* counts was noticed. Similar effect was observed also at 21°C as the isolate could not withstand the same a_w value of 0.869 and started to decline with specific rate $\mu = -0.023$ h^{-1}. On the contrary, the growth of *S. aureus* at a_w = 0.867 and 19°C was noticed with the high probability that highlights the differences between strains [41]. At 37°C, *S. aureus* was able to grow up to almost 20% of NaCl (a_w = 0.860) in the nutrient media. Only if the water activity reached 0.855, the decline of *S. aureus*

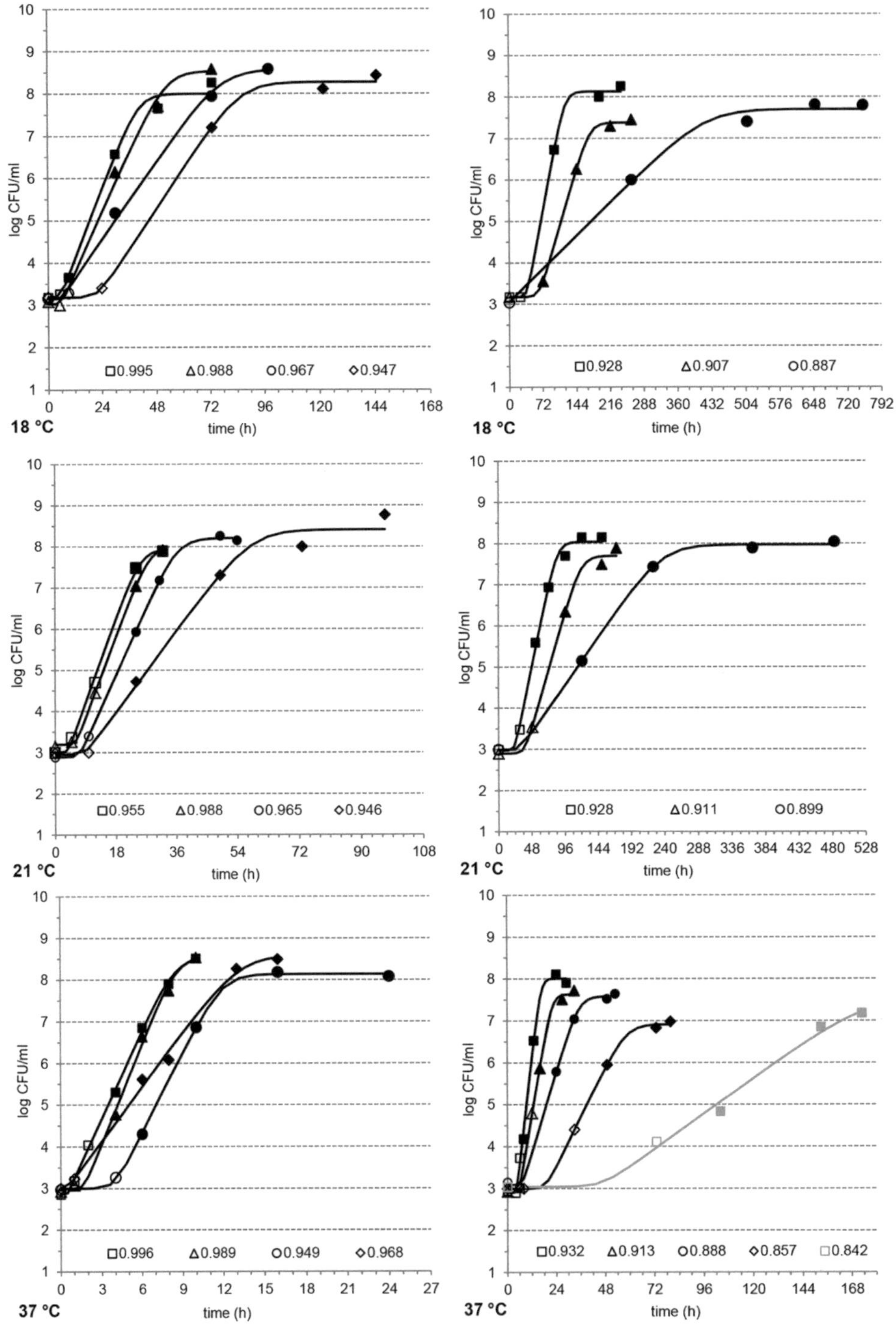

Figure 1. Growth dynamics of *S. aureus* 14733 in nutrient broth at 18, 21 and 37°C in dependence on water activity (♦, ■, ▲, ● counts of *S. aureus* 14733, no SED; ◊, □, Δ, O counts of *S. aureus* 14733, SED detected).

was observed with rate $\mu = -0.025\ h^{-1}$. It grew at 37°C much faster compared to strain ATCC 13565 in BHI broth [42]. Specific growth rates of isolate 14733 and strain ATCC 13565 at $a_w = 0.997$ were 1.796 h^{-1} and 0.970 h^{-1}, respectively. At $a_w = 0.960$, the following specific growth rates were calculated, 1.558 h^{-1} and 0.240 h^{-1}, respectively. On the other hand, the growth rates of 14733 isolate in nutrient broth at 18, 21 and 37°C were comparable with isolates 2064 and D1 grown in both milk and nutrient broth [43] and also with the isolate used by Fujikawa and Morozumi [44]. The average values of growth rates of *S. aureus* 14733 were slightly lower than those predicted by Combase Predictor or Pathogen Modelling Program [45, 46].

It was also noticed that except for cases when *S. aureus* 14733 population was inhibited by high salt amounts, it reached 7 log counts in stationary phase. At all studied temperatures, counts higher than 7 log were reached up to a_w 0.890 (approx. 13% NaCl). Thirty per cent glucose in LB broth resulted in a decreased maximal cell densities in stationary phase of about 0.5–1 log [47].

The range in which the SED was (full markers) or was not (empty markers) detected during the growth of *S. aureus* 14733 in nutrient broth at 18, 21 and 37°C is also shown in **Figure 1**. It is assumed that the minimal concentration of *S. aureus* of 10^5 CFU/ml is needed for SEs production [35, 48, 49]. However, in our case, *S. aureus* 14733 was able to produce SED also at lower cell counts. At 18°C, the SED was detected at a_w 0.995 after only 9 h, even if the *S. aureus* concentration was 4.6 × 10^3 log CFU/ml. Surprisingly, also at such a low water activity value as a_w 0.907 (13.05% NaCl), the SED was detected after 73 h if the *S. aureus* concentration was only 3.6 × 10^3 log CFU/ml. Although the isolate was able to grow at a_w 0.887 with the specific growth rate of $\mu = 0.025\ h^{-1}$, the SED was detected only after 11 days of incubation and counts higher than 6 log CFU/ml. There were also some evidences of lack of the SEs production at counts higher than 10^5 CFU/ml [11].

At 21°C, the SED was not produced as sooner as after 24 h of incubation and even not at almost optimal water activity value (a_w 0.988) and *S. aureus* densities of 2.8 × 10^4 log CFU/ml. On the other hand, at a_w 0.946 the SED was detected in 24 h at 1.4 × 10^4 log CFU/ml and also at 1.4 × 10^5 log CFU/ml at a_w 0.899 after 121 h of incubation. Production of SEA seems to be more dependent on *S. aureus* counts [50]. They detected SEA in tryptone soy (TSB) broth at 20°C after 30 h of incubation and if *S. aureus* counts were higher than 6.04 log CFU/ml.

The most rapid SED production was naturally observed at 37°C. At the higher water activity values, a_w 0.996 and 0.989, the SED was produced after only 4 h of incubation. The *S. aureus* counts needed for the SED production reached concentrations of 2.0 × 10^5 log CFU/ml and 5.9 × 10^4 log CFU/ml, in order. Also at $a_w = 0.949$, 0.932 and 0.913, the SED was produced when *S. aureus* 14733 reached minimal counts of 4 log CFU/ml. Moreover, at 37°C the SED was also detected at such low water activity values as a_w 0.857 or 0.842, when *S. aureus* counts were only 5 log CFU/ml. Higher minimal *S. aureus* counts (5.65 log CFU/ml) were needed for SEA production in TSB broth that was detected after 9 h of incubation [50].

Further, the Gibson's model secondary model Gibson et al. [51] was used to characterise the influence of water activity and temperature on the specific growth rate of S. aureus 14733. Growth of S. aureus 14733 in nutrient broth was positively determined with the increasing value of water activity, resulting in shortening of the lag phase duration and more intensive growth in exponential phase. The growth of S. aureus in dependence on water activity at 18, 21 and 37 °C can be characterised by equations summarised in **Table 2** and it is depicted in **Figure 2a**. The lag phase was described by means of the model by Daughtry et al. [52] according to equation summarised in **Table 2** which graphical representation is shown in **Figure 2b**.

For the Gibson's model, the discrepancy factors ranged from 9.6% to 17.5%, so the model can be considered as very consistent. This model can be also used for the determination of optimal water activity value at each temperature. So, the optimal growth of S. aureus 14733 in nutrient broth at 18 °C can be expected at aw = 0.994, at 21°C at aw = 0.980 and at 37°C at water activity value of 0.986. The prediction of lag phase duration would be estimated with 22-33 % error according to Davey's model. Taking into account that 12-37% of the bound of reliability during cultivation methods is tolerable; these finding demonstrate that the duration of lag phase and also the growth rate of S. *aureus* can be predicted with a defined degree of reproducibility.

With regard to the EU Commission Regulation 1441/2007 [53], the total *S. aureus* numbers in raw milk cheese should not exceed the process hygiene criterion of 4 log CFU/g. Based on a total of 23 examinations of SED presence in nutrient broth with different NaCl concentration at temperatures 18, 21 and 37°C, in 8.7% of cases *S. aureus* 14733 was able to produce SED even if the cell concentration was lower than 4 log CFU/ml. In further 22% of cases, the SED was detected if the *S. aureus* 14733 counts were lower than 5 log CFU/ml, considered as a safe limit of mentioned EU regulation. It is well documented in **Figure 3**, where the pro-

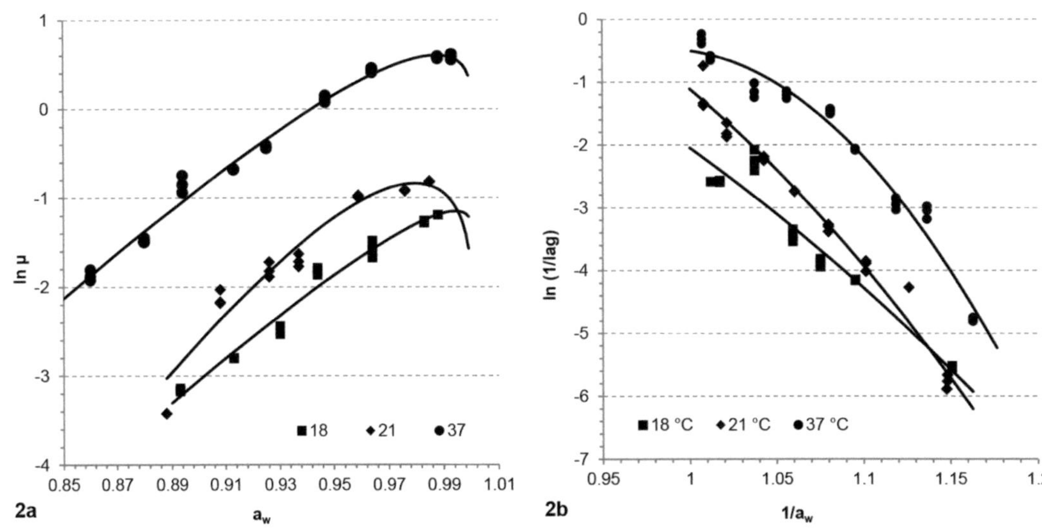

Figure 2. Plots of natural logarithm of specific growth rate (2a; *ln μ*) and reciprocal lag phase (2b; *ln 1/lag*) of *S. aureus* in nutrient broth at 18 (■), 21 (♦) and 37°C (•) in dependence on water activity. Symbols indicate values calculated from growth curves at each incubation conditions. The continuous lines indicate the fitted of *ln μ* (or *ln 1/lag*) versus a_w function, where $\ln\mu = A.b_w^2 + B.b_w + C$, $\ln \frac{1}{lag} = \frac{A}{a_w^2} + \frac{B}{a_w} + C$ and $b_w = \sqrt{1 - a_w}$; A, B and C are the estimated parameters.

http://dx.doi.org/10.5772/66736

Model equation/validation coefficients							
A_f	B_f	$\%D_f$	R^2	$\%V$	RSS	RMSE	%SEP
$\ln \mu_{18} = -32.829 \cdot \mathbf{b}_w^2 + 4.961 \cdot \mathbf{b}_w - 1.338$							
1.117	1.001	11.7	0.974	96.9	0.0038	0.0142	9.2
$\ln \mu_{21} = -59.491 \cdot \mathbf{b}_w^2 + 16.983 \cdot \mathbf{b}_w - 2.048$							
1.175	1.000	17.5	0.942	93.0	0.0121	0.0252	12.8
$\ln \mu_{37} = -35.936 \cdot \mathbf{b}_w^2 + 8.010 \cdot \mathbf{b}_w + 0.159$							
1.096	0.999	9.6	0.988	98.6	0.0782	0.0538	8.2
$\ln(1/lag_{18}) = -24.835 \cdot \mathbf{a}_w^2 + 29.858 \cdot \mathbf{a}_w - 7.068$							
1.327	1.003	32.7	0.921	90.3	1.4436	0.2832	0.8
$\ln(1/lag_{21}) = -49.760 \cdot \mathbf{a}_w^2 + 76.322 \cdot \mathbf{a}_w - 27.672$							
1.217	0.999	21.7	0.980	97.7	0.8456	0.1961	1.3
$\ln(1/lag_{37}) = -129.915 \cdot \mathbf{a}_w^2 + 255.970 \cdot \mathbf{a}_w - 126.570$							
1.246	0.999	24.6	0.973	96.9	1.3102	0.2203	5.1

Table 2. Result of validation of Gibson's model describing the effect of water activity on specific growth rate and Davey's model describing lag phase duration of *S. aureus* 14733 in nutrient broth.

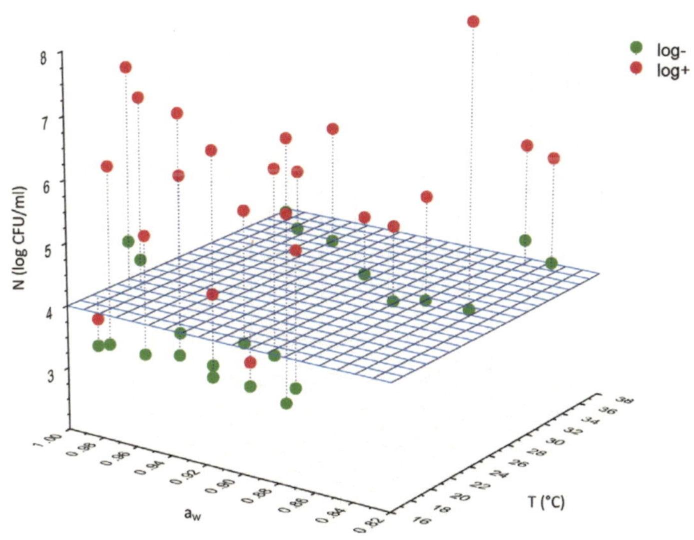

Figure 3. Mutual effect of water activity and temperature on the production of SED in nutrient broth in dependence to *S. aureus* 14733 counts. The green dots represent samples negative for SED presence and blue dots represent positive SED samples.

cess hygiene criteria are depicted with the red net, green dots represent samples negative for SED presence and blue dots represent positive SED samples at each water activity and temperature.

Based on the results, *S. aureus* 14733 can be considered as a strong SED producer, and the SED production is not limited with the incubation temperature and the NaCl addition (up to 15% at 18 and 21°C and up to 20% at 37°C). This complies with the study of Sihto et al. [47] who also observed that glucose stress (in 30% addition) had no statistically significant effect on *sed* expression during all phases of *S. aureus* growth in LB broth. Moreover, Valihrach et al. found that the fat content of milk, origin of milk (cow, goat and sheep), had only an insignificant effect on the SEC production by different *S. aureus* strains [54]. On the other hand, some strain-dependent differences were observed and the higher SEC production was achieved by strains originated from ewes' milk indicating a better adaptation of such a strain on the host environment. Naturally, the highest amounts of SEs are produced at 37°C, as an optimal temperature, compared to lower temperatures. However, SEs production is significantly decreased in milk compared to synthetic nutrient medium. It is worth mentioning also the faster growth of *S. aureus* in liquid culture compared to solid food matrices indicating that the higher growth rate may stimulate enterotoxin gene expression. On food matrix, *S. aureus* cells must attach, adapt, and substantially grow under food condition, while in the nutrient broth the bacteria are planktonic and produce enterotoxin earlier than on solid medium [50]. Also, the expression of SEs is coordinated by many regulatory elements, including *agr* regulatory system. The *agr* positively regulates expression not only of SEs and this expression increases simultaneously with increasing cell density [55].

2.2. Effect of temperature, pH value and water activity on the growth dynamics of *S. aureus* and enterotoxin D production

As it was mentioned above, the traditional artisanal production of "Bryndza" cheese includes fermentation in the presence of LAB, ripening at temperatures from 18 to 21°C and salting with 2–5% NaCl resulting in final soft cheese [1, 2]. In this context, the growth and the production of SED by *S. aureus* 14733 in nutrient broth at 18 and 21°C and optimal temperature of 37°C were observed in relation to pH value (adjusted by lactic acid to values 6.0, 5.5, 5.0 and 4.5). Subsequently, the mutual effect of lactic acid (pH 6.0, 5.5 and 5.0) and water activity (a_w = 0.99; 1.7% NaCl and a_w = 0.97; 5% NaCl) at the same temperatures on the *S. aureus* growth and the SED production in the nutrient broth was analysed.

As it is shown in **Figure 4**, the combination of reduced pH value (to values 6.0 and 5.5) and water activity value (0.99 and 0.97) did not inhibit the growth dynamic of *S. aureus* 14733 almost at all. However, further decrease of pH value down to 5.0 led to the lag-phase prolongation, slowing of the growth rate in exponential phase and to the decrease of the maximal cell concentration in stationary phase at 18 and 21°C. In accordance to these results, it can be supposing that during cheese ripening at 18–21°C, the *S. aureus* growth inhibition can be expected only if the rapid decrease of pH is achieved. But in the case of optimal temperature, even the pH 5.0 is not sufficient to slow down its growth dynamic.

http://dx.doi.org/10.5772/66736

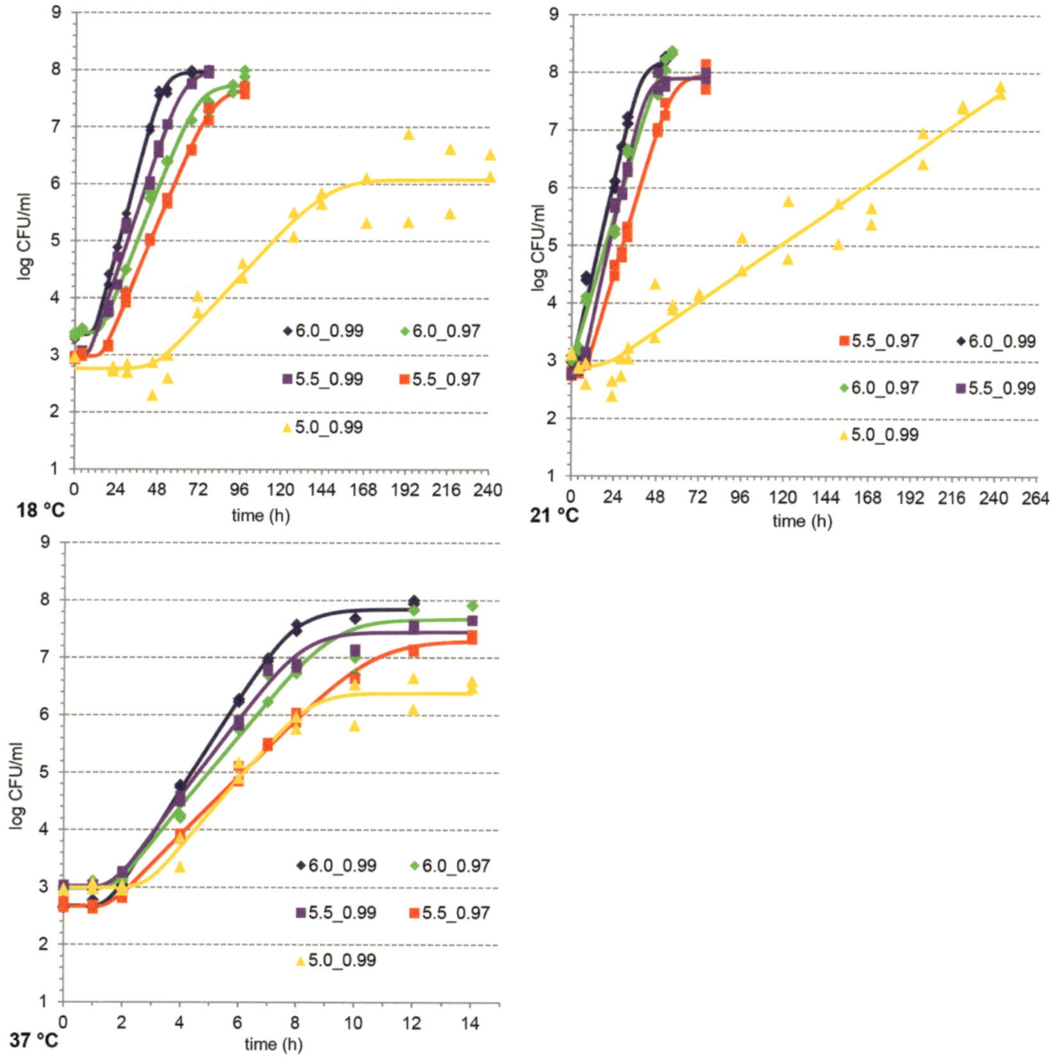

Figure 4. Growth dynamics of *S. aureus* 14733 in nutrient broth at 18, 21 and 37°C in dependence on water activity and pH value (♦ value 6.0, water activity 0.99, ■ pH value 5.5, water activity 0.99, ♦ pH value 6.0, water activity 0.97, ■ pH value 5.5, water activity 0.97, ▲ pH value 5.0, and water activity 0.99).

Taking into account the SED production by *S. aureus* 14733 in dependence to pH and water activity, the strong inhibitive effect of pH down to 4.5 or the combination of pH 5.5 and a_w 0.97 was observed(**Table 3**). The SED was not detected at any temperature if the pH of 4.5 was adjusted by the lactic acid. Compared to the experiments when no NaCl was added to the nutrient broth at pH 6.5, the minimal *S. aureus* counts for SED production of 4.6 × 10^3 CFU/ml (at 18°C) were needed. In the case of pH decreased to 6.0, the minimal *S. aureus* counts increased to 6.3 × 10^5 CFU/ml. Also, the prolongation of the time when the SED was detected from 9 to 28 h was observed at 18°C. And even the minimal *S. aureus* counts did not increase

T (°C)	pH	a_w	μ (h^{-1})	(+) log CFU/ml
18	6.0	–	0.221	5.8 (28 h)
	5.5	–	0.320	5.7 (42 h)
	5.0	–	0.119	4.9 (42 h)
	4.5	–	–0.016	–
	6.0	0.99	0.246	5.5 (28 h)
	6.0	0.97	0.239	4.9 (28 h)
	5.5	0.99	0.364	5.4 (28 h)
	5.5	0.97	0.216	–
21	6.0	–	0.392	6.2 (22 h)
	5.5	–	0.375	6.3 (22 h)
	5.0	–	0.306	6.1 (32 h)
	4.5	–	0.007	–
	6.0	0.99	0.378	6.1 (22 h)
	6.0	0.97	0.295	6.5 (32 h)
	5.5	0.99	0.389	6.0 (22 h)
	5.5	0.97	0.258	6.2 (32 h)
37	6.0	–	2.287	5.2 (4 h)
	5.5	–	2.057	3.9 (4 h)
	5.0	–	1.064	3.3 (6 h)
	4.5	–	0.039	–
	6.0	0.99	1.847	4.8 (4 h)
	6.0	0.97	1.534	3.6 (4 h)
	5.5	0.99	1.403	3.9 (4 h)
	5.5	0.97	1.073	4.9 (6 h)

μ, specific growth rate of *S. aureus* 14733; (+), SED detected in specific time of incubation.

Table 3. Effect of pH value and water activity on the growth parameters and production of SED by *S. aureus* 14733 in nutrient broth at 18, 21 and 37°C.

with the decreasing pH value; the time of positive SED determination extended to 42 h at pH 5.5 and 5.0. The longer time required for SED production in the presence of only lactic acid, compared to combination of lactic acid and NaCl presence, was observed also at 21 and 37°C, although that at 37°C the SED was detected at pH 5.0 after 6 h of incubation.

In the term of SEs production inhibition during cheese manufacture, a rapid decrease in pH value down to pH 5.0 as fast as possible within first 6 h of cheese production is strongly recommended. This was also emphasized by Delbes et al. [48]. They observed that the critical phase of exponential phase of staphylococci occurs mainly within the first 6 h and the rapid pH decrease within this phase significantly contributed to the inhibition of staphylococci in

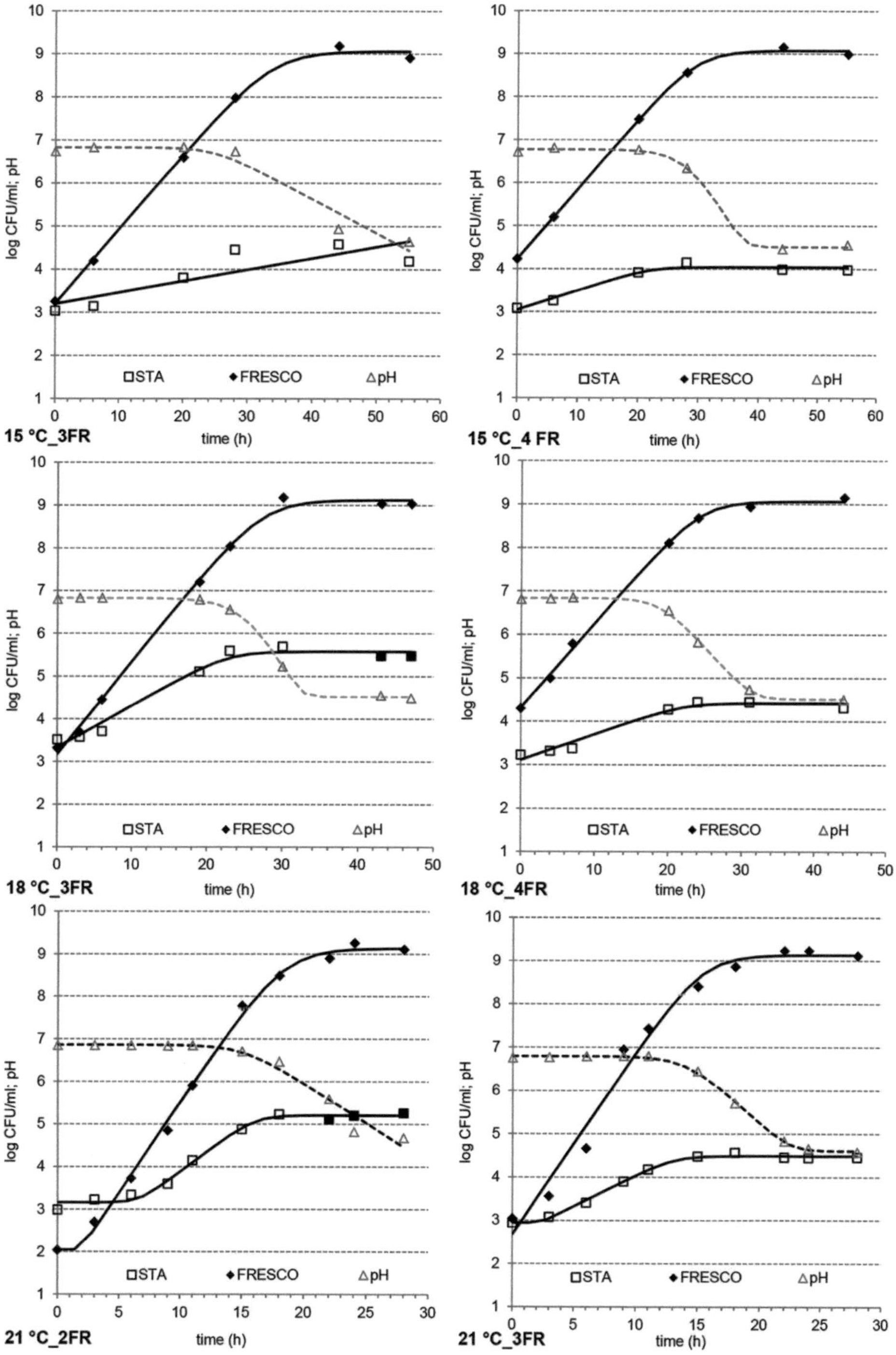

Figure 5. Growth dynamics and pH value changes during co-cultivation of *S. aureus* 14733 and Fresco culture in milk at 15, 18 and 21°C. ♦ presumptive LAB on M17 agar, □ counts of *S. aureus* 14733, no SED, ■ counts of *S. aureus* 14733, SED detected, Δ pH value.

young cheese. Moreover, if pH exceeded 6.3 within the first 6 h, also the SEs production was detected in cell concentration higher than 5 log CFU/g.

With regard to the study of Valihrach et al. [54], based on a total of 24 examinations of SED presence in the nutrient broth in dependence to mutual effect of water activity (a_w 0.99 and 0.97) and pH value (6.0 and 5.5) or pH value (6.0, 5.5, 5.0 and 4.5) at temperatures 18, 21 and 37°C, in 17% of cases *S. aureus* 14733 was able to produce SED even if the cell concentration was lower than 4 log CFU/ml. In further 17% of cases, the SED was detected if the *S. aureus* 14733 counts were lower than 5 log CFU/ml.

2.3. Effect of lactic acid bacteria addition and temperature on the growth dynamics of *S. aureus* and enterotoxin D production

In dairy practise, the initial numbers of *S. aureus* play an important role especially at the beginning of the milk fermentation within the first 6 h or in 24-h-old cheese. As we presented in our previous works [43, 56], one of the most effective tools to inhibit *S. aureus* growth is to add a sufficient amount of active dairy starters, which are able to produce lactic acid very rapidly. Thus, inhibiting the growth of *S. aureus* also, the production of SEs may be inhibited. This effect can be also seen in **Figure 5**, where the growth of *S. aureus* 14733 in the presence of two different Fresco starter culture additions was studied at 15, 18, and 21°C in milk. Those temperatures represent temperatures during ripening of original ewes' lump cheese from raw milk and 15°C is the minimal temperature for proper fermentation process.

During co-cultivation of *S. aureus* 14733 with Fresco culture in milk, the cessation of *S. aureus* growth was observed before the drop of pH observed could significantly affect the growth of *S. aureus* (**Table 4**). In the experiment at 18°C, inhibition occurred at pH values of 6.55–6.55. At 21°C, cessation of growth was observed for pH values around 6.45. As it was shown previously, *S. aureus* 14733 was able to grow under much more acidic stress. When only lactic acid was present in the nutrient media, the specific growth rate of *S. aureus* 14733 of 0.119 h^{-1} was calculated at pH 5.0 and 18°C. At 21°C, the growth at pH 4.5 with very low specific growth rate (0.007 h^{-1}) was noticed, but at pH 5.0, specific growth rate 0.306 h^{-1} was reached by *S. aureus* 14733. Results also showed that *S. aureus* could grow at much lower pH values

T (°C)	$N_{0, FR}$ (log CFU/ml)	pH_{lag} (h)	$N_{max, STA}$ (log CFU/ml)	$N_{max, STA} - N_{0, STA}$ (log CFU/ml)	μ_{STA} (h^{-1})	μ_{FR} (h^{-1})
15	3.26	24.7	4.20	1.16	0.061	0.397
	4.23	28.6	3.98	0.90	0.104	0.375
18	3.32	25.7	5.48	1.56	0.226	0.500
	4.30	19.0	4.32	1.09	0.135	0.447
21	2.04	15.2	5.26	2.27	0.215	0.426
	3.04	14.2	4.46	1.52	0.144	0.421

Table 4. Growth parameters of *S. aureus* 14733 and the pH lag phase in dependence to Fresco culture addition and incubation temperature.

in liquid media (pH 5.25 and 4.48 at 15 and 30°C, respectively) [36]. On the other hand, they did not observe its growth during co-culture with starter cultures at pH 6.8, assuming that the *S. aureus* growth inhibition cannot be attributed only to a drop in pH.

So, even pH and lactic acid play only a minor role in growth inhibition, we may suppose that the expression of genes responsible for SEs production may be influenced negatively. In addition, the *S. aureus* growth inhibition may be accounted to the accumulation of antistaphylococcal substances produced by the LAB present in the Fresco culture [56]. As reported by Charlier et al. [49], several parameters were proposed as involved in *S. aureus* inhibition by LAB, including bacteriocin and hydrogen peroxide production, and competition for nutrients.

During co-cultivation of 14733 isolate with Fresco culture, the SED was produced only after reaching *S. aureus* late stationary phase, however, only if its concentration was higher than 5 log CFU/ml. The minimal starter culture addition needed for *S. aureus* growth and SEs production inhibition at temperatures related to raw milk cheese manufacture should be at least 4 log CFU/ml. Taking into account Commission Regulation 1441/2007 [53], the presence of active starter culture of LAB is able to not only inhibit the growth of *S. aureus* but mainly prevent from SEs production. On top of that, the addition of starter culture can support the growth of natural LAB present in raw milk. Their inhibitory potential, involving not only acidification, can be used actively in safe cheese preparation. Moreover, the starter cultures not only effectively inhibit the growth of *S. aureus* during the fermentation of milk and raw milk cheese but also improve the sensorial properties of prepared cheese [57]. Certainly, these findings do not mean to overestimate the role of LAB and on the other hand to underestimate hygiene control. Minimizing the initial *S. aureus* numbers in raw milk down to 10^2 CFU/ml is of utmost importance in preventing from *S. aureus* population to reach densities necessary for SEs production during cheese manufacture. Our experiments were not focused on the inhibition of staphylococcal isolates with higher NaCl concentrations as salt generally inhibits LAB and support undesirable salt-tolerant bacteria, including staphylococci.

3. Conclusion

Based on this study focusing on the effect of temperature, pH, water activity and initial numbers of lactic acid bacteria on the growth and the ability of *S. aureus* 14733 to produce SED, we may consider it as a strong SED producer. The SED production was not limited with the incubation temperatures and the NaCl addition related to traditional cheese manufacture. As this isolate comes originally from such an artisanal cheese production, we can expect that also other enterotoxin-producing *S. aureus* strains could be able to produce SEs within the population under 10^4 CFU/ml or g in practice. It is absolutely necessary to apply strict prerequisites approach in hygiene to reach the initial number of *S. aureus* as low as possible.

In terms of SEs production inhibition during cheese manufacture, a rapid decrease in pH value down to pH 5.0 as fast as possible within the first 6 h of cheese production is strongly recommended. The minimal starter culture addition needed for *S. aureus* growth and SEs production inhibition at temperatures related to raw milk cheese manufacture should be at least 4 log CFU/ml.

Artisanal raw milk cheese production poses a few critical factors limiting its safety. With reference to the growth of *S. aureus*, commonly present in raw milk, many factors should be taken into consideration. From them, quantitative growth data, cheese type, NaCl content, nature, activity and type of the starter culture and mutual relation between *S. aureus* and lactic acid bacteria populations are predominant. Inhibitory starters producing bacteriocins may also be used. Thus, adding of a starter culture in artisanal cheese production is strongly recommended. This can be the only capable way of assuring the initial dominance of lactic acid bacteria and also supporting the growth of the natural LAB present in raw milk in competition with other undesirable bacteria.

Acknowledgements

We thank MSc. Zuzana Sirotná, MPH, and her co-workers for the SED detection. The results of the research in this chapter were supported by the Slovak Research and Development Agency, project no. APVV-15-0006.

Author details

Alžbeta Medveďová, Adriana Havlíková and Ľubomír Valík*

*Address all correspondence to: lubomir.valik@stuba.sk

Department of Nutrition and Food Quality Assessment, Faculty of Chemical and Food Technology, Slovak University of Technology in Bratislava, Bratislava, Slovakia

References

[1] Valík Ľ, Görner F, Polka PS. Fermentation of ewes lump cheese in sheep farm manufacture. Sheep Goats. 2004;**24**:23–24.

[2] Görner F, Valík Ľ. Applied Microbiology of Foodstuffs. Bratislava: Malé Centrum; 2004. 524 p.

[3] Ote I, Taminiau B, Duprez J-N, Dizier I, Mainil JG. Genotypic characterization by polymerase chain reaction of *Staphylococcus aureus* isolates with bovine mastitis. Veterinary Microbiology. 2011;**153**:285–292. DOI: 10.1016/j.vetmic.2011.05.042

[4] Garzoni C, Kelly W. *Staphylococcus aureus*: new evidence for intracellular persistence. Trends in Microbiology. 2009;**17**:59–65. DOI: 10.1016/j.tim.2008.11.005

[5] Halpin-Dohnalek M, Marth E. *Staphylococcus aureus*: production of extracellular compounds and behavior in foods – a review. Journal of Food Protection. 1989;**52**:267–282.

[6] Baird-Parker A. The staphylococci: an introduction. Journal of Applied Bacteriology Symposium Supplement. 69: 1990;**69**:1S–8S.

[7] Arbuthnott J, Coleman D, DeAzavedo J. Staphylococcal toxins in human disease. Journal of Applied Bacteriology Symposium Supplement. **69**: 1990;101S–107S.

[8] Deurenberg R, Nieuwenhuis R, Driessen C, London N, Stassen FR, van Tiel FH, Stobberingh EE, Vink C. The prevalence of the *Staphylococcus aureus* tst gene among community- and hospital-acquired strains and isolates from Wegener's granulomatosis patients. FEMS Microbiology Letters. 2005;**245**:185–189. DOI: 10.1016/j.femsle.2005.03.002

[9] Bhatia A, Zahoor S. *Staphylococcus aureus* enterotoxins: a review. Journal of Clinical and Diagnostic Research. 2007;**3**:188–197.

[10] Hu DL, Nakane A. Mechanisms of staphylococcal enterotoxin-induced emesis. European Journal of Pharmacology. 2014;**722**:95–107. DOI: 10.1016/j.ejphar.2013.08.050

[11] Rajkovic A. Staphylococcus: food poisoning. In: Caballero B, Finglas PM, Toldrá F, editors. Encyclopedia of Food and Health. 1st ed. Oxford: Academic Press; 2016. pp. 133–139. DOI: 10.1016/B978-0-12-384947-2.00655-3

[12] Ono HK, Omoe K, Imanishi K, Iwakabe Y, Hu DI, Kato H, Saito N, Nakane A, Uchiyama T, Shinagawa K. Identification and characterisation of two novel staphylococcal enterotoxins, types S and T. Infection and Immunology. 2008;**76**:4999–5005. DOI: 10.1128/IAI.00045-08

[13] Orwin PM, Leung DY, Tripp TJ, Bohach GA, Earhart CA, Ohlendorf DH, Schlievert PM. Characterisation of a novel staphylococcal enterotoxin-like superantigen, a member of the group V subfamily of pyrogenic toxins. Biochemistry. 2002;**41**:14033–14040. DOI: 10.1021/bi025977q

[14] Wilson Gj, Seo KS, Cartwright RA, Connelley T, Chuang-Smith ON, Merriman JA, Guinane CM, Park JY, Bohach GA, Schlievert PM, Morrison WI, Fitzgerald JR. A novel core genome-encoded superantigen contributes to lethality of community-associated MRSA necrotizing pneumonia. PLoS Pathogens. 2011;**7**(10):1002271. DOI: 10.1371/journal.ppat.100227

[15] Argudín MA, Mendoza MC, Rodicio MR. Food poisoning and *Staphylococcus aureus* enterotoxins. Toxins. 2010;**2**:1751–1773. DOI: 10.3390/toxins2071751

[16] Omoe K, Hu DL, Takahashi-Omoe H, Hanane A, Shinagawa K. Comprehensive analysis of classical and newly described staphylococcal superantigenic toxin genes in *Staphylococcus aureus* isolates. FEMS Microbiology Letters. 2005;**246**:191–198. DOI: 10.1016/j.femsle.2005.04.007

[17] Jin W, Yamada K. Staphylococcal enterotoxins in processed dairy products. In: Kotzekidou P, editor. Food Hygiene and Toxicology in ready-to-eat Foods. 1st ed. London: Elsevier; 2016. pp. 241–258. DOI: 10.1016/B978-0-12-801916-0.00001-7

[18] Balaban N, Rasooly A. Staphylococcal enterotoxins. International Journal of Food Microbiology. 2000;**61**:1–10. DOI: 10.1016/S0168-1605(00)00377-9

[19] Baird-Parker T. *Staphylococcus aureus*. In: Lund B, Baird-Parker T, Gould G, editors. The Microbiological Safety and Quality of Food. 1st ed. Gaithersburg: Aspen Publisher; 2000. pp. 1317–1330.

[20] Smyth DS, Hartigan PJ, Meaney WJ, Fitzgerald JR, Deobald CF, Bohach GA, Smyth CJ. Superantigen genes encoded by the egc cluster and SaPIbor are predominant among *Staphylococcus aureus* isolates from cows, sheep, rabbits and poultry. Journal of Medical Microbiology. 2005;**54**:401–411. DOI: 10.1099/jmm.0.45863-0

[21] Thomas DY, Jarraud S, Lemercier B, Cozon G, Echasserieau K, Etienne J, Gougeon ML, Lina G, Vandenesch F. Staphylococcal enterotoxin-like toxins U2 and V, two new staphylococcal superantigens from recombination within the enterotoxin gene cluster. Infection and Immunity. 2006;**74**:4742–4734. DOI: 10.1128/IAI.00132-06

[22] Pinchuk IV, Beswick EJ, Reyes VE. Staphylococcal enterotoxins. Toxins. 2010;**2**:2177–2197. DOI: 10.3390/toxins2082177

[23] Bania J, Dabrowska A, Bystron J, Korzekwa K, Chrzanowska J, Molenda, J. Distribution of newly described enterotoxin-like genes in *Staphylococcus aureus* from food. International Journal of Food Microbiology. 2006;**108**:36–41. DOI: 10.1016/j.ijfoodmicro.2005.10.013

[24] Le Loir Y, Baron F, Gautier M. *Staphylococcus aureus* and food poisoning. Genetics and Molecular Research. 2003;**2**:63–76.

[25] Hu DL, Zhu G, Mori F, Omoe K, Okada M, Wakabayashi K, Kaneko S, Shinagawa K, Nakane A. Staphylococcal enterotoxin induces emesis through increasing serotonin release in intestine and it is downregulated by cannabinoid receptor 1. Cell Microbiology. 2007;**9**:2267–2277. DOI: 10.1111/j.1462-5822.2007.00957.x

[26] Ono HK, Nishizawa M, Yamamoto Y, Hu DL, Namane A, Schinagawa K, Omoe K. Submucosal mast cells in the gastrointestinal tract are a target of staphylococcal enterotoxin type A. FEMS Immunology and Medical Microbiology. 2012;**64**:392–402. DOI: 10.1111/j.1574-695X.2011.00924.x

[27] Normanno G, LaSalandra G, Dambrosio A, Quaglia NC, Corrente M, Parisi A, Santagada G, Firinu A, Crisetti E, Celano GV. Occurrence, characterisation and antimicrobial resistance of enterotoxinogenic *Staphylococcus aureus* isolated from meat and dairy products. International Journal of Food Microbiology. 2007;**115**:290–296. DOI: 10.1016/j.ijfoodmicro.2006.10.049

[28] Rosengren Å, Fabricius A, Guss B, Sylvén S, Lindqvist R. Occurrence of foodborne pathogens and characterization of *Staphylococcus aureus* in cheese produced on

farm-dairies. International Journal of Food Microbiology. 2010;**144**:263–269. DOI: 10.1014/j.ijfoodmicro.2010.10.004

[29] Rall VLM, Vieira FP, Rall R, Vieitis RL, Fernandes Jr.A, CAndeias JMG, Cardoso KFG, Araújo Jr. JP. PCR detection of staphylococcal enterotoxin genes in *Staphylococcus aureus* strains isolated from raw and pasteurized milk. Veterinary Microbiology. 2008;**132**:408–413. DOI: 10.1016/j.vetmic.2008.05.011

[30] Aydin A, Sudagidan M, Muratoglu K. Prevalence of staphylococcal enterotoxins, toxin genes and genetic-relatedness of foodborne *Staphylococcus aureus* strains isolated in the Marmara Region of Turkey. International Journal of Food Microbiology. 2011;**148**:99–106. DOI: 10.1016/j.ijfoodmicro.2011.05.007

[31] Akineden Ö, Hassan AA, Scheider E, Usleber E. Enterotoxinogenic properties of *Staphylococcus aureus* isolated from goats' milk cheese. International Journal of Food Microbiology. 2008;**124**:211–216. DOI: 10.1016/j.ijfoodmicro.2008.03.027

[32] Mørk T, Kvitle B, Mathisen T, Jørgensen HJ. Bacteriological and molecular investigations of *Staphylococcus aureus* in dairy goats. Veterinary Microbiology. 2010;**141**:134–141. DOI: 10.1016/j.vetmic.2009.08.019

[33] Bremer PJ, Fletcher GC, Osborne C. Staphylococcus aureus. In: Christchurch, New Zealand; 2004:1–6.

[34] Jay J. Staphylococcal gastroenteritis. In: Jay J, editor. Modern Food Microbiology. 6th ed. Gaithersburg: Aspen Publisher; pp. 441–459.

[35] Asperger H, Zangerl P. *Staphylococcus aureus*. In: Roginski H, Fuquay J, Fox P, editors, editors. Encyclopedia of Dairy Science. 1st ed. San Diego: Academic Press; 2003. pp. 2563–2569.

[36] Sutherland JP, Bayliss AJ, Roberts TA. Predictive modelling of growth of *Staphylococcus aureus*: the effects of temperature, pH and sodium chloride. International Journal of Food Microbiology. 1994;**21**:217–236. DOI: 10.1016/0168-1605(94)90029-9

[37] Notermans S, van Hoeij K. The food safety file: *Staphylococcus aureus*. Woerden: Food Doctors; 2008. 39 p.

[38] Ertas N, Gonulalan Z, Yildirim Y, Kum E. Detection of *Staphylococcus aureus* enterotoxins in sheep cheese and dairy desserts by multiplex PCR technique. International Journal of Food Microbiology. 2010;**142**:74–77. DOI: 10.1016/j.ijfoodmicro.2010.06.002

[39] Ewald S, Notermans S. Effect of water activity on growth and enterotoxin D production of *Staphylococcus aureus*. International Journal of Food Microbiology. 1998;**6**:25–30.

[40] Baranyi J, Roberts TA, McClure P. A non-autonomous differential equation to model bacterial growth. International Journal of Food Microbiology. 1993;**10**:43–59. DOI: 10.1006/fmic.1993.1005

[41] Valero A, Pérez-Rodríguez F, Carrasco E, Fuentes-Alventosa JM, García-Gimeno RM, Zurera G. Modelling the growth boundaries of *Staphylococcus aureus*: effect of tempera-

ture. International Journal of Food Microbiology. 2009;**1333**:186–194. DOI: 10.1016/j.ijfoodmicro.2009.05.023

[42] Rodriguez-Caturla MY, Díaz AV, Reyes Vallejo JL, García-Gimeno RM, Zurera Cosano G. Effect of pre-incubation conditions on growth and survival of *Staphylococcus aureus* in sliced cooked chicken breast. Meat Science. 2012;**92**:409–416. DOI: 10.1016/j.meatsci.2012.05.003

[43] Medved'ová A, Valík Ľ. *Staphylococcus aureus*: characterisation and quantitative growth description in milk and artisanal raw milk cheese production. In: Eissa AA, editor. Structure and Function of Food Engineering. 1st ed. Rijeka: InTech; 2012. pp. 71–102. DOI: 10.5772/48175

[44] Fujikawa H, Morozumi S. Modelling *Staphylococcus aureus* growth and enterotoxin production in milk. Food Microbiology. 2006;**23**:260–267. DOI: 10.1016/j.fm.2005.04.005

[45] ComBase – Combined Database for Predictive Microbiology. Available from: http://www.combase.cc/index.php/en/

[46] Pathogen Modeling Program (PMP), US Department of Agriculture-Agricultural Research Service (USDA-ARS). Available from: http://pmp.errc.ars.usda.gov/PMPOnline.aspx

[47] Sihto H-M, Tasara T, Stephan R, Johler S. Growth behaviour and temporal enterotoxin D expression of *Staphylococcus aureus* strains under glucose and lactic acid stress. Food Control. 2016;**62**:69–73. DOI: 10.1016/j.foodcont.2015.10.008

[48] Delbes C, Alomar J, Chougui N, Martin J-F, Montel MCH. *Staphylococcus aureus* growth and enterotoxin production during manufacture of cooked, semihard cheese from cows' milk. Journal of Food Protection. 2006;**69**:2161–2167

[49] Charlier C, Even S, Gautier M, LeLoir Y. Acidification is not involved in the early inhibition of *Staphylococcus aureus* growth by Lactococcuslactis in milk. International Dairy Journal. 2008;**18**:197–203. DOI: 10.1016/j.idairyj.2007.03.015

[50] Tango Ch-N, Hong S-S, Wang J, Oh D-H. Assessment of enterotoxin production and cross-contamination of *Staphylococcus aureus* between food processing materials and ready to-eat cooked fish paste. Journal of Food Science. 2015;**80**:M2911–M2916. DOI: 10.1111/1750-3841.13143.

[51] Gibson A, Baranyi J, Pitt JI, Eyles MJ, Roberts TA. Predicting fungal growth: the effect of water activity on Aspergillus flavus and related species. International Journal of Food Microbiology. 1994;**23**:419–431. DOI: 10.1016/0168-1605(94)90167-8

[52] Daughtry B, Davey K, King K. Temperature dependence of growth kinetics of food bacteria. Food Microbiology. 1997;**14**:21–30. DOI: 10.1006/fmic.1996.0064

[53] Commission Regulation (EC) No. 1441/2007 amending Regulation (EC) No. 2073/2005 on microbiological criteria for foodstuffs. Official Journal of the European Union. 2007;322: 29 pp.

[54] Valihrach L, Alikayov B, Demnerova K. Production of staphylococcal enterotoxin C in milk. International Dairy Journal. 2013;**630**:103–107. DOI: 10.1016/j.idairyj.2013.01.003

[55] Novick RP, Geisinger E. Qourum sensing in staphylococci. Annual Review in Genetics. 2008;**42**:541–564. DOI: 10.1146/annurev.genet.42.110807.091640

[56] LeMarc Y, Valík Ľ, Medved'ová A. Modelling the effect of the starter culture on the growth of *Staphylococcus aureus* in milk. International Journal of Food Microbiology. 2009;**129**:306–311. DOI: 10.1016/j.ijfoodmicro.2008.12.015

[57] Medved'ová A, Studeničová A, Valík Ľ, Ondruš L. Microbial and sensory quality of raw milk cheeses from the milk vending machines. Acta Chimica Slovaca. 2013;**6**:49–54. DOI: 10.2478/acs-2013-0009

Chapter 10

Surface Proteins of *Staphylococcus aureus*

Janet Jan-Roblero, Elizabeth García-Gómez,
Sandra Rodríguez-Martínez,
Mario E. Cancino-Diaz and Juan C. Cancino-Diaz

Additional information is available at the end of the chapter

http://dx.doi.org/10.5772/65976

Abstract

Staphylococcus aureus is a commensal bacterium that causes infections such as sepsis, endocarditis, and pneumonia. *S. aureus* can express a variety of virulence factors, including surface proteins. Surface proteins are characterized by presence of a Sec-dependent signal sequence at the amino terminal, and the sorting signal domain. Surface proteins are covalently attached to peptidoglycan and they are commonly known as cell wall–anchored (CWA) proteins. CWA proteins have many functions and participate in the pathogenesis of *S. aureus*. Furthermore, these proteins have been proposed as therapeutic targets for the generation of vaccines. In this chapter, different topics related to CWA proteins of *S. aureus* are addressed. The molecular structure of CWA proteins and their role as virulence factors of *S. aureus* are described. Furthermore, the involvement of CWA proteins in the processes of adhesion, invasion of host cells and tissues, evasion of the immune response, and the formation of biofilm is discussed. In addition, the role of CWA proteins in skin infection and the proposal to use them as potential vaccine antigens are described. The information contained in this chapter will help the readers to understand the biology of CWA proteins and to recognize the importance of surface molecules of *S. aureus*.

Keywords: *Staphylococcus aureus*, CWA proteins, surface proteins, vaccines, skin

1. Introduction

Staphylococcus aureus has been widely studied due to their ability to cause infections such as sepsis, endocarditis, and pneumonia. Therefore, it is relevant to find new therapeutic targets against this bacterium; since the treatments with common antibiotics are seldom effective due to the acquisition for multidrug resistance, such as methicillin-resistant *S. aureus* (MRSA) strains [1, 2]. *S. aureus* expresses a variety of virulence factors and some of them are found in the bacterial surface (surface proteins). The surface proteins of *S. aureus* are covalently attached to the peptidoglycan, and for that reason, they are named as cell wall-anchored (CWA) proteins. Within the genus *Staphylococcus, S. aureus* has an average of 24 different CWA proteins, whereas *Staphylococcus epidermidis* and *Staphylococcus lugdenensis* have less CWA proteins. Not all strains of *S. aureus* have the same 24 CWA proteins on their surfaces, there are differences according with their genotypes. With regard to the expression of CWA proteins, it is dependent on the bacterial growth phase and growth conditions; for example, some proteins are expressed only under limited iron concentration [3, 4], while others are expressed predominantly in the exponential phase [5], or in the stationary phase of bacterial growth [6]. The CWA proteins are classified into four families according to a structure-function analysis and to their different motifs. Currently, the CWA proteins have taken great interest due to their multiple functions during the pathogenesis of *S. aureus*.

2. Structure of CWA proteins

All CWA proteins contain a Sec-dependent signal sequence at the amino terminal and at the carboxyl terminal a sorting signal and a hydrophobic domain (wall-spanning W). The sorting signal domain contains the characteristic motif for breaking by the sortase LPXTG (Leu-Pro-X-Thr-Gly; wherein X represents any amino acid). The hydrophobic domain retains the protein in the bacterial membrane during secretion, so that the sortase can join and carry out its transpeptidase function. Between the amino and carboxyl terminal domains, there are different regions or functional domains. Based on its molecular structure and arrangement, the CWA proteins of *S. aureus* have been classified into four families: the MSCRAMM family, the NEAT motif family, the three-helical bundle family, and the G5-E repeat family (**Table 1**).

2.1. The MSCRAMM family

The main feature of this family of proteins is its structural similarity and its mechanism for binding the ligand. The general structure of these proteins is a domain A at the amino terminal and a region R. The A domain is divided into subdomains: NI, N2, and N3, which integrate the ligand-binding domain. The N2 and N3 subdomains form folding structures IgG-like [7] that are important to form the ligand-binding site. With respect to ligand-binding mechanism of these proteins, they bind to fibrinogen through the mechanism "dock, lock, and latch" (DLLs) by N2 and N3 subdomains. The DLL mechanism occurs when the ligand dock to the open apo form and conformation changes create a closed form, in which the ligands are locked into a place [8]. Clumping factor A (ClfA) and ClfB proteins of *S. aureus* and serine-aspartate repeat-containing protein G (SdrG) of *S. epidermidis* are representative proteins of this family.

The R region of the Sdr- and Clf proteins is composed by repeated Ser-As, known as the SD region. However in the fibronectin-binding protein A (FnBPA) or (FnBPB), the R region contains repeated fibronectin-binding, which have the function of mediating ligand binding. The SdrC, SdrD, SdrE, and bone sialo-binding protein (BBP) proteins, which are MSCRAMM of *S. aureus*, have two or more repeated subdomains named as B_{SDR}, ranging from 110 to 113 amino

http://dx.doi.org/10.5772/65976

Protein family	Structural motifs and domains[*]	Proteins	Function during infection
(1) MSCRAMM Clf-Sdr	N-terminal A region (comprises subdomains N1, N2, N3); B_{SDR} repeats (in SdrC, SdrD and SdrE); R region (known as SD region, contains serine-aspartate repeats)	ClfA[a]	Adhesion to fibrinogen; degradation of C3b. Immune evasion
		ClfB	Fibrinogen, keratin and loricrin binding. Nasal colonization by adhesion to desquamated epithelial cells
		SdrC	β-Neurexin binding. Adhesion to desquamated nasal epithelial cells
		SrdD	Adhesion to desquamated nasal epithelial cells
FnBp	A region (subdomains N1, N2, N3); R region (contains fibronectin-binding repeats)	FnBpA	Fibrinogen, fibronectin and elastin binding. Adhesion to extracellular matrix; cell host invasion.
		FnBpB	Fibronectin-binding. Adhesion to extracellular matrix; cell host invasion
Cna	A region (subdomains N1, N2, N3); B_{CNA} repeats	Cna	Collagen binding. Adhesion to extracellular matrix
(2) NEAT	Near iron transporter motif; C-terminal hydrophilic stretch (in IsdA)	IsdA	Heme, fibrinogen, fibronectin, cytokeratin and loricrin binding. Heme capture and iron uptake; nasal colonization
		IsdB[a]	Heme, hemoglobin and 3β integrins binding. Heme capture and iron uptake; invasion of non-phagocytic cells
		IsdH	Heme, hemoglobin binding. Heme capture and iron acquisition; immune evasion by C3b degradation
(3) Three helical bundle	Tandemly linked triple-helical bundle domains (known as EABCD); repeat-containing Xr region; nonrepetitive Xc region	Protein A	IgG, IgM and TNRF1 binding. Evasion of immunity; increased inflammation during pneumonia and skin infection
(4) G5-E	A region; alternating repeats of G5 and E domains	SasG	Adhesion to desquamated epithelial cells; formation of biofilm

[*]All CWA proteins share an N-terminal signal sequence and a wall-spanning region and sorting signal at the C-terminal region.
[a]Antigens as potential vaccines.

Table 1. Structure-function of CWA proteins.

acids and that are located between the region A and the SD region. The repeated B_{SDR} are folded separately and form a rigid bar and it is Ca^{2+} dependent for structural integrity [9, 10].

An atypical MSCRAMM protein is collagen adhesin (Cna). This protein binds to collagen, also has a domain A in its N-terminal and it is divided into three subdomains N1, N2, and N3. The Cna differs from the other members MSCRAMMs because its ligand-binding domain (IgG-folded) is composed of the N1 and N2 subdomains, and not composed of the N2 and N3 subdomains as other MSCRAMMs typical. Furthermore, the space between domain A and the cell wall-spanning W domain consists of a variable number of repeated B_{CNA} domains, which are different from B_{SDR} subdomains. Another difference is that the Cna has a different ligand-binding mechanism named as collagen hug.

2.2. NEAT motif family

The main feature of this family is the presence of near iron transporter (NEAT) motifs, which recognize and bind to heme or hemoglobin. Proteins iron-regulated surface (Isd) A, B, and H contain NEAT motif (one NEAT motif for IsdA, two NEAT motif for IsdB, and three NEAT motif for IsdH) and these proteins are involved in the capture of heme from the hemoglobin. Isd is important for the survival of the bacterium into the host, where the iron is limited. Besides, Isd is involved actively in the metabolism of heme. Heme binds to Isd, and then heme binds to a membrane transporter protein, which transfers heme into the cytoplasm. In the cytoplasm, the iron is released from heme by hemoxygenases [4, 11]. The structure of the NEAT domain has been elucidated and the molecular mechanism of ligand-binding was determined [12]. Other Isd proteins can bind different ligands to the heme group, as the case IsdA that binds to fibrinogen, fibronectin, cytokeratin 10, and loricrin; and IsdB that binds to 3β integrins.

2.3. Three-helical bundle family

The main feature of this family is the presence of several single separately-folded three-helical bundles. Protein A of *S. aureus* is the common prototype of this family. Protein A has five homologous modules in its amino terminal, known as EABCD (each module has a folding three -helical bundles) which can bind to different ligands; then there is a Xr region composed by repeated octapeptides, which are highly variable number, and finally in the constant Xc region [13, 14]. Protein A is a multifunctional CWA protein ubiquitous in *S. aureus* and frequently it is used to subtype strains, based on the variation of the DNA sequence-encoding Xr.

Other proteins of *S. aureus* containing three-helix bundles are: the binder protein IgG (Sbi) with four three-helix bundles which is not covalently linked to the cell wall [15, 16], and the proteins that have a single three-helix bundle, the staphylococcal complement inhibitor (SCIN) and the extracellular fibrinogen binding protein (Efb) [17], which are involved in the immune evasion.

2.4. The G5-E repeat family

The basic structure of this family is G5-E repeat domain. Each domain G5 has five conserved glycine residues, which adopt a folding of β-triple helix-β-like structure. Currently, it is unknown whether this domain is involved in the ligand-binding function. The region E is known as the spacer region and is composed of a sequence of 50 amino acid residues [18, 19]. The domain G5 and the region E form the structure of this family. The G5-E unit is repeated in a tandem arrangement. In addition, proteins of this family have a domain A in the amino terminal. The surface protein G (SasG) of *S. aureus* and the accumulation-associated protein (Aap) of *S. epidermidis* are closely homologous and are members of this family; both proteins are involved in biofilm formation. The G5-E repeated of Aap and SasG are exposed on the surface of the bacterium. For both proteins become functional that must be processed; in the case of Aap, the domain A of the amino terminal is removed by proteolytic processing and in the case of SasG occurs by limited breaking within G5-E domains [20].

2.5. Other CWA protein families

There are other CWA proteins with different functional domains such as the legume lectin and the nucleotidase. These two groups of CWA proteins are classified outside the four families mentioned above, because they are not exclusive of *S. aureus*. CWA proteins with a legume lectin domain are represented by the serine-rich adhesion of platelet SraP [21]. SraP is composed of a BR region and a short serine-rich region (SSR1). The BR region is formed of three different structural domains: the legume lectin-like, the β-grasp fold (β-GF) and the cadherin-like (CHLD). It has been observed that the function of the BR region is to recognize Neu5Ac-containing glycoproteins of mammalian cells; such as the salivary glycoprotein gp340 [22]. In addition, the SraP is involved in bacterial adhesion and the invasion of mammalian cells. On the other hand, the nucleotidase domain has been identified in CWA protein SasH of *S. aureus*. The nucleotidase motif is enzymatically active and contributes to evade the host immune response [23, 24]. It has been shown that when *S. aureus* is phagocytosed, the SasH (also named as synthase adenosine, AdsA) dephosphorylates intracellular ATP to adenosine, where the adenosine is immunoregulatory because the adenosine inhibits the oxidative burst and promotes the survival of *S. aureus* within neutrophil [25, 26].

3. Posttranslational modifications of CWA proteins

The MSCRAMMs proteins achieve proteolytic posttranslational modification in the domain A. Proteases that remove subdomain N1 of MSCRAMMs are located on the bacterial cell surface. Proteolytic processing is conducted by a staphylococcal protease, called aureolysin, which cleaves between the subdomains N1 and N2 of ClfB and ClfA. For FnBPA, there is not a staphylococcal protease, the responsible of this processing is the thrombin of the host. Removal of N1 of ClfB can decrease the length of the protein and cause lack of binding fibrinogen [5]. It is thought that the elimination of N1 subdomain reduces the ability of *S. aureus* to adhere to fibrinogen, loricrin, and cytokeratin 10. The biological importance of the elimination of the subdomain N1 of ClfA and FnBPA is unclear, since experiments suggest no reducing biofilm formation by FnBPA; or no decrease in adhesion to fibrinogen by ClfA and FnBPA processed proteolytically [27, 28]. However, it has been reported that under certain conditions, FnBPs are degraded by the *S. aureus* V8 protease, reducing the ability of the bacterium to adhere to fibronectin [29].

Another posttranslational modification is the glycosylation of proteins Clf-Sdr. It has been shown that the glycosyltransferases SdgB and SdgA of *S. aureus* are responsible to modify the SD region of the Clf-Sdr family. This modification involves adding N-acetylglucosamine residues in the region SD protecting it from the degradation by neutrophil serine protease, cathepsin G [30]. Thus, the glycosylation of repeated SD is crucial for functional maintenance of MSCRAMMs on the surface of *S. aureus*.

4. CWA proteins as virulence factors

The generation of mutants is a useful tool to know the function of a gene; however, the study of CWA proteins has been complicated because the generation of defective mutants of CWA protein had generated, in some cases, unexpected results due to functional redundancy. For example, *S. aureus* expresses some CWA proteins that bind to fibrinogen, and most of the strains can produce two proteins with the same function; in consequence, a mutant protein could be replaced by a protein with the correct function. Another difficulty that occurs in the study of CWA proteins is to obtain mutants in the isolates of clinical relevance, since the studies have been conducted with laboratory strains; such as *S. aureus* Newman and derivatives of NCTC8325 strains. Finally, there is the problem of species because some CWA proteins have a specific function in mice but in humans have different functions or behavior [31].

Despite the difficulties mentioned above, the role of CWA proteins in virulence has been studied. Human population (20%) is permanently colonized by *S. aureus* in the nasal cavity [32], where the bacterium is able to grow exponentially and to express high levels of mRNA encoding CWA proteins [33]. ClfB [34] and IsdA [35] contribute in the nasal colonization in rodents, and ClfB also in humans [36]. ClfB is capable of binding to keratin 10 of mouse and human [37]. Keratin 10 is the largest component of squamous cells. ClfB also binds to the loricrin protein [38]. Some other CWA proteins (such as SdrC, SdrD, SasG, and SasX) can promote adhesion to squamous cells but the ligand or ligands involved are not known [39–42].

4.1. CWA proteins in the invasion of epithelial and endothelial cells

Recently, *S. aureus* was recognized as an intracellular pathogen and its ability to survive inside neutrophils. *S. aureus* can be taken directly by nonphagocytic cells and host cells; subsequently, it can cause damage to the above mentioned cells by the production of cytotoxins. In addition, intracellular bacterium is protected against the attack by the host because *S. aureus* acquires a state of semidormancy known as small colony variants, which yields intrinsic resistance to antibiotic therapy [43].

In the case of FnBPA and FnBPB proteins, the binding of these proteins to fibronectin facilitates *S. aureus* internalization [44–46]. Fibronectin is composed of three different types of structural modules, called 1, 2, and 3, of which the modules type 1 contain two β sheets involved in interactions with the binding domains of FnBPs [47]. In addition, an arginine-glycine-aspartate sequence of one of the modules type 3 of fibronectin is recognized by integrins. Particularly, the interactions of fibronectin with FnBPs and integrin $\alpha5\beta1$ initiate the activation of a signaling cascade that triggers a cytoskeletal rearrangement in the host cell, which causes endocytosis of *S. aureus* [48].

4.2. Immune system and inflammation

The CWA proteins are involved in immune evasion. Protein A binds to the Fc region of IgG, this binding leads to an incorrect orientation of IgG antibody, preventing the recognition of the bacterium by neutrophils and the activation of the classical complement pathway [49].

Furthermore, it has been demonstrated that in pulmonary epithelial cells, protein A is capable of interacting with tumor necrosis factor receptor 1 (TNFR1), triggering the production of interleukin-8 (IL-8) and the neutrophil recruitment, promoting inflammation and tissue damage [50]. Also it has been reported the involvement of protein A in the production of interferon β (IFNβ) and IL-6 in a mouse pneumonia model [51].

ClfA and Can are involved in evading the immune system by recruiting regulators of complement pathway [52]. Furthermore, ClfA is involved in bacterial survival by binding to fibrinogen, because in a sepsis model this interaction reduces the probability of *S. aureus* to be eliminated by neutrophils [53]. It has also demonstrated the importance of modifying ClfA by glycosyltransferases, which add N-acetylglucosamine to the SD region, thereby preventing the proteolysis by cathepsin-B from human neutrophils [30].

4.3. Biofilms

One of the major virulence factors of *S. aureus* is its ability to form biofilms on implanted medical devices, which favors resistance to antibiotics, survival, and dissemination [31]. In the formation of biofilms, a polysaccharide matrix is involved, particularly the molecule poly-N-acetylglucosamine (PNAG) or also called adhesin intercellular polysaccharide (PIA), whose production depends on the proteins encoded by the operon *icaADBC* (intracellular adhesion) [54, 55]. Furthermore, the CWA proteins of the cell-wall are also involved in biofilm formation, such as Bap, ClfB, FnBPs, SasC, SasG, and protein A [31]. It has been shown that Bap and SasC are involved in adhesion of *S. aureus* to polystyrene surfaces and the bacterial accumulation in biofilm formation [56, 57]. In the case of FnBPs, it has been proposed that N2 and N3 subdomains of the domain A are required to promote the bacterial accumulation in biofilm formation [27]. The mechanism of biofilm formation involving SasG consists of an array of loop structures, which are capable of interacting with other SasG located on the surface of another bacterium, thus allowing the accumulation of *S. aureus* [18].

5. Involvement of CWA proteins in skin infections

The study of the participation of CWA proteins in skin infections and abscess formation has been achieved mainly in animal models with CWA protein mutant strains of *S. aureus* (**Table 2**). *S. aureus* strains deficient in sortase proteins, which lost all CWA proteins, are unable to form abscess in mice [58, 59]. Mice inoculated with *S. aureus* strain Newman, deficient in ClfA, showed a lower bacterial load in skin abscesses compared with the wild-type strain [60]. The ClfA protects the bacterium from phagocytosis by neutrophils because ClfA recruits fibrinogen to the surface of the bacterium, thereby preventing the opsonization and recognition by receptors of phagocytic cells.

In a murine skin abscess model, infected with *S. aureus* LS-1 strain, mutant in FnBPA and FnBPB, the bacterial load decreased [60]. FnBPs is also able to adhere and invade the skin keratinocytes [61], thus contributing to the development of skin infection. SasX contributes to skin infection, which was demonstrated in a murine skin infection model in challenge with a SasX-deficient

Infection model	Mutant CWA in *S. aureus*	Result
Murine kidney abscess	Sortase	No abscess formation in the kidneys
Murine skin infection	ClfA	Decreased CFU in the skin abscess
Murine skin infection	FnBPA and FnBPB	Decreased CFU in the skin abscess
Murine skin infection	SasX	Smaller abscesses in the skin
Mice inoculated subcutaneously	Protein A	Decreased CFU in the skin abscesses
Rabbit skin infection	Wild-type	High transcription level of the *isdB* gene in abscesses

Table 2. CWA protein infection models.

strain of *S. aureus*, who produced smaller abscesses compared with those infected with the wild-type strain. In mice inoculated subcutaneously with the *S. aureus* Newman mutant strain, protein A-deficient, the bacterial load on the skin abscesses was significantly lower than abscesses infected the wild-type strain. The role of protein A during skin infection by *S. aureus* is probably by evading the immune response, since protein A binds to IgG and decrements B cells, prolonging the time of bacterial binding with the ligand of the skin. Protein A leads a proinflammatory response in the skin, because the protein A binds to TNFR1 of human keratinocytes and upregulates the expression of COX-2 and IL-8, driving shot downstream of the kinases, which results in the activation of NFkB and AP-1 [62]. IsdA has a function of resistance against the mechanisms of human innate immune defense and its presence on the surface of *S. aureus* causes that the bacterium to be more hydrophilic and is negatively charged [63, 64]. In a rabbit skin infection model, transcription levels of *isdB* were increased 24 h post infection [65], suggesting that it may have a role during infection of the skin. The Isd proteins bind to the ligands on skin cells, and it is probably Isd that is involved in the skin infection.

6. CWA proteins as vaccines

Currently, there is a proposal to use recombinant CWA proteins as potential vaccine antigens. In animal models, the use of CWA proteins has induced immunological protection against *S. aureus* through the production of anti-*S. aureus* antibody [66–68]. However, it has been documented that IsdB vaccine produced immunity in animals, but not in patients with severe infections after cardiothoracic surgery (phase III test) [69, 70]. A strategy to increase vaccine efficacy is to develop multiple vaccines, a vaccine containing four antigens of CWA proteins resulted in greater protection in mouse [68] compared to a single antigen vaccine. Furthermore, the stimulation of humoral immunity is insufficient for protection in humans; subsequently adjuvants that trigger an immune response mediated by T helper 1 (Th1) and/or T helper 17 (Th17) cells, as well as recruit of neutrophils by IL-17 and IFNγ would be important.

6.1. CWA proteins such as T-cell antigen

Up to date, the mechanism of immune system activation by CWA proteins is unknown except for the protein A that binds to TNFR1 and induces the production of interleukin-8 (IL-8) and the neutrophil recruitment [50]. The anti-*S. aureus* vaccines are capable for activating the effector T-cell subsets [71, 72]; however, the epitopes of *S. aureus* that recognize T-cells are unknown. T-cells not activated (virgin) increase their cellular proliferation and production of cytokines (phenotype of activated T-cells) when they are stimulated with extracellular proteins of *S. aureus*, but not when they are stimulated with intracellular proteins of *S. aureus* [73]. Stimulation of virgin T-cell with membrane proteins from *S. aureus* produces a high activation of T-cells, the same takes place when they are stimulated with ClfA [74]. ClfA triggers immunity antibody-mediated in a murine model of *S. aureus* arthritis [67]. On the other hand, ClfA nanoparticle applied to the nasal cavity of mice results in a significant protection against systemic infection by *S. aureus*, and an increase cellular immune response Th1 and Th17 [68]. Immune cellular response type Th17 has an important function in systemic protection against *S. aureus*, because knockout mice to IL-17 cytokine are not immunized with ClfA [75]. These studies suggest the potential role of ClfA as the major antigen to activate T-cells.

Currently, ClfA protein is used in multivalent vaccines. Thus, the vaccine designed by Pfizer, with the status of Phase II clinical trials, is made with ClfA antigens, capsular polysaccharide MNTC, and two proteins (CP5 and CP8) [76, 77]. This vaccine induces a high production of antibodies; however, there are no studies on its cellular immunity. NovaDigm I developed a vaccine with homologues of ClfA and Als3p [78]; in phase I clinical test, the vaccine showed an increase in the production of specific antibody titer and induced Th1 and Th17 cell response in humans [77]. ClfA is emerging as a potent stimulator of T-cells and it is a promising antigen vaccine development; however, there is little research on the potential of other CWA proteins to activate T-cells. Therefore, studies to determine which CWA proteins cause a high T-cell response should be performed to identify potential proteins for future vaccines.

7. Conclusions

Although it has recognized the role and ligands for some CWA proteins of *S. aureus*, there are other CWA proteins whose function in humans is unknown. The structural analysis of CWA proteins is a powerful tool to determine their role in *S. aureus*; however, the use of molecular techniques and animal models are essential for discovering new ligands and/or functions of the CWA proteins, which could be relevant in *S. aureus* pathogenicity.

On the other hand, the immune response of the CWA protein also requires more studies, since the mechanism by which CWA proteins interfere with the host innate immune response is unknown, in particular regulation of complement activation. In addition, determining CWA proteins causing a cellular immune response is crucial for the generation of new vaccines.

Most studies of CWA proteins have been conducted with laboratory strains. These studies should be extended in clinical isolates, where the variation of ligand binding of the CWA proteins is considerable. Additionally, the regulatory system of the expression of CWA proteins is still insufficient, because the expression of CWA proteins depends on the strain understudy.

Surface proteins have a wide range of functions that are essential for colonization and survival of *S. aureus* in the host. Although the structural analysis of the CWA proteins has been crucial to define the mechanism of these processes and has provided the classification of the

CWA proteins, there are many questions to understand completely the functions of the CWA proteins in the pathogenesis of *S. aureus*.

Acknowledgements

This work was supported by the Grant SIP20160325, SIP20161111, and SIP20160135 from Instituto Politécnico Nacional (IPN). JCCD, JJR, SRM, and MECD appreciate the COFAA and EDI, IPN fellowships, and the support provided by SNI-CONACYT. EGG thanks the CONACYT Postdoctoral fellowship and the support provided by SNI-CONACYT.

Author details

Janet Jan-Roblero[1], Elizabeth García-Gómez[1], Sandra Rodríguez-Martínez[2], Mario E. Cancino-Diaz[2] and Juan C. Cancino-Diaz[1*]

*Address all correspondence to: jccancinodiaz@hotmail.com

1 Microbiology Department, ENCB, National Polytechnic Institute (Instituto Politécnico Nacional), Mexico City, Mexico

2 Inmunology Department, ENCB, National Polytechnic Institute (Instituto Politécnico Nacional), Mexico City, Mexico

References

[1] DeLeo FR, Chambers HF. Reemergence of antibiotic-resistant *Staphylococcus aureus* in the genomics era. Journal of Clinical Investigation. 2009;119:2464–2474. DOI: 10.1172/JCI38226

[2] DeLeo FR, Otto M, Kreiswirth BN, Chambers HF. Community-associated meticillin-resistant *Staphylococcus aureus*. Lancet. 2010;375:1557–1568. DOI: 10.1016/S0140-6736(09)61999-1

[3] Mazmanian SK, Skaar EP, Gaspar AH, Humayun M, Gornicki P, Jelenska J, Joachmiak A, Missiakas DM, Schneewind O. Passage of heme-iron across the envelope of *Staphylococcus aureus*. Science. 2003;299:906–909. DOI: 10.1126/science.1081147

[4] Hammer ND, Skaar EP. Molecular mechanisms of *Staphylococcus aureus* iron acquisition. Annual Review of Microbiology. 2011;65:129–147. DOI: 10.1146/annurev-micro-090110-102851

[5] McAleese FM, Walsh EJ, Sieprawska M, Potempa J, Foster TJ. Loss of clumping factor B fibrinogen binding activity by *Staphylococcus aureus* involves cessation of transcription, shedding and cleavage by metalloprotease. Journal of Biological Chemistry. 2001;276:29969–29978. DOI: 10.1074/jbc.M102389200

[6] Bischoff M, Dunman P, Kormanec J, Macapagal D, Murphy E, Mounts W, Berger-Bächi B, Projan S. Microarray-based analysis of the *Staphylococcus aureus* sigma-B regulon. Journal of Bacteriology. 2004;186:4085–4099. DOI: 10.1128/JB.186.13.4085-4099.2004

[7] Deivanayagam CC, Wann ER, Chen W, Carson M, Rajashankar KR, Hook M, Narayana SV. A novel variant of the immunoglobulin fold in surface adhesins of *Staphylococcus aureus*: crystal structure of the fibrinogen-binding MSCRAMM, clumping factor A. EMBO Journal. 2002;21:6660–6672. DOI: 10.1093/emboj/cdf619

[8] Ponnuraj KA, Bowden MG, Davis S, Gurusiddappa S, Moore D, Choe D, Xu Y, Hook M, Narayana SV. A "dock, lock, and latch" structural model for a staphylococcal adhesin binding to fibrinogen. Cell. 2003;115:217–228. DOI: 10.1016/S0092-8674(03)00809-2

[9] Josefsson E, McCrea KW, Ni Eidhin D, O'Connell D, Cox J, Hook M, Foster TJ. Three new members of the serine-aspartate repeat protein multigene family of *Staphylococcus aureus*. Microbiology. 1998;144:3387–3395. DOI: 10.1099/00221287-144-12-3387

[10] Josefsson E, O'Connell D, Foster TJ, Durussel I, Cox JA. The binding of calcium to the B-repeat segment of SdrD, a cell surface protein of *Staphylococcus aureus*. Journal of Biological Chemistry. 1998;273:31145–31152. DOI: 10.1074/jbc.273.47.31145

[11] Cassat JE, Skaar EP. Metal ion acquisition in *Staphylococcus aureus*: overcoming nutritional immunity. Seminars in Immunopathology. 2012;34:215–235. DOI: 10.1007/s00281-011-0294-4

[12] Grigg JC, Ukpabi G, Gaudin CF, Murphy ME. Structural biology of heme binding in the *Staphylococcus aureus* Isd system. Journal of Inorganic Biochemistry. 2010;104:341–348. DOI: 10.1016/j.jinorgbio.2009.09.012

[13] Deisenhofer J. Crystallographic refinement and atomic models of a human Fc fragment and its complex with fragment B of protein A from *Staphylococcus aureus* at 2.9- and 2.8-A resolution. Biochemistry. 1981;20:2361–2370. DOI: 10.1021/bi00512a001

[14] Cedergren L, Andersson R, Jansson B, Uhlen M, Nilsson B. Mutational analysis of the interaction between staphylococcal protein A and human IgG1. Protein Engineering. 1993;6:441–448. DOI: 10.1093/protein/6.4.441

[15] Smith EJ, Corrigan RM, van der Sluis T, Gründling A, Speziale P, Geoghegan JA, Foster TJ. The immune evasion protein Sbi of *Staphylococcus aureus* occurs both extracellularly and anchored to the cell envelope by binding lipoteichoic acid. Molecular Microbiology. 2012;83:789–804. DOI: 10.1111/j.1365-2958.2011.07966.x

[16] Burman JD, Leung E, Atkins KL, O'Seaghdha MN, Lango L, Bernado P, Bagby S, Svergun DI, Foster TJ, Isenman DE, van den Elsen JM. Interaction of human complement with Sbi, a staphylococcal immunoglobulin-binding protein: indications of a novel mechanism of complement evasion by *Staphylococcus aureus*. Journal of Biological Chemistry. 2008;283:17579–17593. DOI: 10.1074/jbc.M800265200

[17] Lambris JD, Ricklin D, Geisbrecht BV. Complement evasion by human pathogens. Nature Reviews: Microbiology. 2008;6:132–142. DOI: 10.1038/nrmicro1824

[18] Gruszka DT, Wojdyla JA, Bigham RJ, Turkenburg JP, Manfield IW, Steward A, Leech AP, Geoghegan JA, Foster TJ, Clarke J, Potts JR. Staphylococcal biofilm-forming protein has a contiguous rod-like structure. Proceedings of the National Academy of Sciences of the United States of America. 2012;109:E1011–E1018. DOI: 10.1073/pnas.1119456109

[19] Conrady DG, Wilson JJ, Herr AB. Structural basis for Zn^{2+}-dependent intercellular adhesion in staphylococcal biofilms. Proceedings of the National Academy of Sciences of the United States of America. 2013;110:E202–E211. DOI: 10.1073/pnas.1208134110

[20] Geoghegan JA, Corrigan RM, Gruszka DT, Speziale P, O'Gara JP, Potts JR, Foster TJ. Role of surface protein SasG in biofilm formation by *Staphylococcus aureus*. Journal of Bacteriology. 2010;192:5663–5673. DOI: 10.1128/JB.00628-10

[21] Lizcano A, Sanchez CJ, Orihuela CJ. A role for glycosylated serine-rich repeat proteins in gram-positive bacterial pathogenesis. Molecular Oral Microbiology. 2012;27(4):257–269. DOI: 10.1111/j.2041-1014.2012.00653.x

[22] Kukita K, Kawada-Matsuo M, Oho T, Nagatomo M, Oogai Y, Hashimoto M, Suda Y, Tanaka T, Komatsuzawa H. *Staphylococcus aureus* SasA. is responsible for binding to salivary agglutinin, gp340, derived from human saliva. Infection and Immunity. 2013;81:1870–1879. DOI: 10.1128/IAI.00011-13

[23] Thammavongsa V, Kern JW, Missiakas DM, Schneewind O. *Staphylococcus aureus* synthesizes adenosine to escape host immune responses. Journal of Experimental Medicine. 2009;206:2417–2427. DOI: 10.1084/jem.20090097

[24] Thammavongsa V, Schneewind O, Missiakas DM. Enzymatic properties of *Staphylococcus aureus* adenosine synthase (AdsA). BMC Biochemistry. 2011;12:56. DOI: 10.1186/1471-2091-12-56

[25] Berends ET, Horswill AR, Haste NM, Monestier M, Nizet V, von Kockritz-Blickwede M. Nuclease expression by *Staphylococcus aureus* facilitates escape from neutrophil extracellular traps. Journal of Innate Immunity. 2010;2(6):576–586. DOI: 10.1159/000319909

[26] Thammavongsa V, Missiakas DM, Schneewind O. *Staphylococcus aureus* degrades neutrophil extracellular traps to promote immune cell death. Science. 2013;342(6160):863–866. DOI: 10.1126/science.1242255

[27] Geoghegan JA, Monk IR, O'Gara JP, Foster TJ. Subdomains N2N3 of fibronectin binding protein A mediate *Staphylococcus aureus* biofilm formation and adherence to fibrinogen using distinct mechanisms. Journal of Bacteriology. 2013;195:2675–2683. DOI: 10.1128/JB.02128-12

[28] McCormack N, Foster TJ, Geoghegan JA. A short sequence within subdomain N1 of region A of the *Staphylococcus aureus* MSCRAMM clumping factor A is required for export and surface display. Microbiology. 2014;160(Pt 4):659–670. DOI: 10.1099/mic.0.074724-0

[29] McGavin MJ, Zahradka C, Rice K, Scott JE. Modification of the *Staphylococcus aureus* fibronectin binding phenotype by V8 protease. Infection and Immunity. 1997;65(7):2621–2628.

[30] Hazenbos WL, Kajihara KK, Vandlen R, Morisaki JH, Lehar SM, Kwakkenbos MJ, Beaumont T, Bakker AQ, Phung Q, Swem LR, Ramakrishnan S, Kim J, Xu M, Shah IM, Diep BA, Sai T, Sebrell A, Khalfin Y, Oh A, Koth C, Lin SJ, Lee BC, Strandh M, Koefoed K, Andersen PS, Spits H, Brown EJ, Tan MW, Mariathasan S. Novel staphylococcal glycosyltransferases SdgA and SdgB mediate immunogenicity and protection of virulence-associated cell wall proteins. PLoS Pathogens. 2013;9(10):e1003653. DOI: 10.1371/journal.ppat.1003653

[31] Foster TJ, Geoghegan JA, Ganesh VK, Hook M. Adhesion, invasion and evasion: the many functions of the surface proteins of *Staphylococcus aureus*. Nature Reviews: Microbiology. 2014;12(1):49–62. DOI: 10.1038/nrmicro3161

[32] Kluytmans J, van Belkum A, Verbrugh H. Nasal carriage of *Staphylococcus aureus*: epidemiology, underlying mechanisms, and associated risks. Clinical Microbiology Reviews. 1997;10:505–520.

[33] Burian M, Rautenberg M, Kohler T, Fritz M, Krismer B, Unger C, Hoffmann WH, Peschel A, Wolz C, Goerke C. Temporal expression of adhesion factors and activity of global regulators during establishment of *Staphylococcus aureus* nasal colonization. Journal of Infectious Diseases. 2010;201:1414–1421. DOI: 10.1086/651619

[34] Schaffer AC, M. SR, Cocchiaro J, Portoles M, Kiser KB, Risley A, Randall SM, Valtulina V, Speziale P, Walsh E, Foster T, Lee JC. Immunization with *Staphylococcus aureus* clumping factor B, a major determinant in nasal carriage, reduces nasal colonization in a murine model. Infection and Immunity. 2006;74:2145–2153. DOI: 10.1128/IAI.74.4.2145-2153.2006

[35] Clarke SR, Brummell KJ, Horsburgh MJ, McDowell PW, Mohamad SA, Stapleton MR, Acevedo J, Read RC, Day NP, Peacock SJ, Mond JJ, Kokai-Kun JF, Foster SJ. Identification of in vivo-expressed antigens of *Staphylococcus aureus* and their use in vaccinations for protection against nasal carriage. Journal of Infectious Diseases. 2006;193:1098–1108. DOI: 10.1086/501471

[36] Wertheim HF, Walsh E, Choudhurry R, Melles DC, Boelens HA, Miajlovic H, Verbrugh HA, Foster T, van Belkum A. Key role for clumping factor B in *Staphylococcus aureus* nasal colonization of humans. PLoS Medicine. 2008;5:e17. DOI: 10.1371/journal.pmed.0050017

[37] Walsh EJ, O'Brien LM, Liang X, Hook M, Foster TJ. Clumping factor B, a fibrinogen-binding MSCRAMM (microbial surface components recognizing adhesive matrix molecules) adhesin of *Staphylococcus aureus*, also binds to the tail region of type I cytokeratin 10. Journal of Biological Chemistry. 2004;279:50691–50699. DOI: 10.1074/jbc.M408713200

[38] Mulcahy ME, Geoghegan JA, Monk IR, O'Keeffe KM, Walsh EJ, Foster TJ, McLoughlin RM. Nasal colonisation by *Staphylococcus aureus* depends upon clumping factor B binding to the squamous epithelial cell envelope protein loricrin. PLoS Pathogens. 2012;8:e1003092. DOI: 10.1371/journal.ppat.1003092

[39] Corrigan RM, Rigby D, Handley P, Foster TJ. The role of *Staphylococcus aureus* surface protein SasG in adherence and biofilm formation. Microbiology. 2007;153:2435–2446. DOI: 10.1099/mic.0.2007/006676-0

[40] Corrigan RM, Miajlovic H, Foster TJ. Surface proteins that promote adherence of *Staphylococcus aureus* to human desquamated nasal epithelial cells. BMC Microbiology. 2009;9:22. DOI: 10.1186/1471-2180-9-22

[41] Li M, Du X, Villaruz AE, Diep BA, Wang D, Song Y, Tian Y, Hu J, Yu F, Lu Y, Otto M. MRSA epidemic linked to a quickly spreading colonization and virulence determinant. Nature Medicine. 2012;18:816–819. DOI: 10.1038/nm.2692

[42] Liu Q, Du X, Hong X, Li T, Zheng B, He L, Wang Y, Otto M, Li M. Targeting surface protein SasX by active and passive vaccination to reduce *Staphylococcus aureus* colonization and infection. Infection and Immunity. 2015;83(5):2168–2174. DOI: 10.1128/IAI.02951-14

[43] Sendi P, Proctor RA. *Staphylococcus aureus* as an intracellular pathogen: the role of small colony variants. Trends in Microbiology. 2009;17:54–58. DOI: 10.1016/j.tim.2008.11.004

[44] Dziewanowska K, Patti JM, Deobald CF, Bayles KW, Trumble WR, Bohach GA. Fibronectin binding protein and host cell tyrosine kinase are required for internalization of *Staphylococcus aureus* by epithelial cells. Infection and Immunity. 1999;67:4673–4678.

[45] Peacock SJ, Foster TJ, Cameron BJ, Berendt AR. Bacterial fibronectin-binding proteins and endothelial cell surface fibronectin mediate adherence of *Staphylococcus aureus* to resting human endothelial cells. Microbiology. 1999;145:3477–3486. DOI: 10.1099/00221287-145-12-3477

[46] Sinha B, Francois PP, Nüsse O, Foti M, Hartford OM, Vandaux P, Foster TJ, Lew DP, Herrmann M, Krause KH. Fibronectin-binding protein acts as *Staphylococcus aureus* invasin via fibronectin bridging to integrin alpha5beta1. Cellular Microbiology. 1999;1:101–117. DOI: 10.1046/j.1462-5822.1999.00011.x

[47] Schwarz-Linek U, Werner JM, Pickford AR, Gurusiddappa S, Him JH, Pilka ES, Briggs JA, Gough TS, Hook M, Campbell ID, Potts JR. Pathogenic bacteria attach to human fibronectin through a tandem beta-zipper. Nature. 2003;423:177–181. DOI: 10.1038/nature01589

[48] Schwarz-Linek U, Hook M, Potts JR. Fibronectin-binding proteins of Gram-positive cocci. Microbes and Infection. 2006;8:2291–2298. DOI: 10.1016/j.micinf.2006.03.011

[49] Smith EJ, Visai L, Kerrigan SW, Speziale P, Foster TJ. The Sbi protein is a multifunctional immune evasion factor of *Staphylococcus aureus*. Infection and Immunity. 2011;79:3801–3809. DOI: 10.1128/IAI.05075-11

[50] Gomez MI, Lee A, Reddy B, Muir A, Soong G, Pitt A, Cheung A, Prince A. *Staphylococcus aureus* protein A induces airway epithelial inflammatory responses by activating TNFR1. Nature Medicine. 2004;10:842–848. DOI: 10.1038/nm1079

[51] Martin FJ, Gomez MI, Wetzel DM, Memmi G, O'Seaghdha MN, Soong G, Schindler C, Prince A. *Staphylococcus aureus* activates type I IFN signaling in mice and humans through the Xr repeated sequences of protein A. Journal of Clinical Investigation. 2009;119:1931–1939. DOI: 10.1172/JCI35879

[52] Hair PS, Ward MD, Semmes OJ, Foster TJ, Cunnion KM. *Staphylococcus aureus* clumping factor A binds to complement regulator factor I and increases factor I cleavage of C3b. Journal of Infectious Diseases. 2008;198:125–133. DOI: 10.1086/588825

[53] Flick MJ, Du X, Prasad JM, Raghu H, Palumbo JS, Smeds EH, M., Degen JL. Genetic elimination of the binding motif on fibrinogen for the *S. aureus* virulence factor ClfA improves host survival in septicemia. Blood. 2013;121:1783–1794. DOI: 10.1182/blood-2012-09-453894

[54] Rohde H, Knobloch JK, Horstkotte MA, Mack D. Correlation of *Staphylococcus aureus icaADBC* genotype and biofilm expression phenotype. Journal of Clinical Microbiology. 2001;39(12):4595–4596. DOI: 10.1128/JCM.39.12.4595-4596.2001

[55] Otto M. *Staphylococcus epidermidis*the 'accidental' pathogen. Nature Reviews: Microbiology. 2009;7(8):555–567. DOI: 10.1038/nrmicro2182

[56] Cucarella C, Solano C, Valle J, Amorena B, Lasa I, Penades JR. Bap, a *Staphylococcus aureus* surface protein involved in biofilm formation. Journal of Bacteriology. 2001;183:2888–2896. DOI: 10.1128/JB.183.9.2888-2896.2001

[57] Schroeder K, Jularic M, Horsburgh SM, Hirschhausen N, Neumann C, Bertling A, Schulte A, Foster S, Kehrel BE, Peters G, Heilmann C. Molecular characterization of a novel *Staphylococcus aureus* surface protein (SasC) involved in cell aggregation and biofilm accumulation. PloS One. 2009;4:e7567. DOI: 10.1371/journal.pone.0007567

[58] Mazmanian SK, Liu G, Jensen ER, Lenoy E, Schneewind O. *Staphylococcus aureus* sortase mutants defective in the display of surface proteins and in the pathogenesis of animal infections. Proceedings of the National Academy of Sciences of the United States of America. 2000;97(10):5510–5515. DOI: 10.1073/pnas.080520697

[59] Cheng AG, Kim HK, Burts ML, Krausz T, Schneewind O, Missiakas DM. Genetic requirements for *Staphylococcus aureus* abscess formation and persistence in host tissues. FASEB Journal. 2009;23:3393–3404. DOI: 10.1096/fj.09-135467

[60] Kwiecinski J, Jin T, Josefsson E. Surface proteins of *Staphylococcus aureus* play an important role in experimental skin infection. Acta Pathologica, Microbiologica et Immunologica Scandinavica. 2014;122(12):1240–1250. DOI: 10.1111/apm.12295

[61] Edwards AM, Potter U, Meenan NA, Potts JR, Massey RC. *Staphylococcus aureus* keratinocyte invasion is dependent upon multiple high-affinity fibronectin-binding repeats within FnBPA. PloS One. 2011;6(4):e18899. DOI: 10.1371/journal.pone.0018899

[62] Classen A, Kalali BN, Schnopp C, Andres C, Aguilar-Pimentel JA, Ring J, Ollert M, Mempel M. TNF receptor I on human keratinocytes is a binding partner for staphylococcal protein A resulting in the activation of NF kappa B, AP-1, and downstream gene transcription. Experimental Dermatology. 2011;20(1):48–52. DOI: 10.1111/j.1600-0625.2010.01174.x

[63] Clarke SR, Mohamed R, Bian L, Routh AF, Kokai-Kun JF, Mond JJ, Tarkowski A, Foster SJ. The *Staphylococcus aureus* surface protein IsdA mediates resistance to innate defenses of human skin. Cell Host Microbe. 2007;1:199–212. DOI: 10.1016/j.chom.2007.04.005

[64] Clarke SR, Foster SJ. IsdA protects *Staphylococcus aureus* against the bactericidal protease activity of apolactoferrin. Infection and Immunity. 2008;76:1518–1526. DOI: 10.1128/IAI.01530-07

[65] Malachowa N, Kobayashi SD, Sturdevant DE, Scott DP, DeLeo FR. Insights into the *Staphylococcus aureus*-host interface: global changes in host and pathogen gene expression in a rabbit skin infection model. PloS One. 2015;10(2):e0117713. DOI: 10.1371/journal.pone.0117713

[66] Nilsson IM, Patti JM, Bremell T, Hook M, Tarkowski A. Vaccination with a recombinant fragment of collagen adhesin provides protection against *Staphylococcus aureus*-mediated septic death. Journal of Clinical Investigation. 1998;101:2640–2649. DOI: 10.1172/JCI1823

[67] Josefsson E, Hartford O, O'Brien L, Patti JM, Foster T. Protection against experimental *Staphylococcus aureus* arthritis by vaccination with clumping factor A, a novel virulence determinant. Journal of Infectious Diseases. 2001;184:1572–1580. DOI: 10.1086/324430

[68] Stranger-Jones YK, Bae T, Schneewind O. Vaccine assembly from surface proteins of *Staphylococcus aureus*. Proceedings of the National Academy of Sciences of the United States of America. 2006;103:16942–16947. DOI: 10.1073/pnas.0606863103

[69] Bagnoli F, Bertholet S, Grandi G. Inferring reasons for the failure of *Staphylococcus aureus* vaccines in clinical trials. Frontiers in Cellular and Infection Microbiology. 2012;2:16. DOI: 10.3389/fcimb.2012.00016

[70] Fowler VG, Allen KB, Moreira ED, Moustafa M, Isgro F, Boucher HW, Corey GR, Carmeli Y, Betts R, Hartzel JS, Chan IS, McNeely TB, Kartsonis NA, Guris D, Onorato MT, Smugar SS, DiNubile MJ, Sobanjo-ter Meulen A. Effect of an investigational vaccine for preventing *Staphylococcus aureus* infections after cardiothoracic surgery: a randomized trial. The Journal of the American Medical Association. 2013;309:1368–1378. DOI: 10.1001/jama.2013.3010

[71] Spellberg B, Ibrahim AS, Yeaman MR, Lin L, Fu Y, Avanesian V, Bayer AS, Filler SG, Lipke P, Otoo H, Edwards JE, Jr. The antifungal vaccine derived from the recombinant N terminus of Als3p protects mice against the bacterium *Staphylococcus aureus*. Infection and Immunity. 2008;76(10):4574–4580. DOI: 10.1128/IAI.00700-08

[72] Misstear K, McNeela EA, Murphy AG, Geoghegan JA, O'Keeffe KM, Fox J, Chan K, Heuking S, Collin N, Foster TJ, McLoughlin RM, Lavelle EC. Targeted nasal vaccination provides antibody-independent protection against *Staphylococcus aureus*. Journal of Infectious Diseases. 2014;209(9):1479–1484. DOI: 10.1093/infdis/jit636

[73] Kolata JB, Kuhbandner I, Link C, Normann N, Vu CH, Steil L, Weidenmaier C, Broker BM. The Fall of a Dogma? Unexpected High T-Cell Memory Response to *Staphylococcus aureus* in Humans. Journal of Infectious Diseases. 2015;212(5):830–838. DOI: 10.1093/infdis/jiv128jo

[74] Fowler VG, Jr., Proctor RA. Where does a *Staphylococcus aureus* vaccine stand? Clinical Microbiology and Infection. 2014;20 Suppl 5:66–75. DOI: 10.1111/1469-0691.12570

[75] Narita K, Hu DL, Mori F, Wakabayashi K, Iwakura Y, Nakane A. Role of interleukin-17A in cell-mediated protection against *Staphylococcus aureus* infection in mice immunized with the fibrinogen-binding domain of clumping factor A. Infection and Immunity. 2010;78(10):4234–4242. DOI: 10.1128/IAI.00447-10

[76] Nissen M, Marshall H, Richmond P, Shakib S, Jiang Q, Cooper D, Rill D, Baber J, Eiden J, Gruber W, Jansen KU, Emini EA, Anderson AS, Zito ET, Girgenti D. A randomized phase I study of the safety and immunogenicity of three ascending dose levels of a 3-antigen *Staphylococcus aureus* vaccine (SA3Ag) in healthy adults. Vaccine. 2015;33(15):1846–1854. DOI: 10.1016/j.vaccine.2015.02.024

[77] Proctor RA. Recent developments for *Staphylococcus aureus* vaccines: clinical and basic science challenges. European Cells and Materials. 2015;30:315–326.

[78] Schmidt CS, White CJ, Ibrahim AS, Filler SG, Fu Y, Yeaman MR, Edwards JE, Jr., Hennessey JP, Jr. NDV-3, a recombinant alum-adjuvanted vaccine for *Candida* and *Staphylococcus aureus*, is safe and immunogenic in healthy adults. Vaccine. 2012;30(52):7594–7600. DOI: 10.1016/j.vaccine.2012.10.038

Chapter 11

Staphylococcus aureus Biofilms and their Impact on the Medical Field

Fany Reffuveille, Jérôme Josse, Quentin Vallé,
Céline Mongaret and Sophie C. Gangloff

Additional information is available at the end of the chapter

http://dx.doi.org/10.5772/66380

Abstract

Despite the discovery of antibiotics, the battle against bacteria is so far in their favor, specifically because bugs are able to develop a superstructure named biofilm, to resist and to survive in the environment. Nosocomial infections, a major health problem, are due at 80% to biofilm-associated infection, and *Staphylococcus aureus* is the leading bacteria species in this domain. Moreover, the antimicrobial resistance of this bacterial community is accentuated when it is formed by superbugs such as methicillin-resistant *S. aureus* (MRSA). In this chapter, the mechanism and the physiology of *S. aureus* biofilm as well as their consequences in the clinical domains are described. To complete the vision on *S. aureus* biofilms, some "anti-biofilm" strategies will be highlighted.

Keywords: *Staphylococcus aureus*, biofilm, antibiotic resistance, anti-biofilm strategies

1. Introduction

Discoveries in microbiology and the setup of aseptically processes in medical science allowed the possibility of high-level surgery over the last century, with the hope of a safe healing. In return, major problems have appeared as nosocomial infections due to bacterial biofilm formations on medical devices [1, 2]. Despite the multiplication of surgical procedures in order to get as close as sterile environment, bacterial contamination remains an important risk. Bacteria could indeed acquire antibiotic resistances and an emergence of multidrug resistant strains is observed [3, 4]. Moreover, the most alarming is that bacteria with regular sensitivity to antibiotics are even able to develop a strategy to survive: the formation of a strong community named biofilm [1, 2, 5]. Biofilm-associated infections represent 80% of nosocomial infections, and *Staphylococcus aureus* is the leading species in this domain [6–8].

Biofilm is defined as a multicellular lifestyle, an organized structure built by almost all bacterial species. Even if the term "biofilm" has been used for more than 60 years, the understanding of this structure started but recently. Fossilized biofilms of 3.5 billion years have been discovered and highlight the hypothesis that biofilm is a survival strategy always used by microorganisms since the dawn of time [5]. Scientists have recently understood that bacteria are not always living as free cells in nature; on the contrary, most of the time, bacteria build a real social life in a resistant community surrounded by a matrix composed of polysaccharides, extracellular DNA, proteins, lipids and other components [1, 2]. Biofilm is present on biotic or abiotic surface and bacteria embedded inside are 10–1000 times more resistant to conventional antibiotics than free-floating bacteria according to the strains, the molecule applied and the model of study [7–9]. Life cycle of biofilm is nowadays well-described. First, bacteria adhere on a surface and they enhance different mechanisms to irreversibly be attached. Then, the program of biofilm starts with a maturation of the multicellular structure. To complete this cycle, dispersion of swimming cells occurs under specific conditions [1, 2, 7–9]. However, the key of biofilm mechanism is the initiation that leads bacteria to form a biofilm and only under specific conditions. This trigger of biofilm mechanism is still an important question. Survival would be the answer, thus biofilm structure allows bacteria to resist to any types of environmental stress including UV, lack of nutrients and presence of antimicrobials [1, 2, 7–9].

All these characteristics lead to major problems in industries as well as in the medical domain. In industry, for example, the presence of multispecies biofilms has a high impact on the processes or on the production and results in high costs. *S. aureus* can be isolated from biofilm found in food industry particularly in dairy process [10], and they are sanitizers resistant [11]. As a consequence, microorganisms can infect the milk or other food products and cleaning the production system is very complicated or impossible. Thus, all the structures need to be replaced representing an important waste of money.

In the medical domain, numerous difficulties to treat biofilm-associated infections are described: resistance to antibiotics and to immune system, spread of infection, sepsis shock and surgical risks to remove infected implant or tissues [1, 6, 8]. *S. aureus* is one of the most frequent germs found in biofilm-associated infections partially resulting from the fact that they are commensal bacteria on the human skin and mucous [12]. Moreover, *S. aureus* multidrug resistant like methicillin resistant *S. aureus* strains (MRSA), is responsible for biofilm infections that are more difficult to treat that need more intensive care and replacement of medical devices as compared to *Staphylococcus epidermidis* biofilm infections, for example. *S. aureus* also embodies an important reservoir of dissemination to other human body sites [12]. Consequently, the development of new therapeutic strategies, through a better understanding of biofilms, is necessary and imperative [4] to fight against this structure resistant to the immune system and antimicrobial drugs.

Here after, to better understand the strength of *S. aureus* biofilms, different aspects relevant to biofilm, its mechanism and its physiology will highlight the aspects that are specific to

http://dx.doi.org/10.5772/66380

Staphylococci and *S. aureus* more precisely. The consequence of *S. aureus* in clinical domain will be described and some "anti-biofilm" strategies will be suggested.

2. Biofilm life cycle

Different steps of biofilm life cycle have been well-described through the study of different bacterial species: reversible adhesion, irreversible attachment, maturation and dispersion [5, 13] (**Figure 1**). First, active bacteria can turn from "swimmers" to "stickers" on a support. A surface is supposed to always be in favor of adhesion because of the prediction that organic substances will concentrate on a surface and microorganisms will easily adhere and be protected from outsider challenges. Adhesion will dependent on the species of bacteria, surface composition, environmental factors, and essential gene products [14]. Microorganisms could adhere on inert or biotic surfaces. Most of the time, interaction between bacteria and abiotic surface involves nonspecific interactions as opposed to active interaction between microorganisms and live tissues [14]. The surface conditioning is quite important through various physiochemical parameters: hydrophobicity, chemical composition of the material, surface energy, eletrostatic charges, temperature, surface roughness and in the case of biotic adhesion: serum and tissue protein adsorption [14, 15]. Hydrophobicity increases bacterial adhesion in most cases [15, 16]. In some environmental conditions, macromolecules adsorption could form a "film" neutralizing excessive charges and surface free-energy facilitating bacteria and surface proximity. It was shown that pH parameters influence *S. aureus* adherence on glass [17].

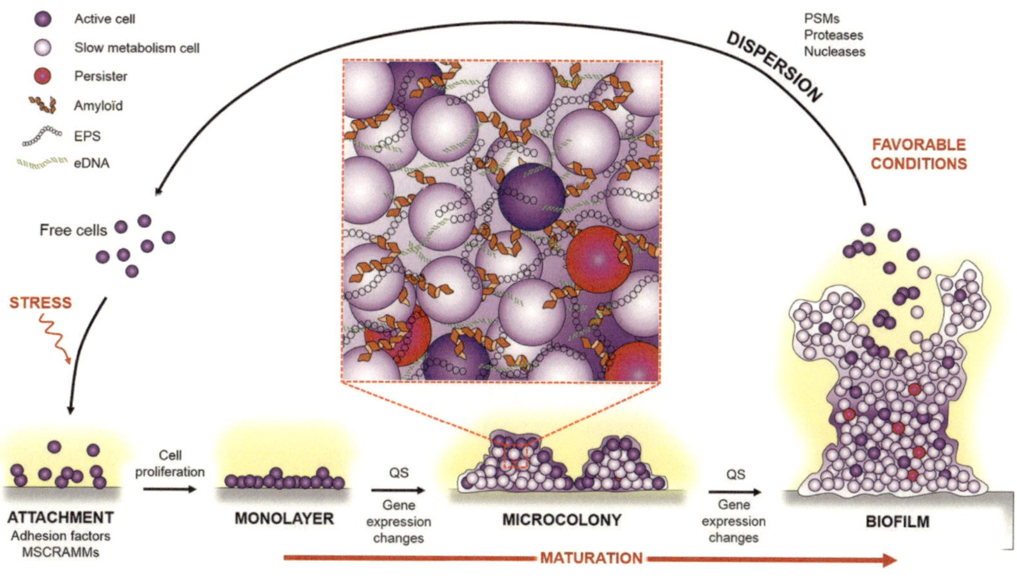

Figure 1. Biofilm life cycle.

As far as *S. epidermidis* is concerned, Sousa et al. [15] have shown that surface conditions influence bacterial adhesion but the cell surface hydrophobicity itself was not linked to adhesion capacity, underlying the importance of other factors as cell wall associated proteins. The first bacteria approaching a surface adhere to it because of good conditioning but afterwards when the rate of cells increases, the following bacteria tend to adhere to previous bacteria instead of the surface [15]. In a case of a bad conditioning of surface and the necessity of adhesion, pili or other bacterial appendices could overcome potential repulsion.

2.1. Attachment on a surface

In any case, the life of a biofilm starts by an adhesion. The latter is reversible but can turn irreversible. Indeed, under specific conditions, events of irreversible attachment tend to increase and lead to the formation of a biofilm. In fact, irreversible attachment is the first step to the maturation of a future biofilm.

At the beginning, adhesion is the fortunate meeting between a good conditioned surface and a bacterium. In any environment, microorganisms can randomly get close to the surface or be attracted by chemotaxis involving their motility system [14]. Very recently, the ability for motility was observed for *S. aureus* even if they do not possess any appendages for movement [18]. This very particular movement is supposed to be a response to very specific conditions.

A surface could be attractive or repulsive for bacteria according to different parameters described above including hydrophobic and electrostatic interactions, hydrodynamic forces and temperature. Hydrophobicity is considered the most important. Bacteria could adhere on a biotic or abiotic surface thanks to the involvement of specific bacterial surface molecules such as the surface protein autolysin or the teichoic acids, altering the physicochemical properties of the bacterial surface rather than mediating the attachment via specific, receptor-mediated interactions [13].

In the human body, *S. aureus* is known to have specific targets in relation with its pathogenesis. Staphylococci attachment to a biotic surface such as human tissue is due to specific interactions with its virulent factors (**Figure 1**). These bacteria possess a large variety of surface-anchored proteins such as the microbial surface components recognizing adhesive matrix molecules (MSCRAMMS). MSCRAMMS are structured in three parts: a binding domain, a cell wall spanning domain and a third part responsible for the covalent or non-covalent attachment of the MSCRAMM proteins on bacterial surface. These adhesins are able to bind to one or several different human matrix proteins (fibronectin, fibrogen, etc.) [13, 19, 20] and are required for biofilm-associated infections on indwelling medical devices covered by host matrix right after insertion [13]. Covalent bonds are catalyzed by sortases recognizing LPXTG motifs. *S. aureus* strains have a high variety of LPXTG-type MSCRAMMs compared to *S. epidermidis* [21]. Other surface proteins involved in adhesion are Sdr proteins (Serin-aspartate repeat family) or Aap (accumulation-associated proteins) [13]. Non-covalently bounds are insured by other proteins such as the autolysin Atl. Autolysins, involved in cell wall turnover, are one of the most abundant proteins on the staphylococcal cell surface and possess binding sites for human matrix proteins [22, 23].

Staphylococci are known for their high ability to stick to plastic surfaces. Teichoic acids, which are not involved in *S. aureus* attachment on biotic surface, are important compounds present in the cell wall and are important for adhesion on plastic surfaces thanks to their interaction with other surface polymers [13, 24]. However, *in vitro* assay over-estimated the interactions between teichoic acids and devices mainly because devices in fluids or in tissue are rapidly covered by host matrix proteins preventing the direct interaction of teichoic acids to plastic. Despite teichoic acids, two other adhesins have a role for adherence on plastic: the cell wall bound surface protein Bap involved in adherence to polystyrene surfaces [25] and SasC a *S. aureus* surface protein involved in attachment on polystyrene that does not mediate binding to fibrinogen, thrombospondin-1, von Willebrand factor or platelets [26]. Also, autolysins facilitate attachment to plastic in addition of their capacity to bind to human matrix and their enzymatic function [23].

2.2. Communication between bacteria

Pseudomonas aeruginosa biofilm is one of the most studied biofilm models. A powerful system of communication between cells was described in *P. aeruginosa* biofilm and named "quorum-sensing" [27]. First the quorum-sensing system was linked to a communication based on cell density. Then, quorum-sensing is virtually connected to biofilm formation and dispersal phenomena. The communication system in *P. aeruginosa* is based on molecules called acyl-homoserine lactones (AHLs) which penetrate bacteria and directly regulate target genes. Quorum-sensing systems have been described in Gram-negative and Gram-positive bacteria. Each quorum-sensing system is composed with different molecules and can activate or inhibit biofilm formation. The most studied system in *S. aureus* is the Agr quorum-sensing system but other systems of communication exist.

For *S. aureus*, only one specific quorum-sensing system was so far described, but most probably, there are other mechanisms for communication. At some point, some genes involved in *S. aureus* virulence were named accessory genes, and an accessory gene regulator (*agr*) was identified as a global regulator of virulence factors genes. Different experimental designs have shown that the Agr system induced by an extracellular ligand, the autoinducing peptides (AIP), is a sensor of population and so considered as a quorum-sensing system. This system can be activated by addition of AIP or by glucose depletion [28]. Briefly, this system is composed of two promoters P2 and P3. P3 transcript encodes RNAIII, the intracellular effector of target gene regulation, answering to *agr* system activation. P2 operon encodes for a two-component system and its autoinducing ligand AIP [29].

During biofilm formation, Agr quorum-sensing system is repressed to stop the expression of *S. aureus* colonization factors [29], and it gets activated during the dispersion of the bacteria [30]. Artificial activation of Agr has also been shown to induce biofilm dispersion [28]. Moreover, Agr quorum-sensing system is necessary for the communication inside mature biofilm to establish the 3D structure through the control of cell dispersion. This probably requires phenol-soluble modulins (PSMs) which are described in the next section and proteases activated by Agr and involved in the degradation of exopolysaccharides (EPS) matrix [31]. However, Agr does not control important biofilm adhesive molecules such as the polysaccharide intercellular adhesions, currently named PIA [32]. In conclusion, Agr system regulation is based on cell density. During the early stage of colonization, cell density is low and as consequences Agr quorum-sensing activity gets weak and the cell wall protein or surface adhesins are not downregulated but highly expressed. In the later stage, Agr activity increases with cell density and thereafter Agr upregulates secreted virulence factors such as lipases, proteases and hemolysin [33]. Not surprisingly, Agr involvement in biofilm formation seems to be under specific environmental conditions as shown by the contradiction of experimental results relevant to the model used in the study [30]. One problem underlined each time is the difficulty to detect *agr* expression due to the very slow bacteria metabolism in the biofilm. During hospitalization, *S. aureus* strains isolated from patients are more frequently Agr-defective strains showing their better ability to turn into a nosocomial infection agent [34]. Some *agr*-defective mutants have been isolated from catheter infections, where they had the capacity to form a compact biofilm with the loss of their capacity to detach and disseminate.

Other regulators have been identified such as Rbf which is involved in *S. aureus* biofilm formation at the maturation stage rather than at the initial attachment [35]. This regulator did not affect *ica* gene locus coding for adhesins; however, a clinical isolate with *rbf* mutation showed a lower capacity to form biofilm. LuxS, another regulator first described in *Vibrio cholerae*, is under the control of the auto-inducer AI-2 and seems to play a role in biofilm formation through the *icaR* expression. However, LuxS is also involved in the S-adenosyl methionine cycle, and its role in biofilm is consequently debated as it could be the result of this metabolic role [36].

In conclusion, production of surfactant molecules dependent of quorum-sensing system appears to be a general mechanism for the biofilm structuring as well as for the detachment of many bacteria. In the specific *S. aureus* quorum-sensing, biofilm is based on the detection of signaling molecules by specific sensors which lead to a chain reaction with different molecular actors and not on a direct communication where the signal molecules enter in the cells and directly regulate different genes. In *S. aureus*, the sensors are numerous and allow a fast answer of the bacteria.

2.3. Maturation

The maturation of biofilm is based on the development of the multicellular structure (**Figure 1**). Biofilm growth is controlled by the increase of bacterial mediators, the slowdown of metabolism and cell cooperation. Maturation starts when bacterial cells induce the biofilm program and create an intercellular aggregation through the production of a "slime" commonly named matrix. The latter sticks bacteria one to each other as well as on surface. The matrix is composed of exopolysaccharides (EPS), proteins and extracellular DNA (eDNA) and is responsible for biofilm maturation that is the result of an organized community construction. This specific 3-dimensional structure appears as a typical mushroom-like shape containing water or fluid channels formed thanks to a disruptive process [37]. Paradoxically, maturation in the construction of the community needs also disruption events. Fluid-filled channels are vital in delivering nutrient into biofilm deeper layers [38]. This kind of structure is species-specific.

Exopolysaccharides are the first molecules discovered in biofilm matrix. In staphylococci, the most described adhesive biofilm molecule is the polysaccharide intercellular adhesion (PIA) or poly-N-acetylglucosamine (PNAG) and represents the major part of the staphylococci biofilm-forming extracellular matrix [39]. PIA has an important role in the biofilm structure and the biofilm-associated infections [40, 41]. Introducing a positive charge in the environment of the bacterial cell surface which is negatively charged, PIA works like a glue sticking the cells together by electrostatic interaction [42]. PIA is encoded by *ica* gene locus and regulated by numerous environmental factors [43]. For example, SarA and SigB upregulate PIA expression and on the contrary LuxS downregulates it [44–46]. PIA is the only factor identified so far as important for staphylococci biofilm formation *in vivo* [13, 43]; however, PIA is not present in all strains isolated from biofilm-associated infections [47]. Therefore, some other compounds like proteins must also play a role.

Numerous specific proteins could be substitute for PIA in biofilm formation as proteins are now recognized as essential for biofilm structure, such as the following proteins: Aap (accumulation associated protein), extracellular matrix binding protein (Embp), protein A, fibrinogen-binding proteins (FnbpA and FnbpB) or *S. aureus* surface protein G (SasG) [48]. This latter mediates intercellular aggregation thanks to hydrophilic interaction with the proteins present on other bacteria [49]. As for *S. aureus* surface protein SasC, which possesses a LPXTG-motif to anchor to cell wall, it is involved in intercellular aggregation and biofilm maturation [26]. Depending on the Staphylococcus, the extracellular Aap protein [50] is involved in PIA-independent biofilm formation in *S. epidermidis* [51] or in the maturation of the biofilm by interactions with PIA like in *S. aureus* [50].

All these results underline the importance of the surfactants in biofilm maturation. Phenol-soluble modulins (PSM) are surfactant peptides found in both *S. aureus* and *S. epidermidis*. Their sequence is species dependant, but they all have an amphipathic α-helix [13]. PSMs are strictly controlled by Agr, with a direct binding of Agr regulator on the *psm* operon promoter, suggesting that Agr-dependent biofilm maturation processes are due to PSMs expression [13]. Moreover, an *agr* mutant strain of *S. aureus* has the same behavior that a completely deleted PSM genes mutant in *in vivo* model [13]. As shown in *S. epidermidis*, the PSM involvement in biofilm maturation is independent of the PIA protein. In *S. epidermidis*, the lack of PSMs leads to biofilms that are more "compact", suggesting that PSM are also involved In biofilm development. Furthermore, as seen in all the *Staphylococcus*, the presence of the PSM peptides is needed for biofilm volume, thickness, roughness and channel formation [52]. Surfactant peptides are therefore the key of the 3-dimensional biofilm structure. PSMs also induce biofilm detachment [52] and are biofilm maturation *in vivo* determinant factors [13].

Amyloid proteins have also been revealed as important for biofilm structure, bringing stability to the matrix [53]. These protein fibers could bind the extracellular DNA. PSMs play also a role as inert fibrils in biofilm, acting as a solid bond, waiting for better conditions to induce their dissociation and promote biofilm dispersion [53, 54]. Bap another cell wall bound surface protein [25, 55–57], involved in adhesion, is also required for biofilm maturation and infection of bovine mammary glands [20, 45]. This protein is a real sensor, responding to environmental conditions (like calcium concentration), and Bap is also a scaffold protein forming amyloid-like aggregates at low calcium concentration and under acidic pH [53].

Under an organized construction, biofilm maturation is based on development and disruption events. Thus, PIA-degrading enzymes (PIAse) are supposed to contribute to biofilm maturating but they have never been found in staphylococci [13]. Anyway other proteases could have an important role in staphylococci biofilm maturation as proven by strains showing PIA-independent biofilm formation [58]. Those proteases are regulated mostly by SarA and more rarely by Agr, but so far no experiments have demonstrated direct evidence for their role on biofilm development or protease-mediated biofilm detachment.

The third important element of matrix composition is extracellular DNA (eDNA). DNA, a polyanionic molecule present in biofilm matrix, is described as a ligand able to link to other molecules present in the matrix such as teichoic acids or PIA. Therefore, DNA has a role in biofilm structure. This presence is based on the involvement of cell death: DNA released from lysed bacteria also called eDNA has a critical involvement during initial attachment and maturation. An increase of cell lysis influences biofilm formation through the Cid proteins [59–61]. Indeed, regulators like CidR which controls autolysis are involved in biofilm development and the formation of the tower mushrooms shapes [62]. Extracellular DNA appears through the bacterial programmed cell death and through the expression of *cidA* gene encoding for a holin responsible for lysis. This system is regulated by the production of an antiholin encoded by *lrgAB* genes which is an inhibitor of cidA-mediated lysis [59, 62]. However, *in vivo*, the importance of eDNA is difficult to assess as well as to understand how a staphylococcal biofilm could survive in the presence of human DNAseI which succeed to disperse a mature biofilm *in vitro* [13].

In conclusion, scientists have realized how important it is to have precise knowledge of the mechanisms involved in the biofilm extend matrix or in the detachment steps to be able to develop anti-biofilm strategies. However, biofilms are also formed by four set of cells: some with an aerobic or fermentative growth, some dormant or dead [63]. This cell heterogeneity within the biofilms has to be kept in mind in the search of anti-biofilm therapy.

2.4. Dispersion

Disruptive processes are vital for biofilm structure and disruption allows the detachment of single cells or large bacteria cluster from biofilm in case of good environmental conditions or in case of expansion of the biofilm (**Figure 1**). This dispersion has important consequences in biofilm-associated infections as it leads to systemic dissemination. It is well known now that detached cells from biofilm could lead to endocarditis or sepsis [13].

Disruption is based on mechanical forces as well as the interruption of the production of the biofilm material and production of enzymes and surfactants that are considered as detachment factors able to destroy the matrix. Agr quorum-sensing system involved in biofilm formation and extracellular protease activity are required to control biofilm dispersal molecules [28, 32, 52]. Expression of *agr* mostly carried out by the bacteria in the outer layers of the biofilm leads to detachment and regrowth [30], but *agr* is also expressed in deeper layers where it is required for channel formations [52]. In fact this dispersal effect linked to Agr system could be due to the involvement of PSMs whose expression is controlled by the Agr quorum-sensing.

Nucleases, the enzymes degrading extracellular DNA are also necessary. The human DNaseI degrades staphylococcal biofilms [64]. Staphylococcal thermonuclease *nuc2* is involved in the biofilm development probably to promote dispersion [65]. A second nuclease *nuc1* showed

http://dx.doi.org/10.5772/66380

the similar dispersal effect as *nuc2* on biofilm *in vitro* [66]. Nevertheless, those effects are not detected so far in *in vivo* models [66].

Other factors, involved in dispersion, have been described such as bacteriophages which have been revealed as important for biofilm development, especially in dispersal stage [31]. Even proteases like Aur metalloprotease and Slp serine protease have been shown to be responsible of dispersal movement [67].

In conclusion, biofilm life cycle starts under the impulse of a stress response (e.g., starvation) and bacteria attach on a surface where cell proliferation is more favorable. A monolayer is formed, and some specific genes are expressed inducing the production of microcolonies. Quorum-sensing system acts as a supervisor, and biofilm is formed in a well-organized structure.

3. Physiology of biofilm

Biofilms seem to be the best strategy for bacteria to survive to any kind of environmental stress. The detection of stress and thus the response needs to be fast enough to survive under those conditions. Therefore, the rapid process of activation of the biofilm program is crucial for the bacteria.

3.1. Program on/off

As described for stress response, the setup of inducible processes is based on the differential expression of an important number of genes [68, 69]. Biofilm bacteria cells are physiologically different from free cells [12]. Indeed, the different steps as adhesion and immobilization need the expression of various genes. More important, the communication between bacteria (quorum-sensing system) controls many metabolic systems and leads to regulation of many genes. The production of the quorum-sensing molecules as an endogenous signal leads to changes according to the detected concentration. Environmental clues trigger genetic and physiological changes also called biofilm transition. As previously described, the matrix is the plinth of biofilm development and is responsible for many processes in the biofilm program. Moreover, biofilm cells show a general downregulation of their metabolism underlining the slow growing cell or the lack of oxygen due to the biofilm structure, like during fermentation. An upregulation of the urease and the arginine deiminase pathway to limit the side effects of the acidic pH during anaerobic growth was also observed in biofilm structure [12]. All those adaptations participate to a general biofilm setup process. The differential gene expressions also lead to antibiotic resistance mechanism. In *S. epidermidis*, some of these antibiotic resistance mechanisms are upregulated during biofilm stage [70]. In *S. aureus*, Agr expression and involvement in biofilm formation depend of the environmental conditions [30]. The *agr* expression shut down has no effect, enhances or inhibits biofilm formation according to the environmental parameters [30].

Biofilm program is a temporary response to stress conditions and this process is able to turn off quite quickly when conditions are more favorable for the bacteria.

3.2. Interactions with the environment and survival strategy

Bacteria have the extraordinary ability to survive in any harsh conditions, and as recently discovered, this is due to their capacity to form biofilm. Many environments can be a source of stress for bacteria. *S. aureus* biofilm have been found in industry and in clinical domain, particularly in biofilm-associated infections. Environmental stresses are supposed to induce biofilm formation. As evidence, sigma B, a protein required for transcription and activated under stress responses due to heat shock, $MnCl_2$, $NaCl_2$ and alkaline shock, is involved in biofilm formation [71, 72].

In *S. aureus*, nutrients like glucose or NaCl can influence biofilm. For example, Rbf regulator is involved in biofilm formation under high concentrations of glucose and NaCl conditions, but not in the presence of ethanol [35]. Nutrient-starvation has been underlined as an important environmental stress which could induce biofilm maturation [61, 73]. *In vitro*, however, the addition of glucose is required for biofilm formation and activation of the *agr* quorum-sensing system [28], even if oldest results showed the contrary [74]. In fact, conditions to form biofilm seem to be very specific, such as a balance between an over-concentration of glucose and a lack of carbon source. The pH maintenance also influences Agr system and, in consequence, probably acts on biofilm formation [74, 75].

Nitrite stress also induces PIA expression, responsible for the major part of the matrix composition [76]. In fact, induction or repression of biofilm formation is due to a balance of concentration of specific nutrients or stress. For example, NO is necessary for biofilm formation until its concentration starts to be too high. Thereafter, NO is involved in the dispersion of the biofilm [77]. It has also been observed that low oxygen, even anaerobic state, like in the heart of the biofilm, increases PIA expression [78].

In human body, the lack of nutrients (e.g., iron, carbon source, etc.) or oxygen, the presence of the immune system or even the antimicrobial molecules are felt by the bacteria as stresses and could induce biofilm program. In *S. aureus*, PIA expression and biofilm maturation are strongly inducible by conditions found *in vivo* as described in a device-related infection model [79]. In *S. epidermidis*, subinhibitory concentrations of tetracycline and quinupristin - dalfopristin induce *ica* gene cluster expression and the increase of Mg^{2+} concentrations increase biofilm production. On the contrary, the addition of EDTA (Ethylenediaminetetraacetic acid) decreases the number of cells on a plastic surface [14]. Zinc concentration might also influence biofilm adhesion through the activity of SasG a surface protein with zinc-dependent mechanical properties [49]. Subinhibitory concentrations of furanone, molecules isolated from red algae, inhibit quorum sensing but also favor biofilm formation [80, 81]. This result reflects the possible inter-species interaction domain and the importance of the specific microenvironment.

In nature, many bacteria live under nutrient-limited conditions, lack of oxygen and under many other dangers like humidity, osmotic pressure and mechanical forces. Biofilm through the presence of the matrix protect all the embedded bacteria from all those environmental variations and pressures.

3.3. Interactions with the host immune cells

During bacterial infection, host immune cells are the defenders of the organism. Through mechanisms such as phagocytosis or release of bactericidal components, these cells are able to fight and neutralize planktonic *S. aureus*. Concerning *S. aureus* biofilm, the general thought is that biofilm structure protects the bacteria against the immune cells, avoiding interaction between both actors. Nevertheless, recent studies reported that polymorphonuclear neutrophils (PMN), macrophages, myeloid-derived suppressor cells (MDSCs) and T lymphocytes can interact with *S. aureus* biofilm in a double-edged interplay (**Figure 2**).

PMNs are the first line of defense in bacterial infections. These cells can phagocyte planktonic bacteria and release bactericidal components such as reactive oxygen species or enzymes [82]. Contrary to the dogma, *in vitro* experiments revealed that PMN can also attack *S. aureus* in biofilm form. PMNs can migrate towards and into the *S. aureus* biofilm and clear it by phagocytosis. The extent of biofilm clearance is apparently depended on its maturation state. Indeed, mature biofilms were reported as more resistant to phagocytosis as young ones [83]. Following phagocytosis, PMNs underwent apoptosis, a programmed cell-death in order to prevent spilling of the bactericidal and cytotoxic entities [84]. In addition to phagocytosis, PMNs can release lactoferrin and elastase through degranulation phenomenon, as well as DNA [85]. Oxygen radical production by the PMNs also participates to biofilm clearance and is depended on the coating of biofilms with IgG, a mechanism termed "opsonization" [86]. In a global manner, PMNs can be considered as an asset to fight against *S. aureus* biofilms.

In parallel to PMNs response, a macrophage response is also triggered during *S. aureus* infections, which is altered in case of *S. aureus* biofilm infection. Indeed, planktonic *S. aureus* normally induces a proinflammatory microbicidal phenotype in macrophages defined as M1. It implies the phagocytosis of bacteria and the production of bactericidal components [87]. In the context of *S. aureus* biofilm infection, *in vitro* and *in vivo* studies reported that invasion of macrophages into biofilms is limited. *S. aureus* biofilms is able to secrete specific toxins

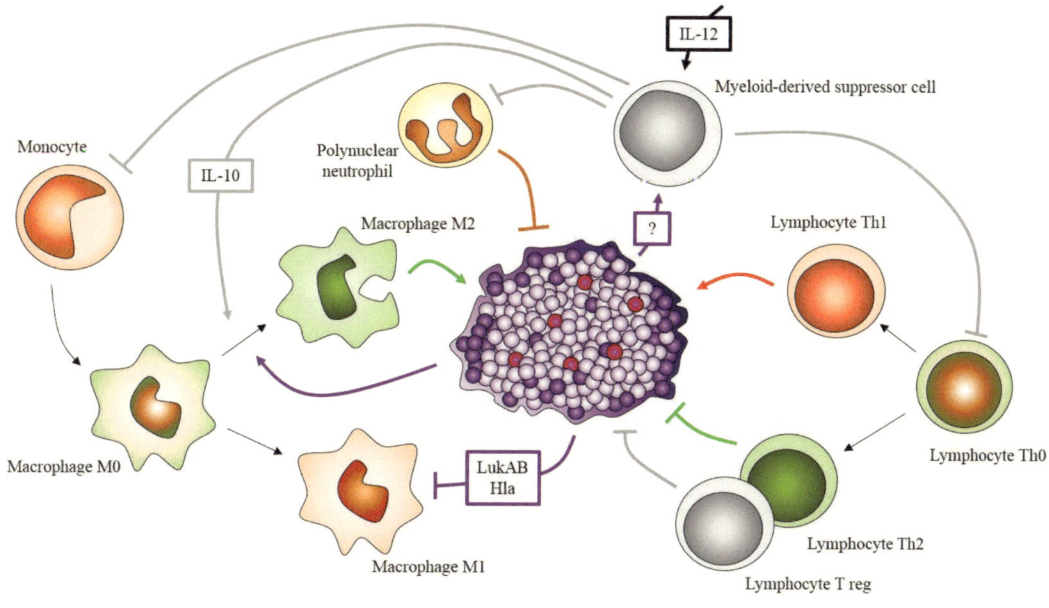

Figure 2. Interplay between *S. aureus* biofilm and host immune cells.

called alpha-toxin (Hla) and leukocidin AB (LukAB) that inhibit macrophage phagocytosis and induce cytotoxicity, promoting macrophage dysfunction and thus facilitating *S. aureus* biofilm development [88]. Moreover, *S. aureus* biofilm can also induce the polarization of macrophages from a proinflammatory microbicidal M1 phenotype to an alternatively activated M2 phenotype, displaying anti-inflammatory properties and limited phagocytosis [33, 89]. A recent study showed that the treatment of established biofilm infections with M1-activated significantly reduced biofilm burdens, supporting that M1 phenotype is unpropitious to *S. aureus* biofilm development whereas M2 polarization favors it [90].

The most recent studies concerning interactions between *S. aureus* biofilms and immune cells focus on the MDSCs, a heterogeneous population of immature monocytes and granulocytes with immunosuppressive properties. In case of *S. aureus* biofilm infection, MDSCs prevent monocyte/macrophage pro-inflammatory activity, inhibit T lymphocytes proliferation and facilitates biofilm persistence [91]. This phenomenon is in part orchestrated by the interleukins IL-12 and IL-10 [92, 93]. IL-12 is a cytokine with both pro- and anti-inflammatory properties that promotes the recruitment of MDSCs whereas IL-10 is an anti-inflammatory cytokine, mainly produced by MDSCs in context of biofilm infection. A recent study reported that IL-10 promotes biofilm growth and anti-inflammatory gene expression in monocytes, which can be assimilated to a polarization to M2 phenotype [93]. MDSCs would in the end be the effectors for the development of the anti-inflammatory environment that favors *S. aureus* biofilm persistence.

Concerning interactions between *S. aureus* biofilm and T lymphocytes, Leid et al. reported that mononuclear leukocytes, especially lymphocytes and in a lesser extend monocytes, can attach to the biofilm but they are not able to phagocyte maturing and fully matured *S. aureus* biofilm [94]. In case of *S. aureus* biofilm infection, early Th1 and Th17 inflammatory responses are increased and Th2 as well as Treg responses seem downregulated [95]. Th2/Treg responses appear as a protection mechanism for the organism as opposed to Th1/Th17 responses, which may favor the development of chronic *S. aureus* biofilm infection [96]. This response, in opposition to what is observed in the macrophage response, reveals the complexity of the interactions between *S. aureus* biofilms and the cells of the immune system.

4. *S. aureus* biofilm-associated infections and antibiotic treatments

4.1. *S. aureus* biofilms are responsible for different types of infection

Different bacteria are involved in infections associated with biofilm development in immunocompromised patients or medical devices. Sadly, the most famous example is *P. aeruginosa* species which develop highly resistant biofilm in pulmonary tract of cystic fibrosis patients.

Biofilm formation is linked to various staphylococcal diseases such as endocarditis, osteomyelitis, skin and soft tissues infections, urinary tract infection, nasal colonization and cystic fibrosis complications as well as implant-associated infections [97–99]. In most of the case, the production of biofilm favors the chronicity of *S. aureus* infections. The colonization of implanted materials by staphylococcal biofilm is one of the highest important issues.

http://dx.doi.org/10.5772/66380

Staphylococcal biofilm can develop on various structures such as catheters, prosthetic joints, prosthetic heart valves, contact lenses, cerebrospinal fluid shunts and cardiac pacemakers [100]. Furthermore, after their implantation in the body, medical devices become coated with host proteins, facilitating the attachment of *S. aureus* and the biofilm formation [101].

4.2. *S. aureus* biofilm-associated infections are more resistant

Biofilms have shown unbreakable structures resistant to antibiotics and many other molecules or environmental stresses. Many hypotheses have been tested to explain this incredible natural invincibility. First, the intrinsic structure of biofilm supposes that antimicrobials could not penetrate inside the biofilm. This hypothesis has been revealed unlikely for most of the antibiotics as the biofilm structure is composed with many water channels. A second hypothesis is based on the fact that the biofilm matrix can accumulate antibiotic-degrading enzymes, and in consequence, antibiotics are quickly destroyed [9]. Then, scientists underline the fact that microorganisms have a very slow metabolism in the biofilm preventing most of the kinetic responses involved in the antibiotic mechanism. The use of antibiotics targeting more specifically those slow growth bacteria was not more successful, even combined with antimicrobial drugs that could target active bacteria present in the biofilm population, known to be heterogenic [63]. Persister cells can also be present in this heterogeneous population and can withstand high concentration of antimicrobial drugs.

Nowadays, it seems that the natural resistance of biofilms comes from the induction of specific biofilm mechanisms [9]. Stress responses, as biofilm formation, lead to the changes of many gene expressions which increase the antimicrobial resistance. Nutrient starvations are now known to favor antibiotic tolerance [61].

Biofilm is the perfect example of an adaptive resistance, not due to a genetic mutation that could be transferred to daughter cells, even if the bacteria proximity in the biofilms increase horizontal transfer gene or mutation that could lead to intrinsic resistance [9].

4.3. Current treatment of *S. aureus* biofilm

Treatment of *S. aureus* biofilm is a therapeutic challenge. Even if everybody has in mind that the embedment of *S. aureus* in slime gives him an increased tolerance to antibiotics, two situations have to be defined concerning the treatment of *S. aureus* biofilm-associated infections.

Firstly, antibiotics can have an inhibitive effect on the formation of biofilm. It is related to the capacity to inhibit the attachment and the initial growth of the biofilm. A recent study specifically evaluated the inhibition of *S. aureus* biofilm formation through the use of a new system the antibiofilmogram® [102]. Based on Biofilm Ring Test® method [103], this system permits to define, for a chosen antibiotic, the minimal inhibiting concentrations (MIC) needed to inhibit biofilm formation (called bMIC). In this study, Tasse et al. reported that the bMIC is equivalent or close to the MIC for planktonic bacteria. Similar values between MIC and bMIC were notably observed for clindamycin, fusidic acid, linezolid and rifampin [102].

The second situation concerns the efficiency of antibiotics on formed/mature biofilm. The sessile community is already organized and persisters can be present. In this case, antibiotic efficiency is defined through the measure of the minimal biofilm eliminating concentration (MBEC) via the use of the Calgary Biofilm Device [104]. MBEC for *S. aureus* biofilms can be 10–1000 times higher than the MIC defined for planktonic bacteria, depending on the investigated strains and antibiotics [105–108].

The difference between bMIC and MBEC is probably due to a lack of penetration/diffusion of antibiotics inside the biofilm, even if this statement still stays controverted. Indeed, a decreased penetration of antibiotics has been observed in *in vitro* models of *S. aureus* biofilm [109, 110]. The penetration inside biofilm varies depending on the type of antibiotics and the structure of the biofilm. On the contrary, other studies, such as the recent one by Boudjemaa et al. reported that the biofilm matrix was not a shield to the antibiotic diffusion. They observed that the concentration inside the biofilm is similar to the one that could be found outside the biofilm. In this case, the resistance to the treatment would be related to a decreased effect of the drug to *S. aureus* [98, 111]. An interesting compromise can be that several factors influence the efficiency of antibiotic treatment against *S. aureus* biofilm. Lack of penetration is one of them but cannot be the only answer by its own.

With regards to this, the combination of antibiotics appears as an interesting solution for an effective treatment. Susceptibility test revealed that rifampin, but also vancomycin and fusidic acid were the most interesting constituent of antibiotic combinations active against the staphylococcal biofilms [112]. In an innovative *in vitro* model, Parra-ruiz et al. demonstrated that the combination of daptomycin or moxifloxacin with clarithromycin is of greater effect than the individual effects of the three agents against a biofilm formed by a methicillin-sensible *S. aureus* (MSSA) strain. Similar observations were made for the combination of linezolid and daptomycin as well as for daptomycin and rifampicin against a MRSA strain [113, 114]. However, recent studies suggested that combination of antibiotics could also have an antagonistic effect on the elimination of *S. aureus* biofilm. It was reported that linezolid can antagonize vancomycin and daptomycin activities [115]. In an infective endocarditis model of biofilm-forming MRSA, Laplante and Woodmansee observed that rifampin and gentamicin antagonized or delayed the bactericidal activity of daptomycin and that daptomycin monotherapy had better *in vitro* activity than vancomycin-containing combinations [116]. Moreover, according to Croes et al., the use of rifampin-containing combinations against *S. aureus* biofilm remains unpredictable, ranging from a tendency toward antagonism to some synergism effects [117]. At the opposite, a recent study, analyzing the antibiotic susceptibility of 58 clinical isolates, emphasized that there are no evidence for advice against the daptomycin/rifampin combination therapy for MSSA/MRSA infection.

The efficiency of antibiotic monotherapies or bi-therapies was most of the time evaluated through the use of *in vitro* models. *In vivo* models of infection are of high importance to comfort and strengthen the results between the bench and the patient bed. In a MRSA joint prosthesis rabbit infection model, the combination of rifampin with daptomycin was observed to be more effective than a treatment of either of these agents [118]. Similar results were reported about the combination of linezolid with rifampin or vancomycin with rifampin in a rabbit model of MRSA foreign body osteomyelitis [119]. Recently, study tested several antibiotics alone and in combination in a murine model of implant-associated osteomyelitis. The authors reported that the most effective antibiotic combinations contained rifampicin and that the combinations containing two nonrifampicin antibiotics were not more active than single drugs [120].

Globally, trying to prevent the biofilm formation appears as the most interesting way to fight this kind of infection. In case of full-formed biofilm infections, using a combination of high-dosed antibiotics containing rifampicin and/or daptomycin seems to be the best option.

In addition to the difficulties to treat biofilm-associated infection, there is also the important delay necessary to spot them. The emergency of finding a technical approach to detect biofilm in the analysis laboratories is huge. Some biomarkers have been searched, especially thanks to qPCR (quantitative polymerase chain reaction) techniques. For example, *ica* genes encoding for PIA can be identified by PCR [47]. However, *ica* operon is not present in all *S. aureus* strains [51], and therefore, it cannot be used as a general biomarker. There still is a lack of tool in the diagnosis of biofilm associated infections. It would be necessary to find either a universal biomarker that defines all biofilm species or at least, a biomarker species-specific detectable in the particular case of the biofilm presence.

5. Future strategies to fight against biofilm formation

Nowadays biofilm existence cannot be ignored anymore. Scientist community has to find new ways of fighting this bacterial social network as to avoid biofilm formation, or to weaken its intrinsic resistance, to disrupt biofilm or to kill bacteria embedded in this structure as detailed by Bjarnsholt et al. [121] and summarized in **Figure 3**.

5.1. Prevention by antiadhesive or anticommunication molecules

Prevention will always be the best strategy to fight against biofilm formation. Moreover, inhibiting the biofilm formation, bacteria stay under "planktonic" form and are much more susceptible to antimicrobial or immune system molecules, and therefore easier to eliminate. Prevention has to be used as a prophylactic strategy, especially for devices implant during surgery [121]. The idea is to avoid bacterial adhesion on material. As a consequence, some anti-adhesive surfaces are developed to be used in implant manufacturing [122]. For example, titan implants

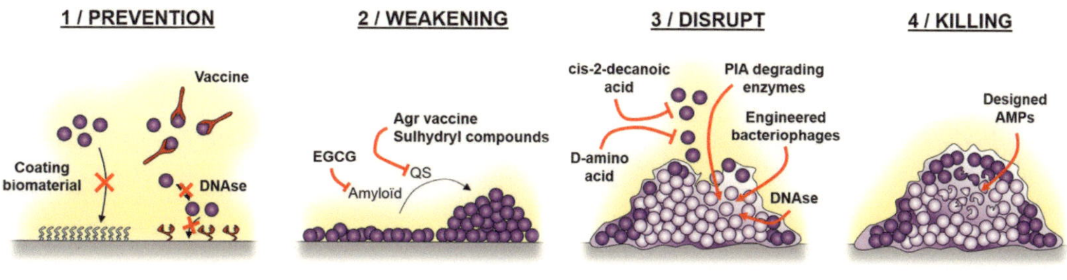

Figure 3. Strategies "anti-*S. aureus* biofilm."

coated with gentamicin showed a local action and a short period release fighting *S. aureus* early infection and decreasing toxic side effect [123]. This strategy could be applied when the infection is not endogenous as the antibiotic release will end at some point and that the implant turns then again into a perfect bacterial support [121]. To prevent bacterial adhesion, it could be interesting to target molecules responsible of initial attachment as adhesins by using neutralizing antibodies [121]. A vaccine was developed based on 4 antigens involved in biofilm formation of *S. aureus*. Its efficiency was proved in chronic osteomyelitis rabbit model but only in combination with vancomycin to kill the free bacteria [124]. Inhibition of biofilm development could be also based on the use of enzymes degrading biofilm matrix components [121] such as DNase which avoid the irreversible attachment step but this strategy does not work in *in vivo* models. Inhibition of biofilm formation could be based on the perturbation of signal like the presence of endogenous nitrite or the addition of exogenous nitrite [76] or D-amino acids which disturb the initial attachment or the maturation. Moreover, surfaces impregnated with those molecules prevent device-related infection [125, 126]. Antiadhesive strategies are often designed for surfaces supporting an antiadhesive molecule which target and antagonized adhesin or other specific attachment molecules [122] avoiding any bacteria adhesion.

To conclude, the conceptualization of molecules interfering with signals responsible for biofilm program induction could be imagined and this could lead to the presence of only free-floating bacteria that are more susceptible to antibiotics.

5.2. Weakening

In case the biofilm prevention fails, other strategies have to be developed. Weakening strategies are based on the idea of avoiding the biofilm properties set up, being efficient only on biofilm in formation not on mature biofilm [121]. Targets of this strategy are virulence factors, communication molecules or specific metabolic pathway involved in biofilm maturation. In *S. aureus,* Agr quorum-sensing system and Agr-regulated PSMs are key controllers of biofilm structure. In consequence, they are the perfect targets for vaccines or drugs [28, 127]. RNAIII-inhibiting peptide negatively regulates quorum-sensing response, and in consequence, it can reduce *S. aureus* biofilms *in vivo* [128].

Molecules interrupting the production or assembly of amyloid fibers could consequently destabilize biofilm structure. The compound (-)-epi-gallocatechine gallate (EGCG) used to fight against amyloid peptides involved in Alzheimer's and Parkinson's diseases is also active to inhibit *S. aureus* biofilm [53]. Another example is the functional micro-domains which have been discovered in bacterial membranes and their inhibition through the application of zaragozic acid avoids biofilm formation [129].

It will be interesting to develop other vaccines or drugs which target virulence factors that enhance biofilm formation.

5.3. Biofilm disruption

As for "weakening" strategies, targeting Agr quorum-sensing system in *S. aureus* will be interesting for triggering disruption [28, 127]. Other molecules have been screened for their ability to disperse biofilm. A fatty acid messenger named *cis*-2-decenoic acid produced during

http://dx.doi.org/10.5772/66380

P. aeruginosa growth has shown a capacity to disperse *S. aureus* biofilm [130]. D-amino acids trigger biofilm disassembly in affecting amyloid fibers and could be a potential strategy to disperse a preformed biofilm [125].

Another target to disrupt biofilm is the matrix, using for example, PIA-degrading enzymes. Two matrix polymers in staphylococcal biofilms poly-N-acetylglucosamine and eDNA could be targeted for their destruction by dispersin B and DNaseI, respectively. Dispersin succeeded in detaching pre-formed *S. epidermidis* biofilm but not *S. aureus* ones, and on the contrary, DNaseI induced a disruption of *S. aureus* structures and not *S. epidermidis* ones [62]. However, nucleases do not impact biofilm-associated infections [66]. Moreover, bacteriophages are known to be involved in biofilm dispersion stage [31]. Therefore, bacteriophages were engineered to produce dispersin B, and biofilm mass reduction was noticed [131, 132].

5.4. Killing

To eradicate a pre-form biofilm is the last chance and this strategy remains the most difficult to fathom. Many molecules have been tested but they have to respect many criteria like the non-cytotoxicity and the non-pro-inflammatory effects. Promising molecules are the "anti-biofilm" peptides inspired by animal antimicrobial peptides (AMPs) which have anti-inflammatory effects and are efficient to destroy Gram-positive or Gram-negative bacteria at very low concentrations [73, 133]. They have also shown their ability to act in synergy with conventional antibiotics, avoiding the use of too high concentrations of each molecule [133].

6. Conclusion

After the revolutionary discovery of antibiotics, the medical community thought that the battle against microorganisms was won. However, the fight had just begun as bacteria can develop resistant structure named biofilm among other strategies. *S. aureus* is one of the most common bacteria found on human epidermis thus when physical barrier such as skin is broken, *S. aureus* could penetrate and adhere to tissue or medical devices. Many *S. aureus* strains are drug-resistant (MRSA), and moreover, *S. aureus* represents the most frequent germ responsible of chronic biofilm-associated infection. The treatment against this kind of chronic infection is useless in most cases, especially against MRSA. *S. aureus* is also present in food infection and responsible of intoxication. For all these reasons, the understanding of *S. aureus* biofilm is necessary in order to develop new strategies to inhibit biofilm formation and/or to eradicate *S. aureus* biofilm. Nowadays, more and more molecular mechanisms are decrypted: bacterial communication, biofilm formation and dispersion. Consequently, new molecules are targeted but so far most of this targeting has revealed inefficient in *in vivo* models. Unfortunately, discoveries on biofilm in general and on *S. aureus* biofilm in particular, represent a drop in the ocean. Bacteria are simple organisms with complex mechanisms. We, scientists and physicians, have to integrate the fact that planktonic bacteria only reflect the optimal conditions of a laboratory environment. `Biofilm is the real enemy, and it changes the all entire picture. New biofilm models have to be developed, especially *in vivo* models.

Acknowledgements

We thank Kevin Delaitre for careful proofreading.

Author details

Fany Reffuveille[1, 2]*, Jérôme Josse[1, 2], Quentin Vallé[1, 2], Céline Mongaret[1, 2] and Sophie C. Gangloff[1, 2]

*Address all correspondence to: fany.reffuveille@univ-reims.fr

1 EA 4691, Biomaterial and Inflammation in Bone Site, Health Pole, University of Reims Champagne-Ardenne, Reims, France

2 UFR of Pharmacy, Microbiology, University of Reims Champagne-Ardenne, Reims, France

References

[1] Høiby N, Ciofu O, Johansen HK, Song Z, Moser C, Jensen PØ, et al. The clinical impact of bacterial biofilms. Int J Oral Sci. 2011 Apr;3(2):55–65.

[2] Costerton JW, Stewart PS, Greenberg EP. Bacterial biofilms: a common cause of persistent infections. Science. 1999 May 21;284(5418):1318–22.

[3] Boucher HW, Talbot GH, Bradley JS, Edwards JE, Gilbert D, Rice LB, et al. Bad bugs, no drugs: no ESKAPE! An update from the Infectious Diseases Society of America. Clin Infect Dis Off Publ Infect Dis Soc Am. 2009 Jan 1;48(1):1–12.

[4] Spellberg B, Guidos R, Gilbert D, Bradley J, Boucher HW, Scheld WM, et al. The epidemic of antibiotic-resistant infections: a call to action for the medical community from the Infectious Diseases Society of America. Clin Infect Dis Off Publ Infect Dis Soc Am. 2008 Jan 15;46(2):155–64.

[5] Hall-Stoodley L, Costerton JW, Stoodley P. Bacterial biofilms: from the natural environment to infectious diseases. Nat Rev Microbiol. 2004 Feb;2(2):95–108.

[6] Bryers JD. Medical biofilms. Biotechnol Bioeng. 2008 May 1;100(1):1–18.

[7] Høiby N, Bjarnsholt T, Givskov M, Molin S, Ciofu O. Antibiotic resistance of bacterial biofilms. Int J Antimicrob Agents. 2010 Apr;35(4):322–32.

[8] Römling U, Balsalobre C. Biofilm infections, their resilience to therapy and innovative treatment strategies. J Intern Med. 2012 Dec;272(6):541–61.

[9] de la Fuente-Núñez C, Reffuveille F, Fernández L, Hancock REW. Bacterial biofilm development as a multicellular adaptation: antibiotic resistance and new therapeutic strategies. Curr Opin Microbiol. 2013 Oct;16(5):580–9.

[10] Shi X, Zhu X. Biofilm formation and food safety in food industries. Trends Food Sci Technol. 2009 Sep;20(9):407–13.

[11] Gibson H, Taylor JH, Hall KE, Holah JT. Effectiveness of cleaning techniques used in the food industry in terms of the removal of bacterial biofilms. J Appl Microbiol. 1999 Jul;87(1):41–8.

[12] Otto M. Staphylococcal biofilms. Curr Top Microbiol Immunol. 2008;322:207–28.

[13] Otto M. Staphylococcal infections: mechanisms of biofilm maturation and detachment as critical determinants of pathogenicity. Annu Rev Med. 2013;64:175–88.

[14] Dunne WM. Bacterial adhesion: seen any good biofilms lately? Clin Microbiol Rev. 2002 Apr;15(2):155–66.

[15] Sousa C, Teixeira P, Oliveira R. Influence of surface properties on the adhesion of *Staphylococcus epidermidis* to acrylic and silicone. Int J Biomater. 2009;2009:718017.

[16] Myint AA, Lee W, Mun S, Ahn CH, Lee S, Yoon J. Influence of membrane surface properties on the behavior of initial bacterial adhesion and biofilm development onto nanofiltration membranes. Biofouling. 2010;26(3):313–21.

[17] Hamadi F, Latrache H, Mabrrouki M, Elghmari A, Outzourhit A, Ellouali M, et al. Effect of pH on distribution and adhesion of *Staphylococcus aureus* to glass. J Adhes Sci Technol. 2005 Jan 1;19(1):73–85.

[18] Pollitt EJG, Crusz SA, Diggle SP. *Staphylococcus aureus* forms spreading dendrites that have characteristics of active motility. Sci Rep. 2015;5:17698.

[19] Patti JM, Allen BL, McGavin MJ, Höök M. MSCRAMM-mediated adherence of microorganisms to host tissues. Annu Rev Microbiol. 1994;48:585–617.

[20] Josse J, Velard F, Gangloff SC. *Staphylococcus aureus* vs. Osteoblast: Relationship and Consequences in Osteomyelitis. Front Cell Infect Microbiol. 2015;5:85.

[21] Gill SR, Fouts DE, Archer GL, Mongodin EF, Deboy RT, Ravel J, et al. Insights on evolution of virulence and resistance from the complete genome analysis of an early methicillin-resistant *Staphylococcus aureus* strain and a biofilm-producing methicillin-resistant *Staphylococcus epidermidis* strain. J Bacteriol. 2005 Apr;187(7):2426–38.

[22] Navarre WW, Schneewind O. Surface proteins of gram-positive bacteria and mechanisms of their targeting to the cell wall envelope. Microbiol Mol Biol Rev MMBR. 1999 Mar;63(1):174–229.

[23] Heilmann C, Thumm G, Chhatwal GS, Hartleib J, Uekötter A, Peters G. Identification and characterization of a novel autolysin Aae with adhesive properties from *Staphylococcus epidermidis*. Microbiol Read Engl. 2003 Oct;149(Pt 10):2769–78.

[24] Gross M, Cramton SE, Götz F, Peschel A. Key role of teichoic acid net charge in *Staphylococcus aureus* colonization of artificial surfaces. Infect Immun. 2001 May;69(5):3423–6.

[25] Cucarella C, Solano C, Valle J, Amorena B, Lasa I, Penadés JR. Bap, a *Staphylococcus aureus* surface protein involved in biofilm formation. J Bacteriol. 2001 May;183(9):2888–96.

[26] Schroeder K, Jularic M, Horsburgh SM, Hirschhausen N, Neumann C, Bertling A, et al. Molecular characterization of a novel *Staphylococcus aureus* surface protein SasC involved in cell aggregation and biofilm accumulation. PloS One. 2009;4(10):e7567.

[27] Davies DG, Parsek MR, Pearson JP, Iglewski BH, Costerton JW, Greenberg EP. The involvement of cell-to-cell signals in the development of a bacterial biofilm. Science. 1998 Apr 10;280(5361):295–8.

[28] Boles BR, Horswill AR. Agr-mediated dispersal of *Staphylococcus aureus* biofilms. PLoS Pathog. 2008 Apr;4(4):e1000052.

[29] Novick RP. Autoinduction and signal transduction in the regulation of staphylococcal virulence. Mol Microbiol. 2003 Jun;48(6):1429–49.

[30] Yarwood JM, Bartels DJ, Volper EM, Greenberg EP. Quorum sensing in *Staphylococcus aureus* biofilms. J Bacteriol. 2004 Mar;186(6):1838–50.

[31] McDougald D, Rice SA, Barraud N, Steinberg PD, Kjelleberg S. Should we stay or should we go: mechanisms and ecological consequences for biofilm dispersal. Nat Rev Microbiol. 2012 Jan;10(1):39–50.

[32] Vuong C, Saenz HL, Götz F, Otto M. Impact of the agr quorum-sensing system on adherence to polystyrene in *Staphylococcus aureus*. J Infect Dis. 2000 Dec;182(6):1688–93.

[33] Thurlow LR, Hanke ML, Fritz T, Angle A, Aldrich A, Williams SH, et al. *Staphylococcus aureus* biofilms prevent macrophage phagocytosis and attenuate inflammation *in vivo*. J Immunol Baltim Md 1950. 2011 Jun 1;186(11):6585–96.

[34] Shopsin B, Drlica-Wagner A, Mathema B, Adhikari RP, Kreiswirth BN, Novick RP. Prevalence of agr dysfunction among colonizing *Staphylococcus aureus* strains. J Infect Dis. 2008 Oct 15;198(8):1171–4.

[35] Lim Y, Jana M, Luong TT, Lee CY. Control of glucose- and NaCl-induced biofilm formation by rbf in *Staphylococcus aureus*. J Bacteriol. 2004 Feb;186(3):722–9.

[36] Le KY, Otto M. Quorum-sensing regulation in staphylococci-an overview. Front Microbiol Internet. 2015 Oct 27 cited 2016 Sep 8;6. Available from: http://www.ncbi.nlm.nih.gov/pmc/articles/PMC4621875/

[37] O'Toole G, Kaplan HB, Kolter R. Biofilm formation as microbial development. Annu Rev Microbiol. 2000;54:49–79.

[38] Costerton JW, Lewandowski Z, Caldwell DE, Korber DR, Lappin-Scott HM. Microbial biofilms. Annu Rev Microbiol. 1995;49:711–45.

[39] Mack D, Fischer W, Krokotsch A, Leopold K, Hartmann R, Egge H, et al. The intercellular adhesin involved in biofilm accumulation of *Staphylococcus epidermidis* is a linear beta-1,6-linked glucosaminoglycan: purification and structural analysis. J Bacteriol. 1996 Jan;178(1):175–83.

[40] Wang X, Preston JF, Romeo T. The pgaABCD locus of Escherichia coli promotes the synthesis of a polysaccharide adhesin required for biofilm formation. J Bacteriol. 2004 May;186(9):2724–34.

[41] Kaplan JB, Ragunath C, Ramasubbu N, Fine DH. Detachment of Actinobacillus actinomycetemcomitans biofilm cells by an endogenous beta-hexosaminidase activity. J Bacteriol. 2003 Aug;185(16):4693–8.

[42] Sadovskaya I, Vinogradov E, Flahaut S, Kogan G, Jabbouri S. Extracellular carbohydrate-containing polymers of a model biofilm-producing strain, *Staphylococcus epidermidis* RP62A. Infect Immun. 2005 May;73(5):3007–17.

[43] Vuong C, Voyich JM, Fischer ER, Braughton KR, Whitney AR, DeLeo FR, et al. Polysaccharide intercellular adhesin PIA protects *Staphylococcus epidermidis* against major components of the human innate immune system. Cell Microbiol. 2004 Mar;6(3):269–75.

[44] Knobloch JK, Bartscht K, Sabottke A, Rohde H, Feucht HH, Mack D. Biofilm formation by *Staphylococcus epidermidis* depends on functional RsbU, an activator of the sigB operon: differential activation mechanisms due to ethanol and salt stress. J Bacteriol. 2001 Apr;183(8):2624–33.

[45] Tormo MA, Martí M, Valle J, Manna AC, Cheung AL, Lasa I, et al. SarA is an essential positive regulator of *Staphylococcus epidermidis* biofilm development. J Bacteriol. 2005 Apr;187(7):2348–56.

[46] Xu L, Li H, Vuong C, Vadyvaloo V, Wang J, Yao Y, et al. Role of the luxS quorum-sensing system in biofilm formation and virulence of *Staphylococcus epidermidis*. Infect Immun. 2006 Jan;74(1):488–96.

[47] Arciola CR, Campoccia D, Baldassarri L, Donati ME, Pirini V, Gamberini S, et al. Detection of biofilm formation in *Staphylococcus epidermidis* from implant infections. Comparison of a PCR-method that recognizes the presence of ica genes with two classic phenotypic methods. J Biomed Mater Res A. 2006 Feb;76(2):425–30.

[48] Corrigan RM, Rigby D, Handley P, Foster TJ. The role of *Staphylococcus aureus* surface protein SasG in adherence and biofilm formation. Microbiol Read Engl. 2007 Aug;153(Pt 8):2435–46.

[49] Formosa-Dague C, Speziale P, Foster TJ, Geoghegan JA, Dufrêne YF. Zinc-dependent mechanical properties of *Staphylococcus aureus* biofilm-forming surface protein SasG. Proc Natl Acad Sci U S A. 2016 Jan 12;113(2):410–5.

[50] Hussain M, Herrmann M, von Eiff C, Perdreau-Remington F, Peters G. A 140-kilodalton extracellular protein is essential for the accumulation of *Staphylococcus epidermidis* strains on surfaces. Infect Immun. 1997 Feb;65(2):519–24.

[51] Rohde H, Burandt EC, Siemssen N, Frommelt L, Burdelski C, Wurster S, et al. Polysaccharide intercellular adhesin or protein factors in biofilm accumulation of *Staphylococcus epidermidis* and *Staphylococcus aureus* isolated from prosthetic hip and knee joint infections. Biomaterials. 2007 Mar;28(9):1711–20.

[52] Periasamy S, Joo H-S, Duong AC, Bach T-HL, Tan VY, Chatterjee SS, et al. How *Staphylococcus aureus* biofilms develop their characteristic structure. Proc Natl Acad Sci U S A. 2012 Jan 24;109(4):1281–6.

[53] Taglialegna A, Lasa I, Valle J. 2016. Amyloid structures as biofilm matrix scaffolds. J Bacteriol 198:2579–2588.

[54] Schwartz K, Syed AK, Stephenson RE, Rickard AH, Boles BR. Functional amyloids composed of phenol soluble modulins stabilize *Staphylococcus aureus* biofilms. PLoS Pathog. 2012;8(6):e1002744.

[55] Cucarella C, Tormo MA, Ubeda C, Trotonda MP, Monzón M, Peris C, et al. Role of biofilm-associated protein bap in the pathogenesis of bovine *Staphylococcus aureus*. Infect Immun. 2004 Apr;72(4):2177–85.

[56] Lasa I, Penadés JR. Bap: a family of surface proteins involved in biofilm formation. Res Microbiol. 2006 Mar;157(2):99–107.

[57] Latasa C, Solano C, Penadés JR, Lasa I. Biofilm-associated proteins. C R Biol. 2006 Nov;329(11):849–57.

[58] Boles BR, Thoendel M, Roth AJ, Horswill AR. Identification of genes involved in polysaccharide-independent *Staphylococcus aureus* biofilm formation. PloS One. 2010;5(4):e10146.

[59] Rice KC, Mann EE, Endres JL, Weiss EC, Cassat JE, Smeltzer MS, et al. The cidA murein hydrolase regulator contributes to DNA release and biofilm development in *Staphylococcus aureus*. Proc Natl Acad Sci U S A. 2007 May 8;104(19):8113–8.

[60] Yang S-J, Dunman PM, Projan SJ, Bayles KW. Characterization of the *Staphylococcus aureus* CidR regulon: elucidation of a novel role for acetoin metabolism in cell death and lysis. Mol Microbiol. 2006 Apr;60(2):458–68.

[61] Nguyen D, Joshi-Datar A, Lepine F, Bauerle E, Olakanmi O, Beer K, et al. Active starvation responses mediate antibiotic tolerance in biofilms and nutrient-limited bacteria. Science. 2011 Nov 18;334(6058):982–6.

[62] Mann EE, Rice KC, Boles BR, Endres JL, Ranjit D, Chandramohan L, et al. Modulation of eDNA release and degradation affects *Staphylococcus aureus* biofilm maturation. PloS One. 2009;4(6):e5822.

[63] Rani SA, Pitts B, Beyenal H, Veluchamy RA, Lewandowski Z, Davison WM, et al. Spatial patterns of DNA replication, protein synthesis, and oxygen concentration within bacterial biofilms reveal diverse physiological states. J Bacteriol. 2007 Jun;189(11):4223–33.

[64] Kaplan JB, LoVetri K, Cardona ST, Madhyastha S, Sadovskaya I, Jabbouri S, et al. Recombinant human DNase I decreases biofilm and increases antimicrobial susceptibility in staphylococci. J Antibiot Tokyo. 2012 Feb;65(2):73–7.

[65] Kiedrowski MR, Kavanaugh JS, Malone CL, Mootz JM, Voyich JM, Smeltzer MS, et al. Nuclease modulates biofilm formation in community-associated methicillin-resistant *Staphylococcus aureus*. PloS One. 2011;6(11):e26714.

[66] Beenken KE, Spencer H, Griffin LM, Smeltzer MS. Impact of extracellular nuclease production on the biofilm phenotype of *Staphylococcus aureus* under *in vitro* and *in vivo* conditions. Infect Immun. 2012 May;80(5):1634–8.

[67] Karatan E, Watnick P. Signals, regulatory networks, and materials that build and break bacterial biofilms. Microbiol Mol Biol Rev MMBR. 2009 Jun;73(2):310–47.

[68] Beloin C, Ghigo J-M. Finding gene-expression patterns in bacterial biofilms. Trends Microbiol. 2005 Jan;13(1):16–9.

[69] Whiteley M, Bangera MG, Bumgarner RE, Parsek MR, Teitzel GM, Lory S, et al. Gene expression in *Pseudomonas aeruginosa* biofilms. Nature. 2001 Oct 25;413(6858) :860–4.

[70] Yao Y, Sturdevant DE, Otto M. Genomewide analysis of gene expression in *Staphylococcus epidermidis* biofilms: insights into the pathophysiology of *S. epidermidis* biofilms and the role of phenol-soluble modulins in formation of biofilms. J Infect Dis. 2005 Jan 15;191(2):289–98.

[71] Pané-Farré J, Jonas B, Förstner K, Engelmann S, Hecker M. The sigmaB regulon in *Staphylococcus aureus* and its regulation. Int J Med Microbiol IJMM. 2006 Aug;296(4–5):237–58.

[72] Rachid S, Ohlsen K, Wallner U, Hacker J, Hecker M, Ziebuhr W. Alternative transcription factor sigmaB is involved in regulation of biofilm expression in a *Staphylococcus aureus* mucosal isolate. J Bacteriol. 2000 Dec;182(23):6824–6.

[73] de la Fuente-Núñez C, Reffuveille F, Haney EF, Straus SK, Hancock REW. Broad-spectrum anti-biofilm peptide that targets a cellular stress response. PLoS Pathog. 2014 May;10(5):e1004152.

[74] Regassa LB, Novick RP, Betley MJ. Glucose and nonmaintained pH decrease expression of the accessory gene regulator agr in *Staphylococcus aureus*. Infect Immun. 1992 Aug;60(8):3381–8.

[75] Regassa LB, Betley MJ. Alkaline pH decreases expression of the accessory gene regulator agr in *Staphylococcus aureus*. J Bacteriol. 1992 Aug;174(15):5095–100.

[76] Schlag S, Nerz C, Birkenstock TA, Altenberend F, Götz F. Inhibition of staphylococcal biofilm formation by nitrite. J Bacteriol. 2007 Nov;189(21):7911–9.

[77] de la Fuente-Núñez C, Reffuveille F, Fairfull-Smith KE, Hancock REW. Effect of nitroxides on swarming motility and biofilm formation, multicellular behaviors in *Pseudomonas aeruginosa*. Antimicrob Agents Chemother. 2013 Oct;57(10):4877–81.

[78] Cramton SE, Ulrich M, Götz F, Döring G. Anaerobic conditions induce expression of polysaccharide intercellular adhesin in *Staphylococcus aureus* and *Staphylococcus epidermidis*. Infect Immun. 2001 Jun;69(6):4079–85.

[79] Fluckiger U, Ulrich M, Steinhuber A, Döring G, Mack D, Landmann R, et al. Biofilm formation, icaADBC transcription, and polysaccharide intercellular adhesin synthesis by staphylococci in a device-related infection model. Infect Immun. 2005 Mar;73(3):1811–9.

[80] de Nys R, Givskov M, Kumar N, Kjelleberg S, Steinberg PD. Furanones. Prog Mol Subcell Biol. 2006;42:55–86.

[81] Kuehl R, Al-Bataineh S, Gordon O, Luginbuehl R, Otto M, Textor M, et al. Furanone at subinhibitory concentrations enhances staphylococcal biofilm formation by luxS repression. Antimicrob Agents Chemother. 2009 Oct;53(10):4159–66.

[82] DeLeo FR, Diep BA, Otto M. Host Defense and Pathogenesis in *Staphylococcus aureus* Infections. Infect Dis Clin North Am. 2009 Mar;23(1):17–34.

[83] Günther F, Wabnitz GH, Stroh P, Prior B, Obst U, Samstag Y, et al. Host defence against *Staphylococcus aureus* biofilms infection: phagocytosis of biofilms by polymorphonuclear neutrophils PMN. Mol Immunol. 2009 May;46(8–9):1805–13.

[84] Guenther F, Stroh P, Wagner C, Obst U, Hänsch GM. Phagocytosis of staphylococci biofilms by polymorphonuclear neutrophils: *S. aureus* and *S. epidermidis* differ with regard to their susceptibility towards the host defense. Int J Artif Organs. 2009 Sep;32(9):565–73.

[85] Meyle E, Stroh P, Günther F, Hoppy-Tichy T, Wagner C, Hänsch GM. Destruction of bacterial biofilms by polymorphonuclear neutrophils: relative contribution of phagocytosis, DNA release, and degranulation. Int J Artif Organs. 2010 Sep;33(9):608–20.

[86] Stroh P, Günther F, Meyle E, Prior B, Wagner C, Hänsch GM. Host defence against *Staphylococcus aureus* biofilms by polymorphonuclear neutrophils: oxygen radical production but not phagocytosis depends on opsonisation with immunoglobulin G. Immunobiology. 2011 Mar;216(3):351–7.

[87] Flannagan RS, Heit B, Heinrichs DE. Antimicrobial mechanisms of macrophages and the immune evasion strategies of *Staphylococcus aureus*. Pathog Basel Switz. 2015;4(4):826–68.

[88] Scherr TD, Hanke ML, Huang O, James DBA, Horswill AR, Bayles KW, et al. *Staphylococcus aureus* Biofilms Induce Macrophage Dysfunction Through Leukocidin AB and Alpha-Toxin. MBio. 6(4 e01021-15)

[89] Hanke ML, Angle A, Kielian T. MyD88-dependent signaling influences fibrosis and alternative macrophage activation during *Staphylococcus aureus* biofilm infection. PLoS One. 2012;7(8):e42476.

[90] Hanke ML, Heim CE, Angle A, Sanderson SD, Kielian T. Targeting macrophage activation for the prevention and treatment of *Staphylococcus aureus* biofilm infections. J Immunol Baltim Md 1950. 2013 Mar 1;190(5):2159–68.

[91] Heim CE, Vidlak D, Scherr TD, Kozel JA, Holzapfel M, Muirhead DE, et al. Myeloid-derived suppressor cells contribute to *Staphylococcus aureus* orthopedic biofilm infection. J Immunol Baltim Md 1950. 2014 Apr 15;192(8):3778–92.

[92] Heim CE, Vidlak D, Scherr TD, Hartman CW, Garvin KL, Kielian T. IL-12 promotes myeloid-derived suppressor cell recruitment and bacterial persistence during *Staphylococcus aureus* orthopedic implant infection. J Immunol Baltim Md 1950. 2015 Apr 15;194(8):3861–72.

[93] Heim CE, Vidlak D, Kielian T. Interleukin-10 production by myeloid-derived suppressor cells contributes to bacterial persistence during *Staphylococcus aureus* orthopedic biofilm infection. J Leukoc Biol. 2015 Dec;98(6):1003–13.

[94] Leid JG, Shirtliff ME, Costerton JW, Stoodley P. Human leukocytes adhere to, penetrate, and respond to *Staphylococcus aureus* biofilms. Infect Immun. 2002 Nov;70(11):6339–45.

[95] Prabhakara R, Harro JM, Leid JG, Harris M, Shirtliff ME. Murine immune response to a chronic *Staphylococcus aureus* biofilm infection. Infect Immun. 2011 Apr;79(4):1789–96.

[96] Prabhakara R, Harro JM, Leid JG, Keegan AD, Prior ML, Shirtliff ME. Suppression of the inflammatory immune response prevents the development of chronic biofilm infection due to methicillin-resistant *Staphylococcus aureus*. Infect Immun. 2011 Dec;79(12):5010–8.

[97] Lebeaux D, Chauhan A, Rendueles O, Beloin C. From *in vitro* to *in vivo* models of bacterial biofilm-related infections. Pathogens. 2013 May 13;22:288–356.

[98] Jacqueline C, Caillon J. Impact of bacterial biofilm on the treatment of prosthetic joint infections. J Antimicrob Chemother. 2014 Sep;69(Suppl 1):i37–40.

[99] Paharik AE, Horswill AR. The Staphylococcal Bioflm: Adhesins, Regulation, and Host Response. Microbiol Spectr. 2016 Apr;4(2)

[100] McCarthy H, Rudkin JK, Black NS, Gallagher L, O'Neill E, O'Gara JP. Methicillin resistance and the biofilm phenotype in *Staphylococcus aureus*. Front Cell Infect Microbiol. 2015;5:1.

[101] Lister JL, Horswill AR. *Staphylococcus aureus* biofilms: recent developments in biofilm dispersal. Front Cell Infect Microbiol. 2014;4:178.

[102] Tasse J, Croisier D, Badel-Berchoux S, Chavanet P, Bernardi T, Provot C, et al. Preliminary results of a new antibiotic susceptibility test against bioflm installation in device-associated infections: the Antibiofilmogram®. Pathog Dis. 2016 Aug;74(6). pii: ftw057.

[103] Chavant P, Gaillard-Martinie B, Talon R, Hébraud M, Bernardi T. A new device for rapid evaluation of biofilm formation potential by bacteria. J Microbiol Methods. 2007 Mar;68(3):605–12.

[104] Ceri H, Olson ME, Stremick C, Read RR, Morck D, Buret A. The calgary biofilm device: new technology for rapid determination of antibiotic susceptibilities of bacterial biofilms. J Clin Microbiol. 1999 Jun 1;37(6):1771–6.

[105] Molina-Manso D, del Prado G, Ortiz-Pérez A, Manrubia-Cobo M, Gómez-Barrena E, Cordero-Ampuero J, et al. *In vitro* susceptibility to antibiotics of staphylococci in biofilms isolated from orthopaedic infections. Int J Antimicrob Agents. 2013 Jun;41(6):521–3.

[106] Revest M, Jacqueline C, Boudjemaa R, Caillon J, Le Mabecque V, Breteche A, et al. New *in vitro* and *in vivo* models to evaluate antibiotic efficacy in *Staphylococcus aureus* prosthetic vascular graft infection. J Antimicrob Chemother. 2016 May;71(5):1291–9.

[107] LaPlante KL, Mermel LA. *In vitro* activities of telavancin and vancomycin against biofilm-producing *Staphylococcus aureus, S. epidermidis,* and *Enterococcus faecalis* Strains. Antimicrob Agents Chemother. 2009 Jul;53(7):3166–9.

[108] Girard LP, Ceri H, Gibb AP, Olson M, Sepandj F. MIC versus MBEC to determine the antibiotic sensitivity of *Staphylococcus aureus* in peritoneal dialysis peritonitis. Perit Dial Int J Int Soc Perit Dial. 2010 Dec;30(6):652–6.

[109] Singh R, Sahore S, Kaur P, Rani A, Ray P. Penetration barrier contributes to bacterial bioflm-associated resistance against only select antibiotics, and exhibits genus-, strain- and antibiotic-specifc diferences. Pathog Dis. 2016 Aug;74(6) pii: ftw056.

[110] Siala W, Mingeot-Leclercq M-P, Tulkens PM, Hallin M, Denis O, Van Bambeke F. Comparison of the antibiotic activities of Daptomycin, Vancomycin, and the investigational Fluoroquinolone Delafloxacin against biofilms from *Staphylococcus aureus* clinical isolates. Antimicrob Agents Chemother. 2014 Nov;58(11):6385–97.

[111] Boudjemaa R, Briandet R, Revest M, Jacqueline C, Caillon J, Fontaine-Aupart M-P, et al. New insight into daptomycin bioavailability and localization in *S. aureus* biofilms by dynamic fluorescence imaging. Antimicrob Agents Chemother. 2016 Jun 13;AAC.00735-16.

[112] Saginur R, StDenis M, Ferris W, Aaron SD, Chan F, Lee C, et al. Multiple combination bactericidal testing of staphylococcal biofilms from implant-associated infections. Antimicrob Agents Chemother. 2006 Jan 1;50(1):55–61.

[113] Parra-Ruiz J, Vidaillac C, Rose WE, Rybak MJ. Activities of high-dose daptomycin, vancomycin, and moxifloxacin alone or in combination with clarithromycin or rifampin in a novel *in vitro* model of *Staphylococcus aureus* biofilm. Antimicrob Agents Chemother. 2010 Oct;54(10):4329–34.

[114] Parra-Ruiz J, Bravo-Molina A, Peña-Monje A, Hernández-Quero J. Activity of linezolid and high-dose daptomycin, alone or in combination, in an *in vitro* model of *Staphylococcus aureus* biofilm. J Antimicrob Chemother. 2012 Nov;67(11):2682–5.

[115] Luther M, LaPlante KL. Observed antagonistic effect of linezolid on daptomycin or vancomycin activity against biofilm-forming methicillin-resistant *Staphylococcus aureus* in an *in vitro* pharmacodynamic model. Antimicrob Agents Chemother. 2015 Sep 14;AAC.01604-15.

[116] LaPlante KL, Woodmansee S. Activities of daptomycin and vancomycin alone and in combination with rifampin and gentamicin against biofilm-forming methicillin-resistant *Staphylococcus aureus* isolates in an experimental model of endocarditis. Antimicrob Agents Chemother. 2009 Sep;53(9):3880–6.

[117] Croes S, Beisser PS, Neef C, Bruggeman CA, Stobberingh EE. Unpredictable effects of rifampin as an adjunctive agent in elimination of rifampin-susceptible and -resistant *Staphylococcus aureus* strains grown in biofilms. Antimicrob Agents Chemother. 2010 Sep 1;54(9):3907–12.

[118] Saleh-Mghir A, Muller-Serieys C, Dinh A, Massias L, Crémieux A-C. Adjunctive rifampin is crucial to optimizing daptomycin efficacy against rabbit prosthetic joint infection due to methicillin-resistant *Staphylococcus aureus*. Antimicrob Agents Chemother. 2011 Oct 1;55(10):4589–93.

[119] Vergidis P, Rouse MS, Euba G, Karau MJ, Schmidt SM, Mandrekar JN, et al. Treatment with linezolid or vancomycin in combination with rifampin is effective in an animal model of methicillin-resistant *Staphylococcus aureus* foreign body osteomyelitis. Antimicrob Agents Chemother. 2011 Mar;55(3):1182–6.

[120] Jørgensen NP, Skovdal SM, Meyer RL, Dagnæs-Hansen F, Fuursted K, Petersen E. Rifampicin-containing combinations are superior to combinations of vancomycin, linezolid and daptomycin against *Staphylococcus aureus* biofilm infection *in vivo* and *in vitro*. Pathog Dis. 2016 Jun 1;74(4):ftw019.

[121] Bjarnsholt T, Ciofu O, Molin S, Givskov M, Høiby N. Applying insights from biofilm biology to drug development—can a new approach be developed? Nat Rev Drug Discov. 2013 Oct;12(10):791–808.

[122] Reffuveille F, Nicol M, Dé E, Thébault P. Design of an anti-adhesive surface by a pilicide strategy. Colloids Surf B Biointerfaces. 2016 Oct 1;146:895–901.

[123] Kittinger C, Marth E, Windhager R, Weinberg AM, Zarfel G, Baumert R, et al. Antimicrobial activity of gentamicin palmitate against high concentrations of *Staphylococcus aureus*. J Mater Sci Mater Med. 2011 Jun;22(6):1447–53.

[124] Brady RA, O'May GA, Leid JG, Prior ML, Costerton JW, Shirtliff ME. Resolution of *Staphylococcus aureus* biofilm infection using vaccination and antibiotic treatment. Infect Immun. 2011 Apr;79(4):1797–803.

[125] Kolodkin-Gal I, Romero D, Cao S, Clardy J, Kolter R, Losick R. D-amino acids trigger biofilm disassembly. Science. 2010 Apr 30;328(5978):627–9.

[126] Hochbaum AI, Kolodkin-Gal I, Foulston L, Kolter R, Aizenberg J, Losick R. Inhibitory effects of D-amino acids on *Staphylococcus aureus* biofilm development. J Bacteriol. 2011 Oct;193(20):5616–22.

[127] Lauderdale KJ, Malone CL, Boles BR, Morcuende J, Horswill AR. Biofilm dispersal of community-associated methicillin-resistant *Staphylococcus aureus* on orthopedic implant material. J Orthop Res Off Publ Orthop Res Soc. 2010 Jan;28(1):55–61.

[128] Giacometti A, Cirioni O, Gov Y, Ghiselli R, Del Prete MS, Mocchegiani F, et al. RNA III inhibiting peptide inhibits *in vivo* biofilm formation by drug-resistant *Staphylococcus aureus*. Antimicrob Agents Chemother. 2003 Jun;47(6):1979–83.

[129] López D, Kolter R. Functional microdomains in bacterial membranes. Genes Dev. 2010 Sep 1;24(17):1893–902.

[130] Davies DG, Marques CNH. A fatty acid messenger is responsible for inducing dispersion in microbial biofilms. J Bacteriol. 2009 Mar;191(5):1393–403.

[131] Hughes KA, Sutherland IW, Clark J, Jones MV. Bacteriophage and associated polysaccharide depolymerases—novel tools for study of bacterial biofilms. J Appl Microbiol. 1998 Sep;85(3):583–90.

[132] Lu TK, Collins JJ. Engineered bacteriophage targeting gene networks as adjuvants for antibiotic therapy. Proc Natl Acad Sci U S A. 2009 Mar 24;106(12):4629–34.

[133] Reffuveille F, de la Fuente-Núñez C, Mansour S, Hancock REW. A broad-spectrum antibiofilm peptide enhances antibiotic action against bacterial biofilms. Antimicrob Agents Chemother. 2014 Sep;58(9):5363–71.